SOUL DOCTORING IS IN T
WHAT THEY SAY

"*Soul Doctoring* captures the future of medicine, in which attention to body, mind, and spirit is the hallmark. Gayle Madeleine Randall, MD brings to this book the expertise of a medical insider and a cross-cultural explorer who possesses an exquisite reverence for non-Western healing traditions. This is a courageous, trail-blazing contribution."

—Larry Dossey, MD, *New York Times* bestselling author, *One Mind*, *Healing Beyond the Body*, *Reinventing Medicine* and *Healing Words*

"*Soul Doctoring* is a beautifully written journey from physician to healer. Dr. Randall reminds us of what matters most: love, compassion, intuition and of course science. Conventional medicine falls short in preventing disease and restoring health. Dr. Randall provides a new framework based on years of experience and practice."

—Mimi Guarneri, MD, FACC, President, Academy of Integrative Health and Medicine, author, *The Heart Speaks*

"Gayle has been able to present the multiple aspects of integrative and functional medicine in a semi-autobiographical and exciting way and weave them into a truly holistic manifesto. I'm not aware of another book that has been able to accomplish this task as well as *Soul Doctoring*. Going through the 25 chapters is not only a journey through Gayle's own life, full of fascinating personal and patient anecdotes, but a comprehensive education of the interested reader about the many dimensions of holistic health and wellness from gut to brain health, and from dreams to planetary health."

—Emeran A. Mayer, MD, *New York Times* bestselling author, *The Mind-Gut Connection: How the Hidden Conversation Within Our Bodies Impacts Our Mood, Our Choices, and Our Overall Health*; Distinguished Research Professor of Medicine, G. Oppenheimer Center for Neurobiology of Stress & Resilience

"In 2017, I found myself in a very physically compromised and frightening time of my life. I had the good fortune to meet the most gifted, kind, knowledgeable and, above all, understanding and honest doctor I have ever spoken to. Dr. Randall literally was an angel sent to me. She has taken care of and looks after my health issues with more compassion and love than I could have ever imagined! She has a true understanding, knowledge and love of the alternative healing practices which is the path I have chosen. I will forever be grateful to her and she is in my prayers every day."

—Olivia Hussey-Eisley, Golden Globe-award winning actress, *Romeo and Juliet;* author, *The Girl in the Window*

"Over the many years as I have followed Dr. Randall's doctoring abilities, I have looked on in amazement at her healing skills. How quickly she finds solutions to patient needs and the chosen designs that she uses for her holistic approaches toward healing, as if the Universe is whispering in her ear. Is Dr. Randall's healing knowingness a genetic gift? Who can know? Perhaps, the Great Spirit loaned her to us so she could teach us how to heal. I recommend *Soul Doctoring*. It is transformative."

—Joseph Rael, American Indian Tiwa and Southern Ute, Sundance chief, teacher and author of *Being and Vibration, Beautiful Painted Arrow: Stories and Teachings from Native American Tradition (Earth Quest), House of Shattering Light: Life as an American Indian Mystic* and *Tracks of Dancing Light*

"Dr. Gayle Randall is an absolute one of a kind being and soul, doing so many things for myself and my family, as well as all of mankind in general, I couldn't be more grateful to have her in our lives really. Anyone who cares about their health and well-being, should do themselves a favor, by reading this incredible book, and make themselves aware of this brilliant and comforting woman."

—India Eisley, actress, *The Secret Life of the American Teenager;* star, *My Sweet Audrina*

"Across the world, people are more aware and devoted to the body rather than to their souls. Unfortunately, the awareness and knowledge about the soul is very low. One has to know about the soul before treating it. Dr. Randall is actively contributing in distributing health and knowledge to people. She has the light to get the information out, and her patients are lucky to have her. I am so happy she has written *Soul Doctoring*."

—Dr. P. N. Awasthi, Ayurvedic medicine master, founder and director, Integrative Medicine Association (in India since 1952)

"Dr. Randall has a deeper connection to the wisdom of the indigenous peoples than any doctor I've ever met and beautifully brings this together with her knowledge of integrative health and medical science. She seeks to truly understand people on the levels of mind, body, and spirit and she also has the (physical and metaphorical) medicine bag to help on all these levels."

—Sage Dammers, cofounder, Addictive Wellness

"Gayle Madeleine Randall, MD is an extraordinary person who has played many roles in my life: physician, teacher, student, colleague, and friend. Her generosity in sharing her story with the world through *Soul Doctoring* is immeasurable. Read it. You'll recognize pieces of your own growth-path, and you'll be inspired to stretch to your own fullest potential. Without giving advice, she advises wisely that each of us is born to deliver a unique message of love to the world."

—Connie Kaplan, author, *The Woman's Book of Dreams*,
Dreams are Letters from the Soul and
The Invisible Garment The Emergence of a New Cosmology

"Gayle Madeleine Randall is generous and wise with her counsel, which begins with a distinguished background in mainstream medicine and then draws on her knowledge of the holistic and Native American traditions. I find it especially important that her philosophy on nutrition is sound and healthy, aimed at longevity and preventing or combating disease, rather than at quick and temporary weight loss. Her advice and encouragement have been invaluable to me."

—The late Roger Ebert, author, *Ebert & Roeper at the Movies*

"'Medical Visionary Futurist' is my description of Gayle Madeleine Randall, MD. Her wide and varied practice has led thousands to much improved and greater health. She leaves no stone unturned in her delving into the secrets of health. She is much to be admired as an open researcher into what is needed in human health. To be advised by her is to be getting the very top advice in medicine today! She is a treasure for all to enjoy and appreciate. Reading this book is an adventure of self and planetary healing led by a Medical Visionary Futurist."

—Howard Wills, well-known healer in Kauai

"I could not put this book down! Dr. Gayle Randall is a true renaissance woman who has given her life to helping others heal on whatever level is needed. *Soul Doctoring* is the stunning compilation of her life's journey and inquiry into the true meaning of physical, mental and spiritual balance. Filled with practical guidelines and spiritual insights, *Soul Doctoring* is one of the most significant books on conscious healing that I have read in years."

—Michele Hébert, Raja Yoga Meditation Guide and author,
The Tenth Door: A Yoga Adventure

"Dr. Gayle Randall has a healing gift unlike any that I've ever seen in my decade and a half of counseling, and her gift is greatly expanded upon in her new book, *Soul Doctoring.* We have collaborated in patient care, and the level of trust in her abilities that my patients have expressed is unparalleled, and I'm beyond excited to partake of and to share her healing modalities with everyone I encounter through this work of art! She has an uncanny way with words, a gentleness with her holistic approach, and I what I consider to be an iron fist in a velvet glove. Dr. Randall doesn't hesitate to "tell it like it is" but does so smoothly & with a kindness and humility that is unusual for such a decorated pioneer in her field, and with razor-sharp intellect. If you are holding her book in your hands, consider yourself extraordinarily lucky, as well as well on your way to healing what ails you. I highly recommend her work as a must-read for anyone and everyone. Place your trust in her, she never disappoints!"

—Dr. Danielle Delaney, ThD, crisis interventionist, author,
and media personality

"Dr. Gayle Madeleine Randall is a medical futurist and holistic pioneer after my own heart. I thoroughly enjoyed getting to know her through her *Soul Stories* podcast featuring people who have changed the world aimed at raising consciousness. Her new book *Soul Doctoring: Heal Yourself, Heal the Planet* is timely, much needed and an exciting healing journey for anyone who reads it. Dr. Randall helps guide us into our own highest potential while healing our Mother Earth. I highly recommend it."

—Dr. Gladys Taylor McGarey, Mother of Holistic Medicine,
cofounder of American Holistic Medical Association,
founder of Living Medicine Foundation, author of five books:
The Physician Within You, Born to Heal, Living Medicine,
Beyond Holistic Medicine, The World Needs Old Ladies

Soul Doctoring

HEAL YOURSELF, HEAL THE PLANET

Gayle Madeleine Randall, MD

Foreword by Olivia Hussey Eisley

Introduction by Emeran Mayer, MD

Transformation Media Books
Saint Louis, Missouri

Published by Transformation Media Books, USA

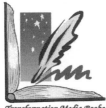

Transformation Media Books

www.TransformationMediaBooks.com
info@TransformationMediaBooks.com

An imprint of Pen & Publish, LLC
www.PenandPublish.com
Saint Louis, Missouri
(314) 827-6567

Print ISBN: 978-1-956897-05-0
eBook ISBN: 978-1-956897-06-7
Library of Congress Control Number: 2022934359

Printed on acid-free paper.

Sundance vision and image: Dr. Gayle Madeleine Randall
Cover Design: Alexa Black
Image Illustration Artist: Moe Sheehan

DEDICATION

My experiences with my American Indian teachers were the most valuable in compelling me forward to fulfill my soul purpose: healing humanity and the planet. They gave me the framework to form my holistic approach, and I will always be grateful to the indigenous peoples for their gifts and regenerative lifestyles. We need to continue to learn from their time-proven wisdom, and understand and remember this knowledge is of equal importance to the scientific contribution to medicine and healing. The real power originates when both come together.

CONTENTS

ACKNOWLEDGMENTS AND THANKS

I have great gratitude and thanks for the many individuals who made it possible for me to write this book. I am grateful to all of my teachers from all walks of life over the years who have helped shape and guide me on my path. I am especially grateful to Joseph Rael, who invited me to dance in his Sun Moon dances that created the space for my vision of this book. Many thanks to my academic teachers and especially Dr. Arthur Schwabe who invited me to become a Gastroenterologist in his division at UCLA. He was the personification of compassionate doctor, professor emeritus at UCLA and a gentleman. Much gratitude to my patients who taught me through their experiences about the importance of self-healing. And special gratitude to Robert Yehling, my editor and collaborator, who has been with me since the beginning; and to his teams at Word Journeys Literary and Write Away Books. Special thanks to Transformation Media Books and Jennifer Geist for her meticulous editorial advice. Also, to my wonderful office team of Toni Campos and Rhonda Wilhite, without whom I could not do half of what I do. Also, Concetta Kirschner and Sara Gepp my social media managers. Also my team of doctors, therapists and trainers that keep me together: Bruce Parker DC, Samantha Binah-Pilates, Larry Greene-Trainer, Sharri Li-Massage. Also my wonderful housekeeper Doris Dominguez and gardener Zesar Gonzalez. And last but not least, my encouraging, loving family: my son Nicolas Perez, daughter-in-law Teresa Perez and granddaughters Madeleine and Vanessa Perez. My many friends who listen to my ideas and passions. You know who you are. My lovely followers who tell me every day there is a dedicated audience for self and planetary healing. And of course, to my beautiful, wonderful horse and soul mate, Tatanka, who is always ready to carry me into the mountains to commune with nature and maintain my spiritual balance.

FOREWORD

By Olivia Hussey Eisley
Golden Globe Award-Winning Actress, *Romeo & Juliet*

Namaste!
It is my pleasure, one filled with love and gratitude, to share about my continuing experience and healing with the most wonderful and "one of a kind" Dr. Gayle Randall.

I was diagnosed with breast cancer in 2008. I chose to have a mastectomy without chemotherapy or radiation. Afterward, I enjoyed nine wonderful years of being disease-free. In 2017, I experienced great difficulty breathing; it turned out to be the darkest and most frightening time of my life! Tests revealed a large metastatic cancerous mass near my heart.

Unnerved, I called my beloved healer and teacher Howard Wills at his healing center in Kauai. He told me to fly to Kauai immediately. After I arrived, I had the good fortune to meet Dr. Gayle Madeleine Randall, who was there for her own healing. I found her to be the most compassionate, knowledgeable and sincere—and above all, the most understanding—doctor I have ever spoken with. Little did I know she would become my new teacher and work along with Howard in my healing process.

I returned from Howard's center and used traditional cancer therapy, which helped shrink the tumor. However, the chemo made me so ill that I sought out Dr. Randall for alternative suggestions. Besides being well-educated and a board-certified practicing doctor of conventional medicine, Dr. Randall has a true comprehension, passion, and wisdom of all alternative healing practices.

At the time I went to see Dr. Randall, I had embarked on a determined life path, one that included alternative medicine. I want you to know that Dr. Randall is not just my healer and friend, but also my teacher—mentally, emotionally and spiritually. She is literally an angel sent to me from God. She has taken care of my health issues and looks after me with more gentleness and love than I could have ever imagined! With her knowledge and love, she has designed my "Path." She continues to travel that path with me as my constant guide.

Thus, I wasn't too surprised to learn that Dr. Randall was one of the first cutting-edge physicians to participate in the groundbreaking work to develop and initiate integrative medicine at UCLA and other facilities. This phenomenon took place in the early 90s, before there was even a name for this type of medicine. In 2000, Dr. Randall also innovated and practiced a form of medicine, ultimately to be dubbed "integrative medicine," at Miraval Life in Balance, which she directed.

Dr. Randall is an integrative and functional medicine doctor with deep, vast knowledge in nutrition, herbology, energy medicine, Ayurveda, and traditional Chinese and Japanese medicine. Mostly, though, it is her heart, compassion and light I admire. I call her my angel, though she is not solely my own; she has taken on the care of my husband, David Glen Eisley, and our darling daughter, India Joy. Not to mention the many who seek her out for care. She always goes the extra mile, whatever it takes to heal that person. Dr. Randall makes us all feel like we are her special patients and insists we let her know our every need.

I believe Dr. Gayle Madeleine Randall is the pinnacle of futuristic medicine, as you can see in the book you are now holding. She excludes nothing and leaves no stone unturned. Her pursuit of excellence is obvious, as she enhances her expertise in areas such as cross-cultural medicines, nutrition and alternative ways to heal outside of the box. She is my friend, teacher, and Soul Doctor.

To her I say, *I am forever grateful. You are in my prayers every day.* I bless the moment we met. Dr. Randall brought me light, guidance and unconditional love . . . and continues to do so. To her I say, "Thank you for your Love, Light and Friendship. And for your knowledge and my continued healing the natural way. You are always in my heart. I love you, Dr. Randall!"

If I had one wish, it would be that everyone could meet Dr. Randall. Since that's not possible, I wish that everyone would read this splendid book, so they too can heal themselves and the planet, and follow the lighted path she has painted for us all.

Blessings!

Olivia Hussey

(Olivia Hussey Eisley is the critically acclaimed and Golden Globe Award–winning actress of Franco Zeffirelli's Romeo and Juliet *and* Jesus of Nazareth *and the author of* Girl on the Balcony.*)*

INTRODUCTION

By Emeran Mayer, MD
Distinguished Professor, UCLA;
New York Times Bestselling Author, *Mind-Gut Connection*

When I first met Gayle Madeleine Randall in 1985, we were part of the Integrated UCLA VA Training program—she was a GI fellow starting her career as a gastroenterologist (and later, a neurologist as well), and I as a junior faculty member who had just finished my specialty training in the same program. Little did we know how our career paths would become intertwined and head in a similar direction.

In contrast to most of our colleagues at the time, we shared interests outside of mainstream medicine and gastroenterology. We had interacted with indigenous healers, and our approach to patients was based on a holistic concept of mind, body and the world, guided by compassion and empathy. Whereas such views of health and disease are becoming accepted by a growing number of physicians in what is now called functional medicine and integrative medicine, our views of health and disease were definitely out of the mainstream in a premier academic institution such as UCLA in the mid-1980s.

That special role didn't keep us from organizing several interdisciplinary workshops at UCLA, where we put together a panel of medical experts with indigenous and traditional healers, providing their assessment of patients with complex chronic diseases. While many of our colleagues considered this an incomprehensible deviation from our academic and clinical mission as gastroenterologists, we kept pursuing this path, wrote a script for a documentary called *The Healing Connection*, and organized a three-day interdisciplinary symposium in Sedona, Arizona, entitled The Biological Basis of Mind Body Interactions.

Gayle has taken this holistic approach to health and chronic disease and transformed it into an amazing career-long journey, in which she has integrated the best of Western medicine with a range of non-traditional approaches. Along the way, she has accumulated a vast experience as a gastroenterologist at an academic institution, intuitive healer, diet and nutrition expert, founder and director of health and wellness spas and integrative healing institutes, and practitioner of integrative and functional medicine at different locations in Southern California. Her book, Soul Doctoring, documents the unique path she has taken and delivers in an easily understandable and entertaining way the many facets of her holistic approach to patients and the world.

In *Soul Doctoring*, much emphasis is given to subjects not taught in medical school and almost universally neglected in medical practice, including trust, love, attitude, intuition, purpose, compassion and worship. These topics refer to the emotional and spiritual dimensions of health, wellness and healing, which have been separated from medicine ever since Rene Descartes decided that these aspects should be addressed by the church, and not by science. While these dimensions of health, wellness and disease have been essential elements of traditional healing practices amongst indigenous people, and amongst traditional Eastern and European medical systems, the West has only recently rediscovered and acknowledged the importance of these factors. In addition, a growing body of science has identified the biological mechanisms underlying these forgotten underpinnings of health and wellness.

Perhaps not surprisingly, since she is a gastroenterologist by training, Gayle also covers the emerging concept of gut health and brain–gut interactions and emphasizes the importance of diet. However, what might surprise you is that we gastroenterologists never received any formal training in nutrition or diet. Transcending this big gap, Gayle has developed extensive experience on her own and views food as medicine. She uses specific nutritional recommendations related to individualized diets and supplements in her treatment plans. Gayle demonstrates her truly holistic view of health and wellness by pointing out that the implications of a healthy diet don't stop at our own health. She acknowledges the intricate relationship between the health of our gut and body, the food that we eat, the soil in which we grow our food, and the health of the environment. Holistic health cannot stop selfishly at our own bodies but has to incorporate the health of all life forms on the planet.

Rather than viewing the mind and emotions as simple functions of the individual brain, Gayle emphasizes that the mind connects not only brain and body, but that it also connects us with the world and all the people around us. The bidirectional interactions between brain, body and the world through our mind provide the theoretical framework for holistic medicine, and recent science supports the crucial importance of these connections for our health. These interacting elements contain our "carbon"-based biological systems, as well as our spiritual dimensions, which go beyond the individual self. While Western medicine continues to focus almost exclusively on a reductionist view and treatment of the body when it fails, integrative and functional medicine have gone an important step forward by recognizing the body and brain as a complex system of interacting parts. Disturbances in these interactions can be diagnosed early before an actual disease becomes manifest, and multidisciplinary treatment approaches are targeted at reestablishing balance within the system.

Gayle has been able to present all these aspects in a semi-autobiographical and exciting way and weave them into a truly holistic manifesto. I am not aware of another book that accomplishes this task as well as *Soul Doctoring*. The book's 25 chapters not only present a journey through Gayle's life, full of fascinating personal and patient anecdotes, but a comprehensive education about the many dimensions of holistic health and wellness from gut to brain health, and from dreams to planetary health.

PROLOGUE
Mending the Sacred Hoop

July 1997

Three days and three nights of the Sundance Ceremony pass. The dancing and fasting from food and water takes its toll on my body during the hottest, driest three days in mid-July I can remember. I surrender to the heat and release my consciousness to fly with the winds of eternity.

A vision gifts me . . .

American Indian elders pass a talking stick around the circle and speak in their native tongue. As one elder begins to speak, an image forms in the smoke from the fire burning in the center of the circle: a woman sitting at a desk, working with a pen, paper and a computer. He passes the talking stick clockwise to the next elder. The talking stick goes around until all have had the opportunity to speak. Each elder discusses this woman seriously, as though evaluating or interpreting her.

She seems familiar, very familiar . . . then I realize the woman is me!

After passing the talking stick for the fourth revolution, the elders seem to come to an agreement. Symbols begin to appear in the smoke as the talking stick reaches each of the four cardinal directions. When the stick is passed to the east, an eagle appears while a golden sun blazes in the background. To the south, a wolf stands by a large, clear blue body of water. To the west, a black bear walks in a lush green forest as the sun sets behind the mountains.

When the stick is passed to the north, a white buffalo appears on a grassy plain beneath large blue skies dotted with puffy white clouds. The buffalo lies down and rolls, then starts to spin, its body becoming round, like the medicine wheel—the most sacred healing symbol in many Native cultures. The wheel changes into a blue-green sphere slowly rotating in space. Our Mother Earth.

Finally, the sphere drops into my arms and transforms into a book that carries an image of me hugging the planet. A book that, the vision speaks, the woman is to write.

That I am to write.

1

Visions come to us carrying deeper messages about our soul purpose. It is our job to understand and manifest them, to see and understand what they tell us about our lives, our health and our way moving forward. This particular vision pushed me forward into integrating my discipline and scientific knowledge, while calling in all of my post-doctoral training. With that came the message of Spirit to look *within*, one of the central premises of *Soul Doctoring*—the book I was tasked to write in the vision.

This Sundance vision in New Mexico guided me to honor spirit, signified by the smoke in the center of the circle. It also reminded me to remember the importance of integrating ancient knowledge into modern health care. The image of the earth depicted the global change in consciousness needed on our planet. If you shift the consciousness of even one individual, it creates the potential for many to change. That shift is even more crucial in today's increasingly hostile world and the climate change, health-care, active pandemic and toxic emergencies we are in. Mother Earth needs us to get it: we have about 10 years to change our consciousness and our ways to save her.

In my vision, the woman arose from spirit smoke, guiding me to keep my spiritual practices for inspiration. The elders discussed and then instructed me to write a book that integrated all I had experienced and learned, to teach others, but more importantly, to encourage all to incorporate it into their own self-care. To follow in the footsteps of the elders who consume only what they need, never waste anything and live in a regenerative way. Giving back to the earth as they take. Thus keeping the planet at the heart of healing.

My experience includes mastery in nearly 30 healing modalities and approaches, built on my foundation as a medical doctor. The vision laid out my work ahead: helping to unite ancient wisdom with modern knowledge, and then teaching the sacred hoop of regeneration.

Upon this realization, the words of my first Native teachers echoed in my heart and mind:

> *Granddaughter, communicate from your heart, see with your heart, speak from your heart, use your mind for knowledge and your heart for wisdom. Honor the Good Red Road. Always remember the value of honoring spirit in treating the body and walking softly upon the earth. Teach about honoring the plants and animals, and things. Teach about living in balance with all things. Do this, my granddaughter, for all the planet!*

I walk and follow these concepts every day in both my life and medical practice at Randall Wellness. They are an integral part of who I am, the very fabric of my nature and soul. I walk them, talk them, live them, breathe them, and teach them.

My teachers have guided me to view all aspects of the individual in my practice. Every aspect is so important in treating "dis-ease" and maintaining wellness—but are often missed by doctors today, rushed as they are to make quick diagnoses, prescribe drugs and push the patient out the door. Their emphasis is on treating only the symptoms, usually with Big Pharma medications. I see it another way. We must consider the whole person, looking beyond the physical body and recognizing the centrality of spirit in any healing endeavor. Thus, my clinical approach to holism overlays the teachings of several modalities at a time, including the medicine wheel and other ancient modalities in which I have been schooled: Chinese and Japanese medicines, Ayurvedic medicine, pranic healing, and many more.

Which brings us to *Soul Doctoring*. This book is the amalgamation of ancient wisdom and modern medicine, and how we can integrate it into our own lives, as presented through my story, life and practice. The goal is to heal ourselves from any dis-ease, dis-order, affliction, or challenge we face, and form the "shoulders" upon which the medicine of the future will stand. What I hope you will find in these pages is a new power: the power to participate fully in your own road to wellness. For that, I provide guidance by example and tools throughout this journey.

My healing and teaching career officially began with Western medicine, with a particular focus on what lies *within*. First, I became an *in*tern, and then I went into *internal* medicine. That led me into gastroenterology, which concerns the inside of people's digestive tracts. I developed a special interest in endoscopic technology, which looks *inside* people's bodies through camera-mounted instruments to diagnose and treat disease. My particular interest was the microbiome of the gastrointestinal tract at UCLA; when I took it up in the 1980s, everyone thought that it didn't matter.

This direction was nothing new for me. In my senior year in medical school, I began studying American Indian theology and philosophy, captivated with the metaphysical approach and how it integrated with my scientific bent. I'm still studying. Among other things, my Native teachers taught me to look within *myself* for God. "There is a little piece of God inside each one of us, and we are all a little piece of God. Fully recognizing and getting in touch with that divinity inside you and in all things is part of healing," they said. They also demonstrated how to live harmoniously with the earth and all animals, plants, and things. They live in a natural regenerative way.

During my evolution as a physician, I've had the great fortune to witness the growth and power of technological science at the prestigious UCLA Medical Center. I've also experienced the magic of "mind-body" medicine through many studies and experiences outside the university. Since that time, colleagues have frequently asked me, "Why did you leave the UCLA faculty?" "Why did you get into holistic medicine?" "What *is* integrative medicine?" "What is functional medicine?"

Before I answer those questions, let's look at what inspired me to enter medical school. I felt an urgent desire to help relieve people's suffering. However, eight arduous years of basic sciences in premedical and medical school separated many of my classmates from their similar humanitarian reasons for joining the medical profession. Lack of sleep, overwork and poor food dissolved once smiling, compassionate expressions. I watched them shift their focus to the diseases their patients suffered, as though disease were independent from the patient's actual distress. Disease became the patient and science the altar from which we invoked our therapeutic actions.

Unlike many of my colleagues, though, I did not lose my fresh, idealistic outlook. I had the positive experience of seeing the person as whole, as taught by my American Indian teachers, who were in my heart to support me.

In the last few years of medical school, we began to see patients at the university hospital, under the tutelage of our supervising (attending) physicians and residents. I was elated at the prospect of working with *people* after years of test tubes and laboratory experiments. *Just what I have been waiting for!* Funding for medical research and National Institutes of Health funding was in its heyday, and many attending physicians were physician-researchers assigned to the hospital wards for a month or two. They often preferred to stay in their labs rather than doing clinical medicine, from which they felt distanced.

Not me. The resident introduced me to the attending physician. He shook my hand out of a sense of duty and called his lab assistant to check on his experiments. So it went. I prepared myself for rounds by reading everything I could find on the diagnoses of each patient. With pertinent medical history carefully outlined on note cards, along with lab results and my own questions, I was definitely pumped up.

4

My presentation began with my most critical patient, a man in his 40s suffering from acute liver failure with no known cause. I didn't even get to finish speaking before the attending physician interrupted me. He went to the whiteboard and made notes while delivering a two-hour lecture on the multiple functions of glutathione in the cellular detoxification of liver cells. I found it very interesting—only to be stunned when he excused himself and hurried to his lab to finish his experiments. My mouth was agape as he ducked out the door.

After this first session of patient rounds, I felt totally deflated. *What about my patient with liver failure?* Is glutathione going to help him? I wish we could have given him a glutathione drip, but the hospital pharmacy did not carry it at the time. I had so many questions, but no time to learn what I needed in order to help this patient. That night, he died in the intensive care unit, comatose and alone. An autopsy showed liver failure from unknowingly ingesting toxins from Jamaican Bush Tea made by a "helpful" neighbor after he came down with the flu. His reaction caused rapidly progressive occlusive disease of his small hepatic veins (which drain deoxygenated blood from the liver to the inferior vena cava of the heart). This reaction manifested in the form of a very large painful liver, jaundice, and ascites (fluid in the abdominal cavity). When I told my supervising resident, he said, "What a great case!" and asked me to present it so everyone in the medical chain could benefit.

While I appreciated his interest, I recoiled at the paradox of describing the *death of my patient* as a "great case." My respect for the human condition made me promise myself I would not grow jaded, nor condone the human indifference and narrowness of this type of thinking. From that moment, I vowed that *the patients and their suffering* needed our closest attention, not the pathology of their suffering to the exclusion of their needs.

I perceived a general lack of concern for the patient as a whole. I felt very alone at times, but I was gratified by the appreciation my patients showed me when I helped them with their personal needs. Doctors rarely considered simple things that were apparent to me, such as allowing food from home or a visit to the hospital garden. Sunlight and fresh air are amazing healers.

Something was lacking: the essential nature of healing, as described by my first Native teachers. *How does it all fit together?* I struggled with the question.

Things began to change in 1982, when I received a highly sought-after position in the UCLA internal medicine residency program. By focusing on the patient, I became an accomplished physician and mastered the art of medicine. I took full advantage of all medical technology available while beginning a journey into holistic medicine. With more freedom to work, I visualized my patients as whole people, connected to body, mind, spirit, community—and the planet. I saw how much time and well-spent attention meant to their outcomes. Something as simple as listening and caring so often made the difference between a lasting cure and a temporary Band-Aid. Many times, I sat by patients' bedsides, comforting them through long painful nights while encouraging them to take a fresh look at their lives. This sometimes gave them renewed hope to overcome their illnesses.

One of my first patients was Carlos Martin, a Hispanic gentleman in his mid-70s. He suffered from sideroblastic anemia, a severe blood disease in which the bone marrow does not make enough white or red cells to fight infections or deliver oxygen to the body. Carlos had been admitted several times for life-threatening pneumonia. After his second admission in two months, he became my patient. I treated him with antibiotics and respiratory therapy, while also giving him intravenous infusions of folic acid; some cases of sideroblastic anemia respond to this vitamin. Although this response is usually seen in children, it could do no harm, I reasoned. We gave it a try.

Yet, I felt there was more to Carlos's condition, something deeper standing between him and the *desire* to heal.

After rounds, I would often visit patients and learn more about their lives. When I visited Carlos, he told me he drank beer and smoked cigarettes every day. I also learned something else: a devout Catholic who attended church weekly with his wife, Rosa, Carlos had not been to mass since her funeral. "I haven't been in almost a year," he said, his face hardening, his jaw set. "I'm mad at God. He took her away."

I reached out and gently touched his shoulder. "Do you want to share what happened?"

"She was so full of love—for everybody and everything. One night she went out to cut some roses for our dinner table. I heard her sweet voice singing to her roses. Can you imagine someone so sweet that she talked and sang to her flowers?" His eyes clouded over, then darkened to pitch black. "Then she was shot—for no reason. Why would God let that happen? She was my reason for living. I loved her so."

Tears spilled over his eyelids like tiny waterfalls, releasing into the deep crevasses of his weathered brown face. "Rosa loved me, too. We didn't have much, but we were wealthier than most people. We had real happiness together. You can't buy that."

"No, you can't," I said softly.

"If you figure out a way, let me know. I'd like to be the first in line."

The twinkle in his eyes returned. I felt an opening in his heart. "If your wife loved you half as much as you loved her, do you think she would want to see you suffering this way?" I asked.

Carlos softened further, a little surprised by my openness and willingness to talk directly. "No, Doctor, I guess not. I don't know why, because she was always healthier than me. But she always said, 'If I go first, you need to remember that Rosa and all of God's angels will be watching over you. So you better take care of yourself.'"

I asked a question he didn't expect from a doctor, let alone a young woman launching her medical career: "Carlos, will you pray with me?"

"Yes." He nodded his head.

Mindful of his theology, we gave thanks to Jesus and Mary, mother of God. We asked that Carlos be healed in his body *and* his heart. "No doctor has ever treated me like you do," he said. "You are not a doctor; you are a good witch the angels and my wife sent to help me."

I chuckled and shook my head. "No, I just work here. If other doctors behaved as I did, then we'd all be doing our sacred work, but we'd still be doctors. Or else we'd *all* be witches. Wouldn't that shock the hell out of the dean?"

We cried and laughed together until sweet tears ran down both our cheeks. We'd built a healing bridge between us. Finally, I asked a question still on my mind: "Carlos, did anyone ever tell you that drinking alcohol and smoking can suppress the immune function in your bone marrow and lungs and make you more susceptible to pneumonia?"

"Rosa always told me it was bad and she kept me from doing it," he replied. "But after she died, I figured, what's the use? But I didn't understand it medically like that." He agreed to stop smoking and drinking if I would be his clinic doctor.

It delighted Carlos that a doctor cared enough to listen to what was really bothering him and explain what he could do to stay healthy. After months of grappling with the effects of a depressed immune system, his white cell count rose from a dangerously low level of 500 to a reassuring 3,500. He was discharged from the hospital and scheduled for follow-up care in my clinic.

I will always remember the joke he played on me when I was still in training at UCLA. He played this joke every time he came to the clinic. First, he would check in with the nurses, who would lead him to my examining room. We would have our session. Afterward, I would leave the room for a customary check-in with the supervising attending physician. Attending physicians would often come to the room so they could meet and observe someone who overcame sideroblastic anemia. "Mr. Martin, you've made quite a remarkable recovery," one said.

"Yes," he replied, with that twinkle in his eye. I was thinking, *No, no, Carlos don't say it! Don't go there . . . you'll ruin my reputation!* I stood behind the attending physician, shaking my head, looking at Carlos with pleading eyes. *Don't say more . . . please.*

The moment spurred him on. With the familiar lilt in his voice, he added, "I am totally healthy and happy again, too. You know . . ." he leaned close to the attending physician's ear, "it is because . . . she is a *weetch*. You need to have more *weetches* like her around this place. You should tell the dean of the medical school to hire more."

Carlos never stopped getting a kick out of that joke.

Later, he wrote a letter to the dean and brought it to the clinic so I could read it. He stressed that all doctors should follow my example and really listen to their patients—and pray with them, too, if that's what it takes to make them better. As I read, I fully appreciated that Carlos was my teacher, as well as my patient. He taught me something very valuable about healing. I remained his doctor for more than a decade until he passed away at 88 from a heart attack in his sleep.

Thanks to patients like Carlos, and facilities like the UCLA Medical Center, my fascination for science and technology continued to grow. So did my intrigue concerning the mysterious nature of healing. Upon finishing my subspecialty training as a gastroenterologist, I was asked to join the department of medicine staff. I conducted research, made innovations in imaging technology and endoscopic surgery, and taught medical students. However, my deepest passion remained patient care. I never lost my close association with patients, nor my passion for studying ancient medicine practices.

In 1988, I delved more deeply into the healing ways of American Indian medicine, reconnecting with a greater perspective of "holism." I embraced and integrated these ancient teachings with my Western medical training. It made me long for an even greater connection with spirit. I took weekend and day trips into the nearby canyon lands or pristine forests of the Angeles Crest National Forest and ran like a wild woman. The earth and her creatures reminded me of the importance of maintaining close relationships with the land, animals and elements. I became involved with keeping the wildlife corridor open in the Santa Monica Mountains, during which I met my now longtime friend, Judy. In her, I found a sister willing to fight the same environmental battles and run wild in the woods with me. Not what you'd expect from a gastroenterologist teaching medical school students!

One day, Judy introduced me to Lewis, a Powhatan man passionate about nature and the sacred purpose of hunting. Lewis showed me a remote area of Red Box Canyon, where humans do not tread. We went to hunt deer but not to kill them. We almost canceled the trip due to the threat of storms. However, when we spoke by phone at 4 a.m., we decided it wasn't going to rain.

When we arrived, the sun was beginning to scatter its first rays over the eastern ridge. We parked our truck near the top of the mountain. Lewis pointed toward a nearly overgrown path, invisible to most passers-by. We ambled down the side of the mountain in our camouflaged clothes, making little crunching noises as we walked on the clear, crisp fall morning. I watched for the wooden cross of sticks that Lewis had left to mark the steep descent into the canyon.

After walking and enjoying the sweetness of the early morning air, Lewis spoke in a low voice. "The deer are the king of the animals in these parts. When the deer go, the people will go, too." An unfathomable sadness dropped over his face like a veil. "When we come upon a group of deer, watch them. The oldest, most feeble doe that will not make it through the winter will stay behind as the rest of the herd scatters. She gives herself away so the others may escape and live. Most gun hunters shoot the biggest, most virile buck. Taking him out hurts the survival of the deer tribe. It doesn't make sense in the natural order of things. Watch carefully for the old doe. She will only give you a moment. She has a bit of gray just under her belly where the front legs meet her body, and she won't be as sleek and fast as the others. There is no more compassionate or noble creature than the deer."

In that moment, a deeper understanding penetrated my heart. I recalled the stories my American Indian teachers had told about the agreement the four-leggeds made with man. "It is an agreement between man and animals made a long time ago," Lewis confirmed. "In return, the humans are to be keepers of the land." We humans would be guardians of the planet, dedicating ourselves to protecting the animals and all living beings . . . and the earth.

Wouldn't that be nice if we all still felt and lived in such a reverent way?

Lewis taught me how to shoot a longbow, track deer and embrace the ceremonial aspects of hunting. I came to see the sacred agreement between animal and man as the ancients must have experienced it. After affirming my observations and memories, Lewis's eyes grew dark. "Mankind has forgotten their part of the agreement."

We came to the crossed sticks and left the path to make our steep descent into the canyon. A snort and rustle of brush arose from the tree line. "They know we're here," Lewis said. "That sounded like the territorial snort of a buck. When you walk into a forest like this, it creates a wave of reaction in the wildlife for miles. They sense your presence and communicate to each other." This led me to reflect on how everything we do creates waves in existence and affects the balance of the earth. If we could only be more cognizant of that in all the ways we live.

When we reached the bottom of the canyon, we found a California bay laurel tree. We rubbed its sweet, pungent leaves all over us to cover our scent. Lewis showed me the deer trails and piles of scat, along with tracks and scat of bear, raccoon, bobcat, coyote and other animals. I learned to tell how many deer are in a band and to distinguish does from bucks by their prints. We saw many deer and played countless hours of "I see you before you see me." After a while, the deer seemed to know we were not going to harm them; some even grew playful. I felt like I had found home.

We headed downstream to explore more of this sacred place, the clear ice-cold waterfalls and pictures within the matrices of stones. It didn't seem possible, but the giant silvery stones populating the river had white crystalline markings that told stories of days gone by, the ancient history of the canyon. One stone carried a perfectly outlined moccasined foot. That became a landmark and prayer spot for me when I later returned to Red Box Canyon. In another stone, a tall brave held a spear above his head.

The stones spoke of the richness of spirit in an old growth forest unchanged by mankind since the beginning of time. Not only is the preservation of such places essential to keep our Mother Earth in balance, but maintaining our connection with nature is an inescapable part of balancing public and planetary health.

As morning turned into afternoon, we returned upstream and saw something new—a few coyotes nibbling on the remains of an old doe. The internal organs had been removed, carefully wrapped inside the tissue sac of the deer's gut and placed in the stream. Her right front leg, chest, neck and head were all that remained, with a long tooth mark in the flesh above her right eye. I could still feel warmth in the remaining parts. I was astounded that this dramatic act of nature could occur so quickly, with no blood anywhere!

Lewis looked around, his eyes widening. "Those coyotes didn't do this," he whispered.

Just then, two amber gleams flashed from the nearby brush. A low, guttural growling sound rose from the same area. We looked down to find the tracks of a large mountain lion and two sets of cub prints. "Don't run, just walk and keep looking behind you," Lewis said in an even, calm but urgent tone. We walked well away from the scene. "It's a good thing that the mountain lion and her cubs just ate, but don't *ever* feel or act like prey, or you *will* be prey. Remember the natural order of things."

Never were the natural laws of survival and respect more apparent to me.

It turned cloudy as we made our way up the stream in silence. Little pieces of round ice began to fall, pinging off the trees and bouncing off our camo-outfits and faces. "I told you it wouldn't rain," Lewis joked.

We both laughed, so happy to be alive, really alive!

When we reached the branch point to ascend the mountain, the sleet turned to snow. As we walked higher and higher, more snow dropped, covering everything with a blissful, quiet blanket of white. A crackle of lightning shattered the silence, followed by a glorious roll of thunder roaring through the canyon below us. It happened again. *Rolling thunder* . . . I now understood the meaning. Behind me, Lewis made happy hooting noises. I thanked the canyon for sharing her magic and respecting me as I so deeply respected her. Not only do we need the earth, but she needs us, I realized.

We arrived at the top. "That is your place now," Lewis said. "It knows you now. It is time for you to be the guardian. Always maintain the balance and never leave a trace of you—not even a footprint."

Months later, while happily rock-hopping downstream on my own, my right foot landed on a loose rock. I slipped and crashed down hard on my right knee; I heard an audible ripping sound. I'd taken my share of dramatic falls, but not like this. I hobbled out of the canyon with the help of a walking stick. I iced my knee, hoping the swelling would just go away by morning. However, at 3 a.m., excruciating pain awakened me. My heart sank. I flipped on the lamp. My knee looked like an over-ripe cantaloupe. I knew my years of running wild with the mountain lions, coyotes and bears had come to a close.

The angst I felt over losing "my church" was worse than the physical pain. I needed to figure out how to bring the mountain to me, but I had no idea how to do that. I have revisited Red Box Canyon many times since, always with the deepest sense of responsibility, awe, respect and gratitude. It has been my honor to watch over that place, and to take my spiritual communion there.

Meanwhile, I prayed for a teacher to help me learn a new way of accessing spirit, one who would also lead me to more deeply integrate the ways of spirit and Oneness with the planet. To strengthen my purpose: to help people heal themselves and the planet.

I have long since moved into my own practice to focus on the cutting edge of integrative and functional holistic healing. My work has truly become my worship and is part of fulfilling my purpose. The resounding success of my patients and my outreach to get my central message across: *heal yourself, heal the planet*. This is what has brought me into the public eye over the past 30 years.

Which leads us to *Soul Doctoring*, the book I envisioned in the New Mexico Sundance Ceremony. Now it is time to share what I have learned in the evolution of a new collaborative vision for health and holism to regenerate humanity and the planet.

CHAPTER 1
A Soul Doctor Is Born

I float in a blue-violet pool of soft maternal comfort, rising and falling on predictable waves that match her quiet breathing. I feel the love of the universe and of my mother. All is as it should be.

Suddenly, orange-coral light floods into my space. I hear voices I recognize, quiet at first, then louder. The closest says, "No Al, not now."

The other voice responds, "Come on, Honey, I miss you."

"No!"

After a little laughing, the voice of my mother says, "Al, be careful!"

I feel apprehensive, frightened. My space becomes smaller, compressing me beyond belief. What is this new feeling? *Pain.* I attempt to cry out, but no sound comes from my open mouth. The fluid of comfort roils like an earthquake of disastrous proportions. A sickening, ripping sound erupts near my body.

My life is in danger. I hear my mother screaming. The fluid is draining. The sounds are so loud they hurt my ears. The lights are so bright. An incessant drum pounds, *boom-boom! Boom-boom! BOOM-BOOM!* I feel sick. I cannot breathe. All of my nerve endings explode at once. Things fade . . . all is black.

I think of leaving my body and begin to move toward the beautiful, soft pink light, but supportive forces around me urge me to stay. They are kind, beautiful, glowing beings of pure light and loving vibration. I want to stay with them. I feel happy and loved and completely sustained in their presence. Even when they return me to my body, I feel their kindness.

Now I know I must stay in my body. It is imperative. I promise them I will stay.

I awaken, my body compressed. It hurts. The loud sounds and rollicking motions have ceased. I hear Mother's breath, much louder than before. Everything is more intense since the blue-violet pool left. For the first time, I feel that I am not welcome in my space. *Mother does not want me here!*

Then I sense a determination build within her. Her muscles tense. Another type of motion begins, a gigantic impact against something hard, like nothing I've ever experienced. It frightens me. A feeling of upward suspension—then *oomph*, again and again, an excruciating pressure against my body.

I move my legs away from the pressure. My little head begins slipping down, outside of my space. "Nurse!" Mother yells.

The impact stops. My position changes. I feel motion. Something is poking my head! I want to recoil, but I cannot. I am pushed down farther, being forced out of my space. *No! It's too soon. Not now!* I am crushed into a small chamber with hard, dense structures in every direction. The only thing to do is surrender.

I emerge into the brightest light. My head nearly explodes. I almost leave my body, the pain so severe. I hear my own voice for the first time, expressed with a sharp cry. It is so loud it reverberates to the core of my existence. I feel anger for the first time.

From a distance, *the other side*, the eternal *kind ones* look over me, pleased. I hear them: "It is alright, little one. Go back . . . promise . . . care, love, compassion. You are here for a purpose to unite and guide others for the benefit of all and the planet." I remember my promise and feel compassion for those who perpetrated this pain upon me. A sacred, eternal law flows through: "No harm shall come to the children." I feel both anger and compassion, experiencing paradox. Another first in my very short life.

Later, the April 30, 1952, *Omaha World Herald* reports:

> *Albert William Randall of Mutual of Omaha and wife Helen Casey Randall are the parents of Gayle Madeleine Randall, born April 29, 1952, at 1:11 PM in Omaha, Nebraska . . . 4 lb., 4oz . . . Due date June 15, 1952. The child is in serious condition at St. Joseph's Hospital. Mother Helen is in good condition.*

The next day, our physician, Dr. O'Donnel, walks into the room. "Helen, we really should consider putting her in an oxygen incubator for a while to be sure," he says.

"How is she doing?"

"She's a fighter, but she's lost almost two pounds since she was born." I only weighed a little over four pounds. Half my body weight is already gone.

"Isn't there a risk, Doctor?" Mom asks.

"Yes, but otherwise, we might lose her."

"Let's wait for Al; he'll be here after work."

"I don't think we should wait that long, Helen," Dr. O'Donnel says.

"OK, I'll call him."

She makes the call. "Hello, Sandra, this is Helen. May I speak with Al?"

"He's taken the Teamsters to one of those long luncheons. I'm not sure where they went or when they'll be back," his assistant says. "I can call Sam and ask him, but I think he went with them."

"No, that's OK. Just have him call me as soon as he gets in."

An hour later, Dr. O'Donnel checks in with Mother. "What did Al say?" he asks.

"I couldn't reach him. How is my baby? Can I see her?"

"She's actually doing quite well. All of the nurses are amazed at how strong that tiny little thing is." The doctor stops and changes directions. "Do you know Amy Jensen?"

"Sure, she is my neighbor."

"Well, we delivered her baby seven weeks early. We're putting the baby in the incubator now. The baby is not breathing well. So when you talk to Al, let the nurse know right away so they can call me at the office, because I have to borrow an incubator from another hospital. All of ours are full; must be something in the air."

"Did Amy have a girl or a boy?" Mom asks.

"A little girl. She named her Pam, I think."

By the time my parents took me home, my weight had increased to four pounds. I could fit inside my dad's size 14 shoe. However, I wasn't tiny for long. I grew with the determination of a true Taurus, topping out the height and weight charts by the time I was two. Generalizations in 1950s America about premature babies being more likely to have lower intelligence, small stature and physical weakness did not hold true for this little bull.

Having a near-death experience and being gifted with the knowing of what comes after and being told I was here for a purpose by *the kind ones* shaped my life and direction from the very first day.

Running with the Horses

A few years later, we moved into our new pink house on a hill, surrounded by cornfields. My mother busily set up the new home, running her errands while carting along my brother and me. Car rides were divine experiences. I kept my nose pressed to the window for any sign of the horses. On one of Mother's usual routes, we passed a vast tract of land where a rich old gentleman kept a small herd of semi-wild ponies, allowing them to run free. His herd included one dominant stallion and a number of mares and younger animals, 15 to 20 horses in all. I felt drawn to them, like they were my brothers and sisters.

I longed to be with my brethren. After seeing the centaurs and Pegasus-like beings in the movie *Fantasia*, I wanted to be a horse. My mother often told me I could be *anything* I wanted when I grew up; I decided that meant becoming a horse. I loved their graceful freedom and high spiritedness. They were the closest beings to me except for my spirit friends, but you couldn't touch them.

By the time we moved into the new house, I'd memorized the way to the ponies. My mother always praised me about how well I behaved in the car, but truthfully, I was off in another world, finding my way "home" to the horses.

I first visited this horse family when I was three. The night before, my parents held a huge party to celebrate the new house. Whenever they threw such big parties, they remained asleep for a long time the next morning. With that in mind, I got up with the first rays of sunlight and walked out the back door. An imaginary thread pulled me toward my horse relatives. I ran down the hill, turned to my right and walked to the street, then walked up another hill. *This is a lot harder and farther than it looks from the car*, I thought. Faltering, I plopped down on my bottom and began to cry.

A whinny reached my ears from a distance. *Horsies!*

I got up and walked until I could see them. They gathered at the fence, waiting for me. I slipped inside easily. They towered over me, nickering low and deep in their throats, like they had missed me, too, and were welcoming me home. I'd dreamt of them so often.

Warm puffs of breathy air caused my hair to fly up. Soft velvety noses explored and soothed my face, the whiskers tickling me into giggling and laughing. I was so joyful that I began to cry. Then I grew very tired. The horses bunched around me, creating shade as I lay down to rest, their tails swishing the air, keeping flies and insects away. I drifted into a deep sleep, exhausted from my long journey. It was the most beautiful, unconditional love I'd felt since *the kind ones* urged me to go back into my body before I entered this world.

As the sun moved in the sky, the horses began to gently nudge me and make little flapping noises with their lips, waking me up. *Am I dreaming?* They were telling me to make my way back home.

I began my journey down the hill, electrified by the nap amongst my loving horse family. My return walk was much easier. I recognized the landmarks, but they looked different from a lower perspective. *Turn at the blue house with the fireplug . . . one last turn up the little hill at the gray house . . .* finally, our pink house.

I walked through the back door just in time. My mother was starting to panic. "Gayle Madeleine Randall, where have you been?"

"Outside."

"Oh." She looked down at my little feet. "Oh God, you stepped in some dog poop! Come here! Were you playing with the neighbor's dog again? You stink!"

She cleaned me up, which I didn't like. It removed the beautiful smell of my horse family. When I laid down for another long nap, I dream-flew over the neighborhood to where my horses galloped, telling each other about a familiar one in a tiny, strange form who visited them that morning.

"Gayle! Gayle Madeleine Randall, where are you?"

Mom burst out of the house. She peered into the tallest tree in our front yard and spotted me. "Didn't I tell you not to climb up into that tree? Get down here!"

I gently swayed back and forth in the top branches, climbing to the tippy-top of that tree. My favorite thing was to get up so high that the weight of my body would make the branches sway. I could see my horse family as little brown, tan and white dots standing or loping majestically against the rolling green landscape. This filled me with endless delight.

Almost two years after my first trip to the horses, they called me again. Now five, I was allowed to play at the neighbors' houses. I knew I needed to see the horses, but my parents would never allow it. I didn't understand the concept of lying, so how was I going to see the horses while getting my parents to think I was with the neighbors? Or somewhere else?

I started to form a different association with lying than the general context. Spirit visitors would come to my bedroom, especially at night, or if I was out in the cornfields alone. These visitors were very loving, like *the kind ones* from before this physical life. Now, they appeared in animal forms. A big black panther would pad down the hall and lay at the foot of my bed while I was sleeping. He was my protector. A rainbow-colored snake would dance on the ceiling to help me get to sleep when my parents hosted friends for parties. Other beings looked like people but were dark-skinned and wore feathers in their hair. They would tell me about the earth and sky. However, my favorite was the tall, beautiful woman that came early in the summer mornings when the corn was tall. I liked to hide in the cornfields before breakfast, hoping to catch a glimpse of her.

I can still hear the screen door slamming as I darted out the door. "Gayle Madeleine! Where are you going?" my mom yelled.

"I'll be right back."

I scooted down the hill and across the road to the cornfield. I loved standing between corn rows or lying on the earth, peering at the cloudless azure-blue sky. If I was really quiet and in tune with my corn plant friends, my tall woman guide would come. She towered over even the tallest plants, her hair golden-white like fresh corn silk. She appeared covered with glitter, moving like the corn when it bent and ruffled in the Nebraska breeze. I never saw anything more beautiful. I thanked her for coming, and she smiled down on me like a mother does her baby. I felt immense love, but if I tried to touch her, she disappeared.

I learned to watch and listen for her messages. She spoke in a smooth whisper about the spirits in plants, how they were our relatives. I would only have to *think* a question, and she would answer. *How can we pick plants and eat them if they feel it?*

"It was the agreement. Always say thank you and give back to the earth and the plants."

After a short time, she disappeared as mysteriously as she arrived. Even when I couldn't see her, I knew she was always *present*, by my side.

One day, I told my mother. "Mommy, I have made the most amazing friends. Did you know that plants have feelings and spirits? The corn lady told me!" I couldn't stop myself; I was so excited. "She is so beautiful. We have to say grace every night, Mom. OK? Oh, also, they can just hear me think. You know, sometimes I can hear other people think, too. Like Charlie the neighbor. I heard him thinking about Lou down the street. You know, he really likes her a lot."

Her clear blue eyes darkened with concern. "We will have to talk with your father when he gets home," she said.

Had I done or said something wrong? Was I in trouble? For what? I so wanted to share the beauty of these friends.

When my father got home, he called me into his den for a talk. That meant one thing: *I'm in serious trouble.* My heart sank into my stomach. I found him in his chair, a cross look on his face. His lips were pursed so tightly they disappeared into his chin. He invited me to sit in the chair opposite, then began to fire questions with the veracity of a prosecutor on *Perry Mason* trying to get the witness to crack.

"Where did you get this idea of plants thinking or talking?" he asked.

"I don't know, Daddy. I thought I saw it."

"You saw a plant talking? Do you want to be put in the nut house?"

I almost started crying. "No."

His voice grew harder, his questions more pointed. "What is this about the neighbors? Where did you get those ideas?"

"Well, I . . ."

"We have to live in the neighborhood and I can't have my kids going around spreading rumors about people! Why don't you use your head? Think of someone other than yourself!"

I was five, and he was brilliant. He could easily disprove everything I said. I felt totally defeated, but for some reason, held to the truth as I knew it.

"But Daddy, they *are* real!" I cried.

He would hear no more. "You are a liar! Go in your room and stay there until you understand what that means."

I spent all afternoon and night in my room, not coming out until the next morning for breakfast. I did as he commanded. I thought lying was not telling the truth. But since I *was* speaking the truth, I came to understand what it meant to be a liar—saying something another person didn't want to hear or believe. That was bad or certainly not desired. I felt that.

"Do you understand what it means to be a liar?" my father asked.

"Yes," I said quietly.

"Good. So don't tell any more lies."

"I won't, Daddy."

Filled with this new revelation, I intended to ask permission to visit my neighbor's house to play. Once my parents said "OK," I would reroute to my beautiful horses instead. This led to several glorious trips, during which I came to know every pony in the herd. They had different colors and personalities, and each held a specific role. I learned their language and moods, much of it telepathic, with body language for emphasis. While I was somewhat limited in my ability to swish or rub my tail against a fence, or flick my ears, I came to understand the neighing and whinnying with ease. The breath language was the most intimate of all.

A white gray-spotted mare was my closest companion. All of the ponies trotted up to the fence when they sensed me approaching, but she was the happiest to see me. I galloped the fields, ate grass and slept with them on the cool, soft green grass, beneath the shade of oak and elm trees during the long hot summer days. The mare would stand close, graze and keep the flies off of us with her long silvery tail. Sometimes, her tail stung my face and eyes if she was particularly irritated with a fly, but I didn't care. I felt so loved and free.

Whenever the sun moved lower in the sky and cast sepia tones across the grassy meadows, a scene like one of my grandma's old pictures, I knew it was time to get home before my mom began to look for me. Sometimes, she would be heading toward the door, but I always arrived in the nick of time. All was well in my secret life as a horse.

A couple of years later, I noticed something happening to White, the name I'd given the mare. Her belly was getting big, and she seemed a little lazy. Some of the others carried big bellies, too. At home, to my surprise, the same was happening to my mother. "I have a baby growing inside me," she said, showing me her belly. Shocked at first, I asked if it hurt. "No." *The horses must have babies growing inside them, too.*

One day, Mom invited her friend Amy and her daughter to the house. "This is Pam, honey," Mom said. "She was born about the same time as you were."

Pam's eyes looked funny, not clear like most. She was very alert, though, and we became good friends. One day, when Pam and I were playing together, I needed to know a few things. "My mom says you're blind," I said. "What does that mean?"

"I can't see."

"What do you mean, you can't see?"

"It means I can hear you and feel you, but I can't see you."

"Oh, you don't believe that, do you? Let's play a game. You teach me to see the way you do, and I'll teach you the way I do."

"OK," she said.

We spent many afternoons playing and laughing together. Sitting side by side in the same chair, we talked for hours about the colors of the sky with clouds and sunsets, and the night sky with the moon and stars. We spent countless hours facedown in the grass or bushes, seeing the earth and grasses and wildflowers. Pam learned the colors of the grass and plants as we rolled in the yard. She "looked" into the faces of the flowers, those smiling faces of the divine, by smelling and feeling them as I described their colors. The things we "saw" in nature became our connection. We even developed a secret code through touch that enabled Pam to see through my eyes. I was able to do much of this languaging, in part, because of the way in which I learned to communicate with my horse friends.

Of all my friends, Pam reminded me of the horses most. She was so sensitive. I felt she saw better than most sighted people. We walked around the neighborhood, pretending I was the blind one and she was sighted. She led me by the hand up to the neighbors' houses and knocked on the door. When someone answered, Pam introduced me as her blind friend and explained she was taking care of me for the day. The person usually invited us in, and I signaled Pam about the color of her dress with hand squeezes. I began squeezing as soon as we entered the door, also stumbling a little, as if I could not see where I was going. Our system was pretty sophisticated. We used a different number of hand squeezes for each color: one squeeze for white, two for purple, three for blue, four for green, five for yellow, six for orange, seven for red, and eight for black.

Pam then complimented the lady on her dress. "What a nice green dress, Mrs. Kroger," she said. She leaned over to me, nodded her head, and added, "You know, that is the color of trees and grass."

This teamwork usually earned us milk and cookies. Sometimes, we walked out of houses with more: hand-me-down dollies, candy, and even roller skates. Our mothers could not figure out what we were up to, but they let it go. We had a lot of fun, and it allowed both of us to develop a greater sense of "vision," along with non-verbal skills we would not have tried otherwise. I never saw blindness as a bad thing.

Little did I know that Pam was the newborn put in the incubator instead of me. Sadly, it didn't work out for her. In the early 1950s, the high concentration of oxygen in incubators caused retrolental fibroplasia, a condition resulting in blindness or retinopathy in premature babies.

Trouble with the Horses

The horses called for me again. Something was not right. It was near suppertime, not the usual time I could slip away unnoticed, but I had to take the chance and get to them. I thought I could hear White neighing wildly, like I'd never heard before. "I forgot something at school, Mom. I'll be right back," I said.

As I ran out the door, I heard her trailing voice. "Your dad's on the way home and dinner will be on the table in an hour. Don't be late!"

I took my brother's bike and rode down the hill, and then up to the fence. Only White was there. She was wild-eyed, screaming in the same pitch I'd heard in my head. "What? What's wrong?" I yelled.

I slipped through the fence. Instead of greeting me, she turned, directing me to follow her. We passed a slope and ran over a huge mound to a part of the land I had never seen; it bordered a little ravine. Blood dripped down the backs of her legs as she trotted ahead. Had she been attacked?

Hurt in some way? When we arrived, I saw a white blood-stained body under a small tree, small and limp. There was no sign of breathing.

I tried to wake it up. "Baby! Little White! Oh no! Wake up! Please, no!"

It was to no avail. White was in pain, pacing back and forth, pawing the ground, unable to hold still. I put my hand on her neck. She was sweaty and tremulous. She pushed me hard with her nose; I fell to my hands and knees. I looked up to see her milk-making parts dripping, about to burst. Not knowing what else to do, I raised my mouth, caught the milk and began scooping it into my mouth. Her milk was hot and rich; it felt like pure love dousing my face and chest. She whinnied, low and deep in her throat; after a few minutes, her shaking stopped. Her eyes gazed at mine with complete and utter defeat and exhaustion. I stayed with Little White for a while, and then covered her with as much dirt and leaves as I could muster the strength to carry. White watched with apathy. I headed home, tears filling my eyes.

A few days later, I came back. Her cheery attitude surprised me. She acted as though nothing tragic happened—like losing her foal—but I sensed her love for me had grown, as mine had for her. White was now my teacher. She and these other beautiful four-leggeds taught me the cycles of life. I learned that even in the throes of the worst kind of loss, life goes on, and that death is not the end, but part of the natural cycle of all things. Goodness and compassion prevail.

One day, one of my mother's friends asked, "What are you going to be when you grow up?"

I tossed my hair as if it were a mane and whinnied. Then I resolutely announced, "A horse!"

Mother and her friends threw their heads back and howled with laughter. I, a proud horse, didn't like it. "Why are you laughing at me, Mommy?" I asked.

"You can't grow up to be a horse, honey," she said.

"But Mom, you said I could do *anything* I wanted!"

Her eyes and demeanor softened. "Well, almost, dear. Little horses grow up to be big horses and little girls grow up into women."

I knew she was right, but it was like finding out there is no Santa Claus for the first time.

From that conversation, a new initiative formed inside me: I would have my own horse. I would ask for a horse every birthday and Christmas. Meantime, I found ways to ride other people's horses until finally, my parents let me rent one.

Becoming a Champion Swimmer . . . and an Independent Girl

In order to keep my mind off of purely horses, my parents introduced me to swimming. I excelled at swim lessons and loved the team spirit and water. Beginning when I was three, they set up an exhibition lane for me during the home swim meets. My brother Gary and I lived in the swimming pool during the hot Nebraskan summers. We would ride our bikes to the pool at 6:30 every morning for practice, swim all day for fun and then enter into swim meets in the evenings. My hair was short and blonde but took on a greenish tint from so much chlorine. The exercise strengthened and hardened my body. I was a tomboy, always in competition with my brother, who was five years older. We would argue about who was faster, stronger or taller. By the time I was 12, my shoulders were broader than most men and I stood six feet tall. I broke the Nebraska state age-group record in the breaststroke and felt destined for the Olympics. Unfortunately, I developed severe swimmer's ear infections, which ended my competitive career.

My parents began to worry. One day, we went to a restaurant for a family meal. My father heard some people whispering, "Is that a boy or a girl?"

The next thing I knew, two years had passed and my mother had enrolled me in finishing school. When she did that, my father at long last agreed to help me buy a horse, because it would be good for my development. They did this to get me out of the pool.

A young man in the area raised an Arabian gelding from a colt but could no longer keep him because he was going away to college. The gelding's name was Sugarfoot, and his markings were identical to White.

Just as I thought I was home free, ready to own my own horse, Father made me agree to a condition—one of several he used to try and control me. He wanted to teach me the value of money, and more importantly, make sure I learned the value of hard work. He had to support himself from a young age, and likewise wanted me to crack down and get tough. He sensed the spiritual, sensitive nature in me, thought it unseemly for my future, and figured some tough discipline would help me grow out of it. "You can have new clothes for school, or you can have a horse," he said. "It is too expensive to get both, and it would not be fair to your sister or brothers. Also, if you decide you are going to get this horse, you need to get a job help to pay for the rent on the stall."

His attitude stunned me at first, but I quickly moved into action. I wanted that horse, the freedom it provided and to reestablish that deeply spiritual connection I felt with horses.

A year later at the age of 15, I began working in a local hospital as a nurse's aide, earning 75 cents an hour. Not only did I need to pay for stall rent, but I needed to think about good clothes, an essential in high school—especially Westside High, also known as "Hollywood High" because of its upper middle–class student body. Showing up without a brilliant wardrobe was a sure ticket to the "out group." Even though it hurt my feelings to be unpopular because of my clothes, I knew clothes did not make a person.

I chose Sugarfoot. He was only three when we bought him for $275—a steal. He quickly became the focus of my existence. Sugar was "green broke" when I got him, not knowing much. He was gentle, but I couldn't ride him at first. I spent every waking moment I could with him. We became best friends. When I walked into the barn, he would nicker and toss his head with anticipation. We loved our time together.

In the beginning, I could not afford a saddle or a bridle, so I first rode him "Indian style" with only a rope, more for me to hang onto than anything else. Training and learning to ride Sugar created true cooperation between us. Besides training him in the typical behaviors, I taught Sugar many tricks such as shaking hands, laying down, rolling over, rearing up and counting. I didn't know any better. It was great fun putting on shows for the little kids that would visit the stables. The kids would ask Sugar to guess their age and to add numbers. He would count by pawing the ground with his hoof until I touched his neck. Then he would stop. Crowds of little kids and their moms piled out of station wagons for the "Sugar Show" on Sundays. We became quite famous in our area.

One full moon night, I stayed late at the stables, and my dad picked me up after a meeting. Nearby, they had graded the pasture where my childhood ponies once roamed for the new Interstate 80, a huge shopping mall and a gated community. I looked up at the stars and moon, daydreaming about my ponies and little girl days, when I ran and ate grass with them, thinking they were full-grown horses because I was so small. I chuckled at the memory. Then an old longing rose from deep in my heart, how I believed I would grow up to be a horse and run free.

My peaceful melancholy was broken by Sugar, who walked up behind me and almost pushed me down with his nose. "What? How did you get out? Never mind," I said, spinning around. "What!" I screeched as he prodded me from the front.

He tossed his head up and down and squealed as he moved beside me. Never had he done that before. I slid easily up on his back and we immediately broke into a trot, heading off trail and down the hill toward the cleared land.

Tension and heat began building in his body. We had no bridle, not even a rope. Sugar would have stopped had I asked him, but I allowed his intuition to lead us. The cleared track was lit up by the silvery moonlight, the stars countless and dazzling in their brilliance. We slid downhill on the loose dirt like a baseball player sliding into home, landing softly upon the flattened area of smooth earth. Sugar hit the ground running. His hooves seemed to barely touch the ground. I crouched forward, becoming one with the powerful movement of his body. We flew over the land with the force of the wind, his mane whipping against my face, the tears in my eyes the only sense allowing me to know we had not merged into one great speeding creature. We sped on for what seemed like time without end.

Finally, we slowed to a lope. Our chests heaved in sync, sweat pouring down, nostrils flared. We both raised our heads, happy to be alive in the body and free. "Thank you, Sugar! I love you!" I yelled. He tossed his head proudly as steam rose from both of our bodies. He trotted us back to the stable.

CHAPTER 2
Medicine Man's Prediction

I was born into this world to be a healer and bridge for medicine, and to do my part to restore it to the whole-body, whole-mind, whole-spirit medicine known to the ancient Greeks, ancient Egyptians, Indians, Chinese, and those before. I was also tasked with restoring vitality to individuals, community and the healing arts, for the benefit of the planet.

To get there, I needed the necessary training through medical school, the most acceptable portal in the Western world to become a practicing physician.

Not surprisingly, my path was different, which became evident during my junior and senior years of medical school at the University of Nebraska. We were allowed to have "out-state," real-world experiences for our clinical training, beyond the academic institution and Lincoln city limits. We had two choices: training at a little practice in rural Nebraska or visiting a remote American Indian reservation. I chose the reservation. In the early 1970s, we *were* the doctors there when we visited. They were happy to have us, and I wanted to practice, not just observe. We could call a licensed physician or physician assistant for support, but we were the front-line physicians in the clinic. We also had a nurse, which led to something I learned early on: if you want to know how to do something, ask the nurse! They almost always know.

When I first arrived at the reservation, I was a little taken aback. I did not expect luxury, or even basic middle-class comforts, but I had no idea how severe the living conditions were. There was a faint smell of sewage, and broken-down cars everywhere. It wasn't unusual to see drunken men wobbling or reaching the point of unconsciousness, then lying alongside the road during the middle of the day. My prefab house with a toilet and kitchenette tucked into a one-room studio quarters was considered upscale. Everybody used the same laundromat.

While I waited, I could smell the scent of the person beside me. What did I smell like to them? Soap? I didn't mind. I wanted to melt into the tribe. I was a good sport who had roughed it before.

I developed a great deal of compassion on the reservation. But the people didn't want my compassion. Sometimes, I got the feeling they didn't want me around at all. They avoided eye contact, though the little kids would stare, point and giggle at my white hair (more on that in a minute). No one talked to me at all until they saw me in the clinic and observed me providing the care that helped their families and themselves.

One morning, I unlocked the clinic, walked through the back door, turned on the lights and headed for the front door. Sometimes, a few early arrivals would be waiting outside. As I opened the door, a woman fell forward into my arms. She smelled like fire. "What happened?" I asked.

"My propane tank blew last night," she wheezed. "It was really bad. I waited as long as I could, but I can't breathe," she panted, "Doc, can you help me?"

About the same time, the nurse arrived for her shift. We got the woman on a gurney and started an IV. I knew enough by her wheezing voice and blue, dusky color that her oxygen was falling, so we administered a breathing treatment and oxygen. I turned to the nurse. "Brenda, see if you can get a chest X-ray. I'm calling the on-call doctor and the ambulance."

There were no helicopters available to ferry reservation patients to the hospital, so we stabilized her and summoned the nearest ambulance. We continued our treatment, giving her intravenous corticosteroids and treating her with furosemide, which extracted fluid from her body to reduce swelling and the edema (fluid buildup) in her lungs.

Thank God for Western medicine, I thought.

However, she wasn't responding well. Even though we gave her pure oxygen, the fluid in her lungs interfered with her body's ability to oxygenate her tissues, and she struggled to breathe. After a few hours, she was still having trouble. The nurse and I looked at each other, deeply concerned, both knowing we'd done everything we could think of.

I got down on my knees beside her bed. I searched through all the prayers in my internal repertoire and began to pray. When I chose to convert to Catholicism in junior high, after a protestant-Unitarian Sunday school childhood, my father insisted I take it a step further and study all the great religions of the world. My mother was the product of a Jesuit Catholic Irish upbringing; the more universal Unitarianism was my father's preference. So, I settled on the Lord's Prayer and a few Hail Marys. While praying, I also began to think of *the kind ones* who accompanied me into my birth, and my childhood spirit friends, the horses and others. I called upon them: "Please help this woman breathe easier. Thank you, God. Amen."

I turned to the nurse. "Can you send someone to find as many of her relatives and friends as possible and bring them back to the clinic?" I asked.

She did. When the relatives arrived, we all gathered around the patient's gurney, chanting, praying and swaying. Their deep beliefs and mine formed a bridge of healing energy over and through our patient. Soon, she began to breathe and feel better. Importantly, her color improved. She began to pink up! The ambulance finally showed up, the answer to our prayers!

Or so I thought. No sooner did we get her into the ambulance and on her way to the hospital than I turned around to face a boy standing in the clinic, his eyes wide and intense. "Are you alright?" I asked.

"The Medicine Man wants *you* at his house at sundown!" he blurted out rapidly and breathlessly.

Just as suddenly as he appeared, the boy disappeared, his words trailing off his back. Stunned, I started to grow frightened. *Oh my God!* I thought. *Have I broken some kind of sacred agreement or made some transgression involving American Indian medicine?*

The Medicine Man

What was about to happen? I had no idea. But, being a brave young woman, I headed for the Medicine Man's house on a dusty, out-of-the-way road, just before sundown.

The entire area is known to us native Nebraskans as "Big Sky Country." The sunrises and sunsets can be magnificent. Like this evening. The sky lit up with reds, oranges and golds so brilliant and extraordinary that my heart lifted, excitement replacing my fear and trepidation. Even the sight of the dead "ponies" (broken-down cars and trucks) by the side of the road seemed in balance with the greater scheme of things. As I walked, I began to attract eager reservation dogs, panting and wagging as they trotted alongside me.

When I reached the Medicine Man's house, I looked up to the porch. He was waiting. With his inside arm, he embraced his mate (the Medicine Woman). Both of their outside arms were outstretched to receive me, their kind eyes and faces beaming. The Medicine Man's back was strong and straight, giving him the appearance of being tall, even though his chest and stomach were shaped like a barrel. His regal profile reminded me of an eagle looking over his territory. His deep brown eyes glinted happy blue light, while the lines in his weathered face spoke of his enormous experience and pain. Immense wisdom and kindness were palpable all around us.

The woman presented the perfect image of the Earth Mother, a sacred, holy sense of the nurturing feminine divine that seemed to extend beyond her role on the reservation. Her squinty eyes burrowed sweetly above the plump cheeks of her wind-tanned face, and her large lap and big bosom spoke of harboring many a child and grandchild. She was full of love, but also no-nonsense.

I stepped onto the porch. They hugged me as if I was their long-lost granddaughter. They invited me into the kitchen, and we shared food and stories at their table. They told me to return the next day. After several visits, they sat me down at the table. "Our ancestor spirits and dreams instructed us to teach you some of our ways so that you can help others," the Medicine Man said. "Not for you to be Indian, but for you to be a bridge between peoples and medicines."

They added I had to continue visiting them, even after I left for training far away. (I had been accepted to UCLA for internal medicine training but did not know it yet. Apparently, they *knew*.) They said to come at least once every season, in order to learn the things I needed to know.

"This may sound strange to you right now but . . . this is your path," said Grandfather, after telling me address him that way. "Remember, it is not so much that you are to become Indian, because if you try to, your people and mine will reject you and even hate you. It is because you are going to do something different for your people. You will teach them something they have forgotten about being whole."

I felt so happy and honored. I wanted to say something profound, but all that came out was, "Thank you, Grandfather."

Grandfather grunted, his eyes sparkling knowingly. He pressed me close to his left side, a fatherly hug.

These grandparents became my first holistic teachers. They taught me about the sacred circle, the universal laws, the cycles of life and many other things. Grandfather was a holy man. He allowed me to observe and even assist with healings when he felt it was right. "You will need to know these things someday. You were born that way—with the gift," he said. "But I can't show preference to you, or people will be jealous. You need to be patient, and you will see in time how medicine works."

At first, I wasn't sure what he meant by "how medicine works." I found out through his method of teaching, which rolled out like a room-length carpet opening slowly. First, I learned that "medicine" is much more than treating and healing. It pertains to the sacred power in all things, which rises from the source of life and earth-based wisdom. The cultures and social structures of most indigenous peoples are based on this universal concept. The "medicine" of which Grandfather and Grandmother spoke exists in everything and everywhere around us—at all times. It is much more than a pharmaceutical, herbal or other treatment. It is the sacred power of life and energy present in all things.

My grandparents shared their herbs and uses of the plants that grew wildly on their land. Grandmother, was a herbalist medicine woman, and taught me that picking the herbs—and knowing when and how to pick them—is a sacred communion forged between plants and humans. She showed me how to identify the leader or guardian of a group of herbs, and how to ask and give back after taking.

As I worked with them, I sometimes thought of the visions, dreams and spirit friends of my childhood. One day, while we were preparing herbal waters for a sweat lodge healing, I remembered the teachings of my beautiful corn lady friend. I told Grandfather, "When I was little, I would run out into the corn fields, and a huge, beautiful corn goddess would appear to me and teach me about talking to the plants and things."

"Yes, the Corn Maiden appeared to you," he said matter-of-factly, like it was no big deal. "She was telling you to follow the natural laws and respect the spirits of the plants and animals and things. In this way, the natural balance and health of the earth is always maintained."

In the fall of 1983, after I began my residency and internship at UCLA, I paid Grandmother and Grandfather a visit. Grandfather told me it was time to watch him perform healing work on a middle-aged woman plagued by insomnia, nightmares and abdominal cramps. Her family, Grandfather, Grandmother and I accompanied her into the house. I noticed dark circles under the woman's eyes as she slumped forward, holding her stomach. Grandfather placed his right hand on her left shoulder and looked her in the face. He reminded her of their previous chat, which I wasn't present to hear, and asked if she was ready. She managed a weak grin. "Yes."

He sat the woman in a comfortable spot, and covered her with a soft, well-worn Pendleton blanket, one of his medicine blankets. Grandmother handed her an herbal tea of burdock, slippery elm, wild rhubarb and white sage. I followed Grandfather outside, where he constructed a small totem doll out of wood and adorned it with hair and clothes that belonged to the woman inside. As he worked, he prayed and sang while cleansing the doll with tobacco and cedar smoke. After about two hours, Grandmother came out and said, "It is done, *Wash-te-loh* (it is good)."

We went back inside. The woman was sleeping like a baby in the easy chair. Grandfather adjusted her blankets, and then drummed and sang over her for another hour. When he finished singing, she opened her eyes.

She looked years younger, renewed. She flashed a large toothy smile and thanked Grandfather.

Grandfather used many methods for his healing work, including sweat lodges, pipe ceremonies and vision work. Grandmother conducted her own kind of healing in the kitchen, where I would sometimes help her make poultices, powders and teas. Grandmother (or sometimes *we*) would administer them to the people while she sang healing chants and waved her feather fan over them.

By watching and studying my grandparents, and later other teachers, I learned that the true "magic" of shamanism is about being a good human being that listens and connects with the soul of another. No matter the instrument, treatment or paraphernalia, soul doctoring shifts the energy for the deep, long-standing healing that can return us to our greatest potential as humans and souls. That is its magic. One people, one planet.

Final Visit with My Grandparents

One spring, about three years after arriving in California and UCLA, I headed for Nebraska to visit my parents—and then, with great excitement, to see my grandparents. I was finishing my internal medicine residency and preparing to begin subspecialty training as a gastroenterologist.

My grandparents received me with open arms and smiles, as always. Right away, I noticed something smelled good on Grandmother's stove. My little living room cot was all set up with a Pendleton blanket and clean, fresh sheets turned down on the corner. *Ah, home!* Great Spirit had gifted me with the grandparents I never experienced in my family life.

The next morning, Grandfather woke me just before dawn, as he often would when I visited. "Get up, girl! Father Sun is not going to wait for ya!"

My spirit tingled with excitement. What would the day bring? Jumping out of bed into my jeans, I hurried and brushed my teeth quickly, then splashed some water on my face. I burst out onto the porch to find Grandfather doing a prayer smoke. My enthusiasm melted into question, and then doubt, when I sensed distance in him. While he was a serious man who frequently feigned sternness to get my attention, this was different.

The air stood heavy as we took a long walk into the surrounding hills. We arrived at a crest as the sun rose over the eastern horizon; we sang the sunrise chant. After we finished our songs and prayers, Grandfather said, "Times are changing, Granddaughter. Things are changing for you and your people, and for our people. You are graduating from more than your medical course work. We are proud of you, because you have graduated from our school as well . . ."

Is this the end of our time together? "Grandfather?"

He interrupted me. "Some things are bigger than we are. Some things do not pertain to us personally." Moisture welled up in his eyes. "Tribal law and politics are strong, and our people need us to stick together. You will have many teachers. It is time for us all to move on. You have come to us for four years; that is the number of completion. Our interaction will always be with you. You cannot tell anyone our names or where we live. It has been a gift for you to carry on."

My heart sank. I was very sad. Had I disappointed them in some way? Not visited often enough?

During this final visit, Grandfather and I sat across the kitchen table from each other, as we had so many times before. He touched me on the crown of my head. My hair had turned completely and prematurely white. "You have been lightning-struck, Granddaughter," he said. "The Great Spirit has given you the gift of doing things differently. Remember that, for all the People. What we have shared together is sacred and we will always carry it with us. That can never be taken away from you. It's not important for you to prove it. What is important is that you *live it*. You must go and walk in your own moccasins over many mounds.

"Do not hold heaviness in your heart. Many teachers will come to you and you have much to learn. One day you will grow into part of a living bridge between worlds. Go now and walk in beauty. Our love is always with you."

My heart shattered with the truth behind his words. He hugged me to his side with his left arm, which I treasured every time. "It's alright, Granddaughter; you know my spirit will never leave you. You have to let go and move on. It is a lesson you will have to face many times. Know your own strength and that you have done well."

I tried not to cry, but tears ran from my eyes like warm rivers. "Thank you, Grandfather, I will try."

Grandmother walked over to my other side and hugged me, crying and smiling at the same time. "Promise me, don't lose your way," she said. "The earth needs you."

"OK, Grandmother, I promise." The softness of her body comforted me.

We spent the rest of the day visiting around the kitchen table, making herbal remedies and doing chores. Just another day of routines. It somehow made the finality of it all a little easier.

The next morning, I left at dawn—never to return.

My first American Indian teachers influenced my development more than I ever could have known during our time. Still, almost every day, I feel or recall a teaching, or realize something they told me that I wasn't equipped to understand at the time. It happened, and happens, through patients. In this way, I have connected with patients on a heart level since day one, so I can listen to more than the scientific clues of their complaints.

Patients have always been much more to me than their diseases. Each is special, with mental, emotional and spiritual layers to their illness—as well as the physical layers. This seemingly new but truly ancient perception of balance was given to me by my American Indian teachers. Even though I still had much science and technology to master, I always attempted to keep sight of the holism my grandparents shared with me. Although my patients were grateful for the advances modern science offered them, the holistic approach gave them most of their comfort.

I parted company with my teachers on the reservation years before I satisfied my quest for spiritual understanding with trips to the Santa Monica Mountains, deep esoteric studies and educational initiatives in "alternative medicine," as we called it then. With the loss of Grandfather and Grandmother as physical presences in my life, I yearned for an embodied spiritual teacher, and felt the time was near.

Joshua Tree

That time arrived in September 1990. I felt compelled to go to Joshua Tree National Forest on the second full moon of the month (blue moon) and do a vision quest ceremony. My decision was abrupt, spur of the moment. I loaded my medicine bags, some ceremonial items, water and a sleeping bag into my Toyota Forerunner and hit the road. One of the medicine bags was for bear medicine, which I made out of chocolate-colored leather and then beaded to honor and exemplify the power of the direction of the west, the earth and her feminine quality.

I placed the bag on the passenger seat and drove to Joshua Tree Monument. The iridescent beaded image of a huge female bear came alive in the light of the setting sun. The stream of water originating from her right front paw literally flowed, feeding a clear blue river below. I've always loved driving through the desert because it creates the environment for spiritual cleansing. This drive from the Santa Monica Mountains to Joshua Tree seemed like a fold in timelessness, the blink of an eye.

I arrived inside the Joshua Tree boundaries shortly after dark as the moon started to peek over the horizon. A cluster of large, rounded stones attracted my attention, ancient giants with expressions of timeless wisdom on their faces. The immense stones seemed purposely stacked and arranged into groupings. The formations held a significance they weren't giving up, a mystery to be revealed at the right time to an appropriate and worthy beholder. Even the Joshua trees seemed to dance and wiggle mysteriously with my arrival, marking the beginning of a great ceremony.

After many minutes of driving through the curving roads of the reserve, I was magnetized to a particular grouping of huge, rounded boulders typical of that sacred land, but with an inexplicable special meaning. Even though I had never been to this spot before, it felt familiar, a gateway to another energetic reality. I pulled over to park. As I collected my things, two owls hooted back and forth in the distance as if to say, "*Whoooo* is this one?"

"*Whoooo?*"

I passed through the gigantic boulder "gateway" just as the moon cast her first beams over the horizon. The huge, honey-colored moon was just rising. She greeted and welcomed me to this shimmering, clear and cold desert land. I walked up to the giant stones and found the perfect altar to support the sacred medicine items I brought along, waiting to be anointed with sage smoke for the ceremony. There I placed the bear medicine bag, my feathers, sweet grass and sage. As the moon rose over the distinctive Joshua trees, I sang, cleansed myself with sage and prayed, giving thanks while asking to be shown the way to my new teacher.

I began. First, as my grandparents taught me, I offered prayers of gratitude to the Great Spirit, the Ancestors and Mother Earth, the Grandfather Sun for awakening my bear medicine, and Grandmother Moon for welcoming and letting me know I was in the right place. I thanked the stone people, the guardians of the gateway through which I consciously passed, and all the people of the desert and guides who led me where I needed to be. I asked the powers of the desert to help me to find my human teacher . . . to show me the way.

The sage and sweet grass smelled especially sweet; it lingered in the air long after I burned it. The scent followed me as I began a long trek into the desert to find my spot for my vision quest. I wove in and out of cactus, yucca and the namesake Joshua trees until I arrived on a mound in the middle of a valley, surrounded by red rocky peaks. Multitudes of Joshua trees populated the entire valley, their arms stretched into the midnight-blue sky, now speckled with millions of sparkling stars. The moon loomed large, her silvery smile beaming down on my progress, approving my power spot.

I worried a little about finding my way back to the car, but let it go and turned my attention to my quest. I made two circles, one clockwise with tobacco, the other counterclockwise with corn meal, large enough to enclose belongings and myself on the mound. The clockwise circle honored the masculine sun while holding the protective space for sending out prayers; the counterclockwise, or moon-wise circle, honored the feminine and the receiving of new information for manifestation. My intent was to stay inside the circle until I received an answer to my quest.

The craggy, mountainous peaks appeared full of ancient images with symbol-filled walls and ancestors from other times and places. Bright, silvery shafts of moonlight illuminated sugary grains of desert sand; it looked like a shimmering dream. Cacti, Joshua trees and sagebrush inhaled the moonlight and became alive with energy all their own.

I sat in my circle for hours and watched this waking nighttime dream, the desert vibrant and full of life. The owls hooted back and forth in the distance while little creatures scurried from place to place nearby. It comforted me. The understanding swept over me that the desert was once an ocean. The brush, trees, cacti and even the glittering sand played tricks on my senses, moving like a sea current. It felt so real that I felt like I was floating outside my circle. I rolled onto my stomach. I could see life everywhere and in everything, grateful the desert had revealed this teeming life from eons gone by. I came to understand the deeper meaning of the line from the song "Horse with No Name," a hit by America during my college years: The desert appeared to be an ocean that erupted into sparkling life under the light of the full moon.

Time passed slowly, almost to a standstill. The desert fell silent. Time became eternal, like it would never move forward. Then I heard faint drumming in the distance. *Am I hearing things? There's no one out here.* It grew louder. *I do hear drumming . . .* It continued to build. *I can hear singing, too! American Indian chanting! Oh my God! I'm not alone here.* I relaxed into the idea that sound carried a long way in the desert.

The calm, even beat of the drum calmed and encouraged the agitation and anxiety to pass through me. Slowly, nodding my head to the beat of the drum, I laid back, pulled my sleeping bag around my shoulders. Well-being permeated my core. Now elevated beyond lower-vibration energies like fear or doubt, I snuggled into my sleeping bag as I laid in my nest of blankets, looking up at the stars and moon, which remained almost straight overhead in the sky. It was if time stopped and the moon would never move. I accepted that and let go of all the preconceived notions within me.

Then I heard a soft padding sound on the desert sand, like walking, soft walking. *Maybe moccasined feet?* They were coming toward me.

An almost imperceptible touch on my left shoulder followed. I looked up. A thin dark American Indian man with deep black eyes looked at me. The light of Universal kindness shone from them. As he leaned over, gently moving closer to me, I could see the cosmos in his eyes. He extended his hand. I practically fell into his eyes, so deep and dark, and the virtual galaxies spinning slowly in space, sparkling inside them.

He took my hand lightly and respectfully and invited me to follow him. We moved effortlessly across the desert toward the sound of the ceremonial music that had first caught my attention. Under the moonlight, I beheld the people dancing in a circle and chanting to the beat of the drummers. We joined and danced tirelessly until the violet haze of predawn began to show in the sky.

When dawn arrived, he led me to a spring-fed pool on the other side of the valley. Water flowed from the rocks, turning muddy and red-brown after it mixed with the red earth. We waded into the red pond. He stood by me and began to chant a beautiful medicine song as he patted the reddish mud all over my body. His voice was so familiar, resonating through my soul . . . where and when would I have heard it before? I could not remember. His energy reminded me of *the kind ones*. I looked down and noticed my body was small and brown, my hair black and straight.

Now, you are initiated into the people of this tribe, he told me telepathically. *You will be a dancer for all the people . . .*

Without warning, a howl 10 feet away pierced the darkness. I lurched up from a lying to sitting position, astounded to find myself still inside my circle on the mound as coyote after coyote began to run in a circle around my spot in the desert.

I looked behind me. A coyote howled from the depths of his lungs. He ran toward me and then joined the circle, accompanied by maybe 20 others yipping and running around me in a clockwise direction. My heart was about to pound out of my chest when I realized they were *dancing* with me. I let out a huge howl and laugh, and they scattered in all 360 degrees, running to the mountains rimming the valley. Grandmother Moon was still straight overhead, chuckling with us!

For several hours, I listened to the songs of the coyotes howling back and forth to each other about the tall white-haired two-legged, who became their dancing companion, until finally I drifted off into a deep sleep.

Violet predawn light began to paint the sky. I struggled to bring my awareness into my body and put some order or sense into my experience. I found the ring of coyote tracks about 10 feet from the perimeter of my circle, blurring my sense of reality. What was of this world . . . and what was beyond it? Or did it even matter? Then I realized I was in our physical world, and everything else I'd experienced was my vision. Which was more real?

Most of all, I wondered about the man with the galaxies in his eyes. Was he my teacher?

A New Teacher Arrives

About a year later, a girlfriend came to my Hollywood Hills house on a rainy afternoon and gave me a VHS tape. "Watch this," she said.

I sat down and tried to watch the scratchy, snowy static and listen to the garbled voices on the poorly copied tape. It took a few tries. Finally, I could focus on the content. The tape was from a show called *Thinking Allowed*, and host Jeffery Mishlove was interviewing a man named Joseph Rael, who he described as a world-renowned shaman, storyteller and visionary. When I heard Joseph's voice, it sounded strongly familiar. In the interview, Joseph spoke of the importance of metaphor in understanding how everyday life works. He shared how he was raised and trained as a holy man by his grandfather in Picuris Pueblo, New Mexico, a people whose ancient Tiwa language is a living metaphor right down to the very word, action and sound. His name with the people, *Tslew-teh-koyeh* (Beautiful Painted Arrow), carries the metaphorical meaning of the sacred arrow that hits its target and releases healing vibration to the entire planet.

Jeffery asked Beautiful Painted Arrow if he would sing. He rose from his chair. "I'm going to sing a medicine song I rarely sing. Somehow, this is the song that is called for right now," he said.

He began to chant his medicine song. I listened, mouth open, dumbstruck, covered in goose bumps. It was the song the Medicine Man sang to me in my Joshua Tree vision! *When the student is ready, the teacher will come.*

My next question roared through, urgent and strong: *How am I ever going to find him?*

The next morning, the phone rang early. Another girlfriend excitedly informed me of a special meeting to be held at Connie Kaplan's house. (Connie would later become my Sundance sister and dream teacher.) The speaker? Joseph Rael. "Do you want to go?" she asked.

"I wouldn't miss it for the world!"

I met Joseph at Connie's, listened to his talk and gifted him with traditional tobacco and sweet grass. A week later, I called him at his home in New Mexico. As I dialed, I wondered, *is he even going to remember who I am? Will he accept me?* There were so many people there vying for his attention. *What if he says no?* I fought off the doubt and followed my heart.

The phone only rang once. "Hello?" It was his familiar voice.

"This is Gayle Madeleine Randall. Is this Joseph?"

"Yes, I know you. I've been waiting for you," he said. "When I was in Germany two years ago, I saw your face in a vision during a sweat lodge ceremony. You asked me if you could be my apprentice and I said 'yes.' I've been waiting for you ever since. So . . . what took you so long?"

"I'm not sure. I think I was trying to find you."

"You think too much," he said. "But that's OK. You'll get over it. You need to come here and get started. How about February?"

My heart sang. My vision was unfolding before me!

The following February, I saw Joseph, beginning a long apprenticeship and friendship that lasts to this day. He's a highly educated man who merges modern thought and ancient mysticism into his evolutionary philosophies. Joseph initiated me into his tribe and asked me to become a Sundancer. I eventually danced in four Sun-Moon dances, and helped Joseph facilitate the first Sun-Moon Dance in Germany in 1995.

My work with Joseph gave me the final push for creating an integrative model for infusing Western medicine with the spiritual perspective of the ancients.

CHAPTER 3
Every Body Is Special

"Each individual's body is uniquely different from another, and yet when the essences of our consciousness are combined, we are all One."

—Purnanand Awasthi, MD

As I learned more tools from the Native and Eastern traditions, and understood the spiritual purpose behind the healing, I incorporated them into my practice at the UCLA Digestive Diseases Center. The word got out, and a long line of patients formed to seek alternative care. Many came only after standard medicine failed them, their problems sometimes unrelated to digestive systems.

Our patients had reached a dead end—from a Western medicine point of view. I realized this while coordinating *The Healing Connection*, a photodocumentary and the first integrative medicine initiative at UCLA. We decided to branch out and look at the effect of adding other modalities to their treatment regimens. They had nothing to lose, right? We already worked with American Indian and traditional Chinese medicine practitioners, but we really needed another approach to complete the healing circle we envisioned.

In 1993, I "came out," in a medical sense, when I organized *The Healing Connection*. Through this work, I developed close working relationships with George Amiotte, a Lakota Sundance Chief who studied under Frank Fools Crow (a widely loved and respected Lakota medicine man), and Tatsuo Hirano, an exceptional healer and doctor of traditional Chinese medicine. These extraordinary people came into my life at the most appropriate time.

The design for *The Healing Connection* also called for a healer from the Ayurvedic tradition, preferably also a medical doctor. I had trouble finding someone. First, we didn't have any money to pay; we performed these medical services purely for the benefit of what we may learn and carry into the future. It was a very big ask, and my search for a practitioner willing to donate their time for the benefit of humankind proved fruitless.

I let it go and placed my intent on a positive result. I remembered the saying that led Joseph Rael to me: *when the student is ready, the teacher will come.* Would it work for asking for the right healer to help our efforts?

I found out two weeks later. I was attending in-clinic patients at the UCLA Digestive Diseases Center. I saw patients for as long as it took to address their problems. (I did not abide by the prevalent bottom-line blueprint of "see more patients in less time.") I accepted an ever-increasing patient load, yes, but I still took all the time each patient needed. My patients waited, and did not mind for the most part, because when their turn came, they knew I would really listen to them. In my world, every body is special. So is every person. Because of the sacred bond I feel for my patients, I did not allow interruptions during my consultations.

Sure enough, as I was seeing a patient, we heard a knock on the door. I got up, irritated. *Oh boy. This better be good,* I thought.

I opened the door to see the sheepish face of my nurse. "Dr. Randall, you had better come out here and see this for yourself," she said.

I walked into the waiting room. There stood an East Indian gentleman in traditional white clothing, his stark white hair a striking contrast to his dark skin. He stood alongside a younger man. "Dr. Randall," the younger man began, "allow me to present my father-in-law, Dr. Purnanand Awasthi from Mumbai, India."

Dr. Awasthi stood in his traditional white tunic top and white pants, his sandaled feet close together in perfect balance, hands pressed together as if in prayer. "Hello, Dr. Randall," he said. "I am here visiting from India for three months. I have heard you need me, and I have come from India to help you."

I was flabbergasted. *How did he know?* I never contacted him. I never knew he existed.

I looked around. My awaiting patients and staff were riveted by the gentle power of this man's words. He read the question dancing in my widening eyes. "When you consider the physical, each individual's body is uniquely different from another, and yet when the essences of our consciousness are combined—we are all One," he said, my soul drinking in every drop. "What you know . . . we all know." He sounded like a timeless poet out of India's rich Vedic past.

Dr. Awasthi was the medical jewel of an integrated education. He was both a surgeon and an Ayurvedic practitioner. He received full training in Ayurveda, the ancient Indian medicine, as well as Western medicine. In 1952, he became the head of India's Integrative Medical Association, decades before we even started combining the words "integrative" and "medicine" in America. This pioneer had been living my medical dream for as long as I had been on the planet!

I knew exactly what to do with this gift from the heavens. Dr. Awasthi became my teacher and colleague through *The Healing Connection*. He taught me many invaluable lessons and philosophies that, I realized, were similar to those my American Indian teachers had shared. "God is in everyone, and yet everyone is different," he explained. "God takes on individual forms in each of us. Thus our own consciousness is a small particle of the consciousness of God." He also introduced me to the ageless Sanskrit and Hindu greeting, "Namaste," which essentially means, "the God in me honors the God in you."

Can you think of a nicer, more uplifting greeting? To honor how special each and every body is?

Not surprisingly, we continued our correspondence for many years, mostly by email.

A Different View of Our Body and Individuality

Dr. Awasthi offered a far different—and healthier—view of our body and individuality and how its sacredness fits into the world and life. In Western medicine, we have been taught that what is good for most of us most of the time is good for everybody. Fair enough: we all want to live in a healthy society, where we look out for each other's well-being as part of living purposefully, right?

However, your body is different than mine, your mind is different, and so is your medical and health history. I have different nutritional and healing needs, and yours might be more or less urgent than mine. If we are to agree that our body is our temple, as spiritual leaders and visionaries have tried to teach us for thousands of years, then how do you care for *your* body temple in a way that honors who you are, your challenges or healing issues, and your path to healing and wellness?

There are also social matters and expectations that can be impediments to feeling our body is special—especially for women. During our lifetimes, we've been conditioned on different ideas of what makes up a "good body" or a "special body" through advertising, TV shows and movies. We are told what is "attractive"—and not—by others who hold expectations and measures. We're told to go by others' definitions of what "a good figure" means, what "skinny" is. Or "fat." Or "tall." Or "short."

These comparisons drive so much of the beauty and women's care product businesses, and so much self-esteem messaging. But what do they say about the *healthy* body? The body that is well? Your body—and mine?

This troubling dialogue leads to real problems with how we communicate with our bodies. By communication, I mean *think of, talk to, feed, care for* and *nurture*. How do you honor your body? If you have trouble honoring your body, the temple that houses your heart, vital functions, mind and soul, how can you fully participate in your recovery, healing and/or life of well-being? Also, how can you fully participate if you rely on outside experts (health-care professionals) to keep you mobile, upright and able to make it through each day?

Every body is special. If we are all made in God's image (or the Universe, Higher Power, whatever you want to call the Source of all life), then how can our bodies *not* be special? We need to rise up and accept this about ourselves. This truth about your body, and mine, lies at the heart of soul doctoring, personal healing and your right to a happy, healthy life.

Everything begins with taking care of your body—and asking for help when we need assistance. For some, asking for help is easy: you know something I don't, or have something I need, and you ask for it. However, for others, asking for help is the hardest thing in the world—especially when it comes to health. Sometimes, people come into my office with ready-made obstructions to asking for and receiving healing. With these patients, I feel like I'm navigating an iron labyrinth. They are often afraid to reveal how much help they really need, for fear of revealing something "weak" or "dis-eased" within themselves. They keep their real wounds covered and hidden. Also, they might be embarrassed or not want to take responsibility for healing, which typically involves a lot of work.

How do we, as healers, doctors and health-care providers, turn around the patient? The key is to foster *trust*. It allows the patient to open up and reveal their weaknesses, which is a sign of *strength*. We need to show our patients we are there, so they know they are safe and can trust us with their secrets. Along with this comes the challenge of convincing the patient to let down her or his guard and ask for help when they need it—often, if necessary.

Remember how we constantly asked for help or guidance when we were kids? It was a natural part of growing, learning, becoming strong and knowledgeable. It is just as vital to ask when we're adults—but sadly, by then, many of us have been conditioned to believe that asking is a sign of weakness. Undoing this messaging into something right and positive for our ongoing health takes constant guidance and a level stance by the health-care practitioner.

In my 40 years as a practicing physician, I have learned that each patient is special and possesses his or her unique way of processing energy and manifesting disease. This is why every body must be considered unique and special to both practitioner and individual. Two people may receive the same diagnosis, such as high blood pressure. However, they may respond to identical treatment in entirely different ways. The underlying root cause(s) may be completely different. While meditation or yoga may help one alleviate high blood pressure through stress reduction, another might respond better to salt restriction and a gradual weight-loss program.

How Ancient Healing Traditions Work with the Individual

A greater appreciation for working with the uniqueness of each individual's body and healing needs can be found in ancient traditions, in which I'm also certified and experienced. Doctors of Chinese and Japanese medicine will consider the *temperature*, the cold or heat, in a patient's condition. One person might present a viral infection with heat syndrome, while another will show a viral infection with cold syndrome. From there, doctors will consider the *yin* and *yang* of each patient or issue, the essential female and male energies, how we balance energetically. In another ancient healing art, Indian Ayurveda, the body type, or *dosha*, is crucial to determining treatment. All treatments in Chinese, Japanese and Ayurvedic medicine work with and through these individual variations.

Let's return to yin and yang. In Chinese philosophy and medicine, Taoism ("The Way") is represented by the yin-yang symbol, which reflects energetic balance and a holism of body, mind and spirit. When we dance along the spiritual line between light and dark, the ideal and ordinary worlds become one. The two ends of the paradox meet and become one unified whole.

Likewise, when yin and yang are in balance, we are generally very healthy. That is how Chinese and Japanese medicine functions. When they are imbalanced, diseases occur. Health is a physical expression of balance; diseases express imbalances. Doctors of Chinese, Japanese and Ayurvedic medicine look at the symptoms *and* other diagnostic methods to identify patterns of disharmony. They read the body much like a farmer reads the land. Each vital organ system must be in balance microcosmically (within itself) as well as macrocosmically (within its relationship to the other organ systems, whole body-being, and the planet). Ancients knew that individual healing could only be complete with a healed, vibrant environment. That's food for thought—especially in these times when our planet is in distress and we need to regenerate both ourselves and the earth.

Chinese, Japanese and Ayurvedic medicine begins with the degree and depth by which practitioners read signs in our bodies, both obvious and subtle. They determine the level of health through four principal examinations:

- The normal and abnormal organ system functions in your body;
- Your pulse rate and tongue health (which present any number of possible health issues), through a complex diagnostic process;
- Viewing the outer body as a window into the internal organs; and
- Recognizing a two-way connection between the body and the mind.

The laboratory that provides Chinese, Japanese and Ayurveda medicine practitioners with the most significant information is the human body itself.

Cardinal signs of imbalance relate to each of our vital organs, as well as multi-organ disharmonies. Let's look at the effects of a common example, like overeating. Some suffer from extreme fatigue after eating too much. A few may be overcome by sleep. Chinese and Japanese medicine attribute this to the spleen. (The spleen indicates the entire function of the digestive system. Think pancreas, small intestine and large intestine.) If the spleen is out of balance, it can easily affect the lungs. This may result in phlegm accumulation and a stuffy sensation in the chest, nasal congestion, and shortness of breath. Allergies, bronchitis or asthma could also arise. Often, asthma sufferers have skin problems such as eczema. Chinese and Japanese medicine both hold that the skin is closely related to the lung system. Eczema would occur with those suffering from asthma.

By being able to recognize the cardinal symptoms of single organs and organ relationships, healing regimens like acupuncture and herbal treatments are able to get to the root of a problem instead of placing a Band-Aid over the symptoms. That's our goal, always: to eliminate and overcome the symptoms, not just cover them up. Using acupuncture, herbs and other modalities, the practitioner seeks to restore balance. When the body is balanced, and the yin and yang are in harmony, health is restored.

Ayurveda, the "Science of Life"

Ayurveda is a Sanskrit word derived from two ancient roots: *ayur*, or life, and *veda*, knowledge. *Knowledge of life.* "There are many vedas," Dr. Awasthi said, "but this is the one for you to focus your attention."

Knowledge, when arranged systematically with logic, becomes science. During the course of thousands of years, Ayurveda became the science of life, its root in ancient Vedic literature, its reach encompassing body, mind, emotions and spirit. It also incorporates the environment, and how our relationship with it impacts our walk through the world and our health. This is an aspect we need to remember in these daunting times of massive pollution, global warming and climate change, runaway health crises such as the COVID-19 pandemic, and the mass extinction of animals, plants, insects and flying creatures on our planet.

Ayurveda defines health as:[1]

- Sense of well-being;
- Evenly balanced emotional states;
- Good memory, comprehension, intelligence and reasoning ability;
- Proper functioning of the senses (sight, hearing, smell, taste and touch);
- Abundant mental, emotional, physical and spiritual energy;
- Good and efficient digestion of food and drink;
- Normal elimination of waste; and
- Healthy functioning of bodily organs, tissues and other systems.

Ayurveda holds that the structural body is made up of five elements (ether, air, fire, water and earth). The functional body is governed by three doshas: *vata*, which is ether and air together; *pitta*, which is fire and water; and *kapha*, which is water and earth. Vata-pitta-kapha are present in every cell, tissue and organ. Yet, they differ in expression and combination between each person. Proportions of vata-pitta-kapha change according to diet, lifestyle, emotion and spiritual state. And body type. Ayurveda recognizes seven body types: mono (vata, pitta or kapha predominant), dual (vata-pitta, pitta-kapha or kapha-vata), and equal (vata, pitta and kapha in equal proportions).

In Ayurveda, the living body is a mini-universe governed by the same forces that govern the external world. *A mini-universe . . .* that makes you very special, in and of itself! As life enters our material body, our doshas work in harmony to maintain balance or health. Disharmony between the doshas creates disease. A good diet, exercise, proper lifestyle and spiritual practice keep the body and its doshas balanced, enhancing our opportunities for physical and spiritual harmony.

A complete healing art, Ayurveda also works to bring clarity in relationships. Clarity creates compassion, which is another form of love. As Dr. Awasthi taught me, "Love is clarity. Without this clarity, there is no insight. Ayurveda is an art of insight that brings harmony, happiness, joy and bliss in our daily life, our relationships and our daily living. This brings happiness to the one and the planet. Ayurveda can add longevity to life."

This quality of consciousness can enable us to deal with our inner lives, inner emotions, inner pain, grief and sadness.

Native Medicine Addresses Individual Needs

Native philosophy and medicine also account for the needs of each individual. So do most indigenous cultures and practices throughout the world. Shamans, or medicine people, have developed strikingly similar methods, symbology and non-technological capacities for health and healing. How is it that some Tibetan mandalas and Native medicine wheels have nearly identical symbols and forms, when the peoples live halfway across the world from each other? The uniformity of shamanic methods suggests that people arrived at the same conclusions through thousands of years of trial and error.

The centerpiece of ancient healing was a shamanic experience. There's a lot of mystery, dogma and wrong thinking attached to "shaman" and "shamanic experience."

A shamanic experience is a great "body-mind-spirit-emotion" adventure in which both client and shamanic healer fully participate. The shaman guides clients to transcend their ordinary definition of reality, no matter how big or small; maybe it's the notion that they are sick. Shamans call upon the natural energies of the sky above, earth below, and the sacred circle, including all the directions, along with plants and creatures. During the ceremony, the participant experiences shifts and changes in their perspective. Some changes can become 180-degree shifts that flip old feelings or beliefs and remove thought viruses. This is what returns and restores power and healing energy. The shaman shows the client that he or she is not alone in the struggle, and that another human is willing to help them—whatever it takes. This requires the shaman's true expression of love and compassion, as well as a commitment from the client to struggle alongside the shaman, gain understanding of self and overcome the disease. The shaman makes use of a deep understanding and the individual needs of the person being healed. Caring and curing go hand in hand.

Getting Unstuck from the Form

How do we move our special bodies from the Western medical form we know to embrace other modalities? It begins by getting unstuck.

We have become far too attached to techniques and procedures in Western medicine, so attached that doctors often lose sight of the patient—and the patient knows no other way. The concept of a person needing a different technique or approach to treat them, based on their unique needs, is foreign to most Western practitioners. Rather, physicians commonly perform the same "knee-jerk" battery of expensive and highly technical tests on every patient who enters their clinics and expresses similar symptoms. When tests do not reveal a diagnosis, doctors tell their patients that nothing is wrong, or perhaps to see a psychiatrist instead. "Since my tests can't find it, you don't have it," the train of thought goes. And, taken even further, "You might be a bit crazy."

Joseph Rael taught me not to "get stuck in the form." Forms are only good as long as they help you grow from an old practice into a new one. As soon as we release an old form and replace it with a new one, he said, we begin to develop so we can later release the new form. This cyclical process keeps us constantly changing and evolving. It does not discount the value of techniques and tested results, but emphasizes the need for more flexibility when applying scientific techniques to something as dynamic as the life of a human being. Each person owns a unique constellation of needs.

This new approach of viewing our bodies as special, sacred temples of life includes *co-participating*. We need to be fully involved with our own healing and well-being—one of my strongest messages to you! I think of the late mythologist-storyteller Joseph Campbell's classic work, *Hero with a Thousand Faces*.[2] In it, Campbell describes the classic hero's journey as something far different than the 19-year-old basketball phenom who jumps straight into the NBA and becomes an instant "hero" to millions of kids. In Campbell's version, the individual is stripped of all old belief systems and tools. He or she must reach deep to find their essence. The resulting "climb" out of the "dark night of the soul," or "rite of passage," perhaps in co-participation with a Shaman, creates such radical change in the person that they view the world and its people with more love, compassion, detachment and wonder. They also connect with their higher purpose on our planet.

The miraculous saves of Western medicine are not always adequate to effect long-term healing. That's because Western treatment generally amounts to healing the body without healing the mind, emotions or spirit. It does not take into account the family, community or planet. I think of the huge number of cardiac surgery patients who are given a new lease on life, but still can never return to work. They become "cardiac disabled," hobbled also by depression and a broken lifestyle. Why? Because they have not been shown a new way to carry on, nor given the tools to build that new way for themselves.

This trend has led forward-thinking health professionals and patients to seek supplementary healing methods, like our early work at *The Healing Connection* at UCLA. Unfortunately, much of this experimentation has resulted in difficulty distinguishing spurious from effective healing techniques. I was reminded of this when reading *Un Do It! How Simple Lifestyle Choices Can Reverse Most Chronic Diseases*, written by my friend, celebrated physician and author Dr. Dean Ornish.[3] Years ago, Dr. Ornish developed the only system scientifically proven to reverse heart disease without drugs or surgery. It created an entirely different way of treating this huge national problem. In *Un Do It!*, he and his wife Anne follow up with even more comprehensive holistic treatment and healing plans for all patients, regardless of their medical conditions.

The Shamanic Way, for Today

We make strong lifestyle choices and reverse chronic diseases when we view the body as a special, radiant spiritual being. Ancient shamans knew this. Many methods used by awakened healers today are time-tested techniques, thousands of years older than Western medicine and psychotherapeutic approaches. We are deeply grateful for their shared knowledge to increase healing in all peoples worldwide.

The shaman has the ability to move between ordinary and altered states of consciousness at will. The ancient way reaches so deeply into the human mind, heart and soul that one's usual cultural belief systems about reality are essentially, or at least temporarily, suspended. I can speak to that: I have practiced and experienced the merger of shamanic methods with Western and other healing modalities in both North and South America, resulting in effective, more lasting healing. This experience becomes a graceful dance between ordinary reality and shamanic reality, with a sole purpose—to change perspective and initiate the healing response in the subject or patient.

Shamanic methods do not require changes in assumptions about reality in ordinary state of consciousness, nor a change in the unconscious mind. There is no danger of "losing control," as with drugs. Shamanism only awakens what is already deep inside. The basic experience is straightforward and can help to effect healing, though it requires impeccable practice, self-discipline and dedication. One's cultural or religious background does not seem to determine a client's openness to shamanism. Their conscious experience is the fundamental issue.

A scientific basis for shamanism exists in neurochemistry. Consciousness-altering substances such as dimethyltryptamine, or even dopamine and endorphins, exist naturally in the human brain. These chemicals elevate in various situations, such as Tibetan lamas or advanced yogis in altered states of deep meditation, or aboriginal shamans engaging in trance-type states. Often, athletes touch such altered states—the so-called "zone"—while achieving great physical accomplishments.

These levels can be measured after such experiences. Years ago, Richard Davidson and his colleagues at the Health/Emotions Institute in Madison, Wisconsin, asked to study Tibetan monks to practice meditating.[4] They were granted permission to study the Dalai Lama's monks, with the Dalai Lama involved in the analysis. They found increased activity in certain portions of the brain, particularly the left prefrontal lobe, along with increased immunity and changes in neurochemistry. In a corporate setting, they also taught meditation to and studied Westerners who had previously not meditated, and found changes in similar areas. Benefits lasted for up to eight weeks and included increased brain activity in the left prefrontal lobes, similar (though maybe not as profound) to lifelong meditators (the Tibetan monks). This, after just eight weeks of meditating!

The shamanic *experience* effects lasting healing. Shamanism is a strategy for personal learning. Action upon that knowledge is required in order to effect healing.

Power of Healer and Client: Sam's Story

The moving story of Sam illustrates the compelling power of the relationship between shamanic healer and client. After learning of my unique approach to medicine from a friend, Sam came to my Malibu office on a summer afternoon after being hospitalized for seizures. He suffered from metastatic brain melanoma. After being diagnosed three months before, he was receiving the standard treatment—chemotherapy, radiation, intravenous corticosteroids and anti-seizure medications. Metastatic brain melanoma is a very serious condition, often deadly within weeks or months. "I'm willing to continue this poison and radiation because maybe it's keeping it from getting any worse, but I'm afraid. Something is missing and I'm not getting any better," Sam told me.

He began to cry. I sensed the huge disconnect between his tears and the sunshine lighting up the ocean waves beneath my office. I felt a message through the salt in his tears. He stood up from his chair to look out the window. "You see all those people?" He was looking at the busy beach below. "They have no idea what it is like to be alone . . . really alone . . . and have your life threatened by cancer."

I stood and put my right hand on his left shoulder. "You are not alone anymore. Come on, sit down. Let's figure this out together."

We put our heads together and designed a program. "I can do that," he said. "I believe that is going to help me."

Sam had just taken the critical first step in healing: *our own belief we can heal.*

Sam and I added herbal immune enhancers, tonic mushrooms, an organic vegan diet and antioxidants to his other treatment. We tailored it to his limited ability to take supplements. (When people are receiving harsh medical therapies, it is often difficult to take supplements, because they are nauseated and weak.) Most importantly, we developed a personalized meditative visualization, which he described as "seeing the tumors shrinking and disappearing from my body as normal tissues and cells become stronger and fill in the spaces." We created another visualization in which Sam saw himself surrounded by loved ones and embedded with magenta light, which projects unconditional love. We worked on this together, with me setting the intention and guiding him. His homework was to continue the visual meditation once or twice a day between our weekly meetings.

Sam also was dealing with a frayed relationship with his family—not what you want when battling metastatic brain melanoma. Originally from the Midwest, he had not stayed in close contact, because his parents could not understand why he left the family farm to become a writer in Los Angeles.

"Sam, maybe it's time to mend issues with your family and allow them to become involved," I suggested.

"OK, Doc. I guess so," he replied, without much enthusiasm. "If not now, when?" At least he was willing.

It didn't take long. Once Sam swung open the door to his parents, siblings and extended family, they took turns traveling to California to be with him. They started a prayer circle that gave him great encouragement and strength. Soon, his seizures stopped, and he was able to get around and go to movies and dinner.

Three months after our initial meeting, I was struck by how well he looked. "You've put weight on and you have a sparkle in your eyes," I said.

He brought along some amazing news. "Thanks, Doc. My CAT scan showed no evidence of tumors! Can you believe it? The oncologists said this was unheard of in their medical experience."

I smiled and gave him a big hug. "Congratulations. I am so happy."

He wore a wall-to-wall smile. "My family is celebrating and giving thanks to God. Thank you, Dr. Randall. You are amazing!"

Sam far outlived his "weeks or months" prognosis. He survived for more than five years. He learned he was no longer alone, physically or spiritually. When he passed over, he did so surrounded by his family at their Des Moines, Iowa, farm home. They believed that their shift to appreciate Sam's uniqueness, the subsequent love he received from family and friends, our work in God's favor and his own belief in his health combined to allow him an extra slice of life.

Treatments Tailored to Our Own Body Characteristics

One day while at my clinic at UCLA, I saw three consecutive patients with exactly the same symptoms, and nearly identical stories. Teresa, Linda and Barbara were once healthy young adults, but they began to experience abdominal cramping and diarrhea about a year prior to seeing me. Thorough Western physical evaluations, they received the same diagnosis, a "spastic colon or IBS (irritable bowel syndrome) diarrhea prone," and prescribed a bowel relaxant and antidepressant. When they arrived in my clinic, only Barbara was taking the antidepressant; Linda and Teresa had stopped because of side effects and no improvement in their symptoms.

I listened to their individual stories, skeptical about the spastic colon or IBS diagnosis. Not surprisingly, I examined them and learned each suffered from a different ailment. I always felt that irritable bowel syndrome, or spastic colon, was a wastebasket diagnosis, created because of a failure to diagnose and treat the actual root cause more specifically. I used three different tests on the women, and arrived at three different ailments, just from taking *one* extra step per patient:

- After serum antibody allergy testing, it turned out that Teresa had a wheat and gluten allergy. Her symptoms resolved after she removed wheat and gluten from her diet.

- A stool analysis proved Linda's diagnosis was related to a microbiome imbalance. She had dysbiotic (bad invasive) bacteria, complicated with yeast overgrowth and absence of good gut flora (*Lactobacillus* and *Bifidobacter*). Her cramping and diarrhea resolved with three months of herbal therapy to inhibit the pathogenic dysbiotic bacterial growth, along with yeast and a probiotic (friendly gut flora), and restricting sugars and refined carbohydrates in her diet.

  I gave Linda targeted amino acids and adaptogens that helped resolve her symptoms in three more months. Repeat tests showed much healthier levels of all five neurotransmitter biochemicals, and her adrenal curve of cortisol and DHEAS (two other signs of flight-or-fight) normalized. Linda was a happy camper.

- Barbara was different. While her tests were normal, her symptoms were triggered by emotional stress. The antidepressant medication helped her emotions, but not her bowel symptoms. She began to exercise and learned how to reduce her tension with meditative practices. After a few months, her symptoms improved, but not completely. We drilled down deeper. Through a hypothalamus pituitary adrenal (HPA) test, we found alarmingly low levels of serotonin (ST), GABA and dopamine, and high levels of norepinephrine (NE) and epinephrine (E). These are the biochemicals the body releases in a primal fight-or-flight response, and if chronic, result in neuro fatigue pattern.

Every Body Has a Soft Spot

Every body has at least one soft spot. When the going gets tough, the soft spot will let you know. These spots are like *balance barometers*—they let us know when we are tipping the scales and moving into an imbalanced state. Physicians are all too familiar with patients that return repeatedly with the same complaints, such as back pain, headaches, abdominal cramping or recurrent colds. For example, a patient might say, "Every time I get a cold, it goes right to my chest," or "Whenever I am under a lot of stress, I get a migraine."

These conditions could represent diseases that need diagnostic testing to rule out serious illness. However, it is wise to be aware that soft spots talk to us. They warn us of imbalances and imminent danger to our energy, bodies and health if we do not respond to their bidding. If we learn to recognize these early warnings, and listen to our bodies talking to us, we can often use simple, holistic measures to prevent problems with our balance.

Elaine's story illustrates this. A 40-something writer, she came to my office for severe diarrhea, abdominal cramping, weight loss and anxiety attacks. She was working a high-stress job as a creative editor, complete with arduous deadlines and little positive feedback from her workplace. She'd had a tendency toward these symptoms her entire life, she said, but they'd never before presented this severely.

I began with basic diagnostic tests (colonoscopy, stool tests for pathogenic bacteria, parasites, yeast and blood), which affirmed the absence of any serious problems. At another appointment, Elaine revealed that her job was consuming her strength. While she really wanted to work on her own book, she equated leaving work to "leaping off a cliff" and being left without a means of support and benefits.

"Sometimes, in order to make room for something great, one must give away or let go of something," I told her gently.

She wrung her hands. "I know I have to write this book. It's a need, not an option. But I'm afraid. It's like I have to jump over this cliff, but there are no guarantees I'm going to land safely."

"There are no guarantees you'll get home tonight, either, but you have to trust," I said.

"My body is telling me it won't allow me to stay in this job."

I nodded. "Then listen to your body."

Elaine decoded her body's message. She chose to leave her job and work on her own book. Since then, she has gained support from several sources for her writing and has nearly finished her second novel. On occasion, her "soft spot" kicks up with its flash of insecurity, which she handles by meditating and using soothing colonic herbals (such as slippery elm, marshmallow root and glutamine) for calming her colon.

Shortly before her 46th birthday, Elaine had a setback. She returned to square one with no obvious explanation. "I planned a trip to visit my family in Montana," she explained in my office, "but I had to cancel it because I was so ill. There is no way I can go on a plane with these bowel symptoms."

I got right to the point. "You know this is your soft spot, Elaine . . . what is this really about?"

After considering several factors, she replied, "My mother . . . she's such a bitch!"

"OK . . . is that new?"

"No, she was born that way."

"So what do you think your body is trying to get you to pay attention to?" I asked. "Is there something you are supposed to deal with that you've been suppressing, like the work thing? You know your body will find a way to get rid of it, and that is what you are suffering from."

She began to cry uncontrollably. "Oh my God, I thought I'd done this already."

I held her in my arms. "It's alright . . . time to get it out. Let it go."

What Elaine said next stunned me. "When I was still a little girl, my mother told me I was the product of an accidental pregnancy and an unsuccessful abortion... My mother said she never wanted me and was sorry she ever had me. She was very abusive and always favored my sisters." Thankfully, she let it come out.

Although Elaine had dealt with these issues in psychotherapy, the vibration of being an unwanted child still resonated within her system. Her soft spot was screaming out, It's *time to release this attachment!*

"It's not that the work you did before was of no value. No work is ever wasted," I said. "This stuff is like peeling an onion. You came here to do this work, and each time it comes up, it is at a higher or deeper level. Like a spiral. You did the psychotherapy part—the emotional/mental part. Now we need to clear the energy/spiritual body. That will release you from the negative charge of the trauma and heal your body."

I taught Elaine a meditation technique to release unhealthy attachments. We then planned and conducted a shamanic ceremony. Her severe symptoms resolved. She learned a far better way of dealing with her mother's cruelty than burying it deep within herself, which forced her body to cleanse itself through her colon. Painfully. Today, she listens attentively for its messages while doing her regular practice to keep herself cleared from negative energies.

Elbert Hubbard once said, "Every spirit makes its house, but afterwards the house confines the spirit, so you had better build well."

Nothing reflects this more accurately than viewing the body as the house of the soul. In the Tiwa metaphor-language, *Wa Ma Chi* is the "Sound of God." Joseph Rael taught me that all components of the Wa Ma Chi are of equal importance. The *Wa* is the breath of life, and GOD, or the spirit. The *Ma* is the material aspect of form, and the *Chi* is the movement or energetic-etheric aspect.

At the time of conception, the breath of God (Wa) is inhaled into the body (Ma), resulting in the life force that governs our physical existence (Chi). In Chinese medicine, Qi carries a similar meaning to the Tiwa's *Chi*. Likewise for *Ki* in Japan, *Shka* in Lakota and *Prana* in India. All of these words celebrate the life force that courses through our bodies over our meridians, our energy highways. An easy way to think about life force is to envision it as a freeway. Sometimes, freeways get congested and stop traffic flow; the same happens in our bodies. This congestion comes from energy blockages that can present a multitude of different symptoms, such as a stiff neck, stomachache or headache. In Chinese medicine, this congested Chi is called *phlegm*. The movement of energy in our bodies is blocked, out of balance and stuck in a particular area that bothers us. It becomes a "soft spot," such as what Elaine experienced. If left unattended, the congested Chi will work into the Ma (material aspect of the body) and cause illness. In our necks, congested Chi may lead to muscle spasms or arthritis. In our stomachs, it may become ulcers, diarrhea or colitis, while in our heads, it could affect sinus drainage or result in chronic migraines. We must listen to what our bodies are saying and address the issue, every time, before it manifests as illness or disease.

Physicians and healers need to be acutely aware of body messages, so they can read the body's language and suggest the proper course for patients to remove obstructions to their Chi, their energy flow. A complete treatment plan must include tools that patients can use to keep their energy flowing. Medicine is only a temporary remedy; it does very little to remove energetic blocks. It primarily treats pain at brain level. However, it is a good idea to create immediate relief, because that alone may initiate the healing response. Getting out of that painful grip allows us the space to consider other holistic measures. Then we can follow up with a plan that treats the problem by opening up the flow of energy through blocked areas, such as acupuncture, chiropractic massage, salt bathes, ice and other body treatments, or movement.

Next, we honor the spirit, or Wa, by moving within or beyond our personal mythology and belief systems to the true essence of ourselves. Taking care of the body honors the soul housed by it. We honor Chi (life force) through exercise, massage, body work, psychotherapy, meditation, prayer, ceremony, dance and countless other ways of moving energy through the body. We honor Ma, the body that houses our soul and allows us to grow and learn on this earthly plane. We nourish it through good nutrition, exercise and rest.

Finding Our Right Balance

Each of us must find the right balance for our individual makeup. Some of us are vegetarians and vegans, while others prefer meat. These tastes can be easily discovered through tuning into your body's needs, along with some trial and error. Those who have done a great deal of spiritual work know that honoring the spiritual body is just as sacred as the material body. More, actually. They are all part of our wholeness: body, mind, spirit and emotions.

Treating our bodies as special, and keeping them healthy and in balance, requires regular monitoring—even by those who seem to work hard at maintaining balance and living with joy and purpose. Take Steve, who spent nearly 20 years studying and practicing Hinduism. At age 53, he reached the level of priesthood, carried a Hindu name, traveled often to India and enjoyed a close friendship with Mother Amachi (an embodiment of the Divine Mother Energy). Back home in California, Steve lived in a beautiful house with his lovely wife and close family.

Steve arrived in my office complaining of abdominal pain, bloating and diarrhea. His previous test results showed the presence of parasites. We decided to treat him with standard pharmacological anti-parasite medication, since he had failed natural therapies for parasites before he came to me. During treatment, Steve felt poorly, and his symptoms worsened. I suggested we do a colonoscopy or barium X-ray of the colon to look for signs of colitis. However, he did not want to take time away from his spiritual work. We held off. After he finished the pharmacological agents, we followed up with different herbal and probiotics. His symptoms improved, but they were not completely resolved.

Steve planned to return to India very soon, which concerned me because of his battle with parasites. "Steve, you need to protect yourself from getting reinfected when you travel," I told him. "There is an herbal tincture to prevent parasites, and a tonic to balance the 'cold bitter effects' of the tincture when you are in India. Also, if you eliminate breads, pastas and all simple carbohydrates, that will help your symptoms and make you less inclined to become infected."

He looked at me, a bit puzzled. "When I travel, I have no symptoms," he said. "It's only after I return from India that I get any symptoms."

I suspected his elevated spiritual state, especially in India, might account for that. Serving and being in close proximity to the energy of the Divine Mother, through Mother Amachi, kept him well during his travels.

When Steve returned to California, he called me, complaining of being sick again. "I did not take the herbal tincture when I was in India, because I didn't have time to get it before I went," he added.

His news didn't surprise me, though I think his experience after India might have been different had he taken the tincture. "Steve, I'm concerned you might be suffering from another ailment, such as colitis," I said. "If it is colitis, we need to do further testing to diagnose it, and you would need a different treatment regimen."

"I'm much too busy for that. I have several seminars and retreats scheduled and can't break my schedule for any tests."

I found it interesting that, while doing his spiritual work, he was fine. No complaints. He seemed to be protected. However, when he returned home, symptoms plagued him. Why? My intuition told me two things. First, Steve operated with two personalities. When working for "The Mother" and serving, he was truly on his path, taking take of others. However, he was different at home, perhaps not so kind to the mother of his children. Was his body trying to metaphorically point out this dichotomy? Second, Steve was not willing to care for his own body. His only real commitment was to his spiritual work, including the retreats and seminars—and only when he was away from home.

When the time was right, I questioned Steve further. "What is happening at home?" I asked.

"The kids are great, but my wife is never happy," he replied. "She should get a job if she doesn't like staying home with the kids. She doesn't know what she wants."

"Maybe she just wants more of your time with the family," I said. "Let me ask you: how can you be of service to Mother Amachi if you are physically out of commission? Also, isn't honoring the mother of your children reminiscent of honoring the Divine Mother? It most likely will help your wife feel happier and honored, too." Something clicked. A new clarity shone in Steve's eyes. "That rings true. I'll try," he said.

My most important job was to gain Steve's understanding that his body is special. It is his temple. Without it, the spirit cannot reside in this plane of existence—however highly intentioned his spiritual work may be.

We are not just our body, nor just our spirit. We need to care for this temple of our souls to continue having the physical experience we call life—and listen to continue living in great health.

CHAPTER 4
Healing Begins with Trust

I experienced an affirmation of medicine's sacred nature while on call as a key member of the UCLA/CURE Hemostasis team. As a therapeutic endoscopist, I performed technical procedures to control life-threatening gastrointestinal bleeding. Our UCLA/CURE team conducted the research and invented these tools and the technique to stop GI bleeding and avert surgery—now used by every gastroenterologist across the globe to save lives and prevent surgery for GI bleeding.

The call schedule for this role was grueling. Every third night, we were frequently called into the hospital in the wee hours, right through the early morning.

One night, while in a deep dream state, I was awakened by a call from the Veteran's Hospital. "Hello!" I answered after one ring.

"Dr. Randall?" It was a young male.

"Yes?"

"This is the senior resident in the ICU from the Wadsworth VA. We have a John Doe in his forties with a hematocrit of twenty [author's note: normal is forty] and a hemoglobin of five [normal is ten]. We've typed and crossed six units and we're running in FFP [fresh frozen plasma] through a central line and blood through both antecubital and a femoral vein. You better come in—he's putting it out faster than we can put it in. He's a drinker; you can smell it. But we are waiting on his alcohol level."

Most likely, the man was bleeding to death from dilated veins in his esophagus (esophageal varices), a condition that occurs with severe alcoholic liver disease and cirrhosis. I ripped myself from my bed, threw on some jeans and a sweatshirt and left the house. Questioning the sense of this work, I thought to myself, "Why am I torturing myself for a guy who wrecked himself by drinking?"

I never answered that question. Knowing that alcoholism is an illness and he is a fellow human, I instead beat myself up for harboring those thoughts about a person who desperately needed my help. As I drove to the hospital at 3 a.m., the dream in which I was immersed returned to me . . .

The stars sparkle brightly against an indigo-violet sky. I see myself from the outside, as if an observer. I wear a supple deerskin dress that hangs nearly to the ground. My long black shiny hair is worked into two thick braids at either side of my face. I gently walk across a field in beaded moccasins, and pass underneath a large metal bridge, like a freeway overpass. I kneel down to examine a person lying under the bridge . . . a young man, seemingly asleep. His long thick blond eyelashes and a round metal shield beside his head strike me most. I place one hand on his stomach and one on his cheek, and he awakens.

I arrived at the hospital and proceeded directly to the intensive care unit, where I found my patient. The internal medicine team and a young doctor from my team, training to be a gastrointestinal specialist, gave me a report. The patient's blood pressure was dangerously low, as was his blood count, and he was actively bleeding. The intern handling his case told me, "We corrected his clotting factors, but it's coming out faster than we can put it in!" A moment later, he added, "They found him unconscious under a freeway overpass in a pool of his own blood. Someone lost a hubcap and went looking for it, or they never would have found him."

I looked at the patient, a bit amazed. He had the same young face and long thick blond eyelashes as the man in my dream! Then the dream's meaning unfolded: no matter how high-tech and scientific our medicine is, there is still an element of sacredness that remains. "This is sacred work," I must have said out loud. I looked up at the questioning faces of my team. "Let's get this guy cleaned out. We have work to do."

The team lavaged the blood and clots from his stomach as best they could, by using a tube passed through his nose into his stomach, saline and what looks like a turkey baster. We performed a long difficult endoscopic procedure and eventually stopped his bleeding by injecting his dilated veins with sclerosant (a solution of irritating chemicals, including sodium tetradecyl sulfate and absolute alcohol, that coagulates tissue and closes the veins). The bleeding finally slowed down as we struggled to see through the spurting fountains of blood to inject in the proper places.

We finally finished. "Good job, Dr. Randall," the residents said.

"Yes, well, this is the easy part. Let's stabilize him and see if we can get him on the right road to recovery."

For the next few weeks, I followed his progress closely. After the initial stages of his recovery, I spoke with him about what happened and how he almost lost his life. "I know; the other doctors told me—you saved my life. Thank you," he said.

"Well, I'm happy to hear you care. How in the world did you end up under that freeway overpass?"

"Honestly, I don't know, Doc," he said. "I don't remember much since I served in the Persian Gulf War. I found out my wife had left and taken my son to live with another man. I used to be a writer before I entered the service. When I heard about my wife, I was still assigned to duty overseas. I began drinking to dull the pain. It just got worse and worse. I didn't want to face it. I didn't care whether I lived or died. I felt like my whole life was taken away from me."

I told him this was his home now, and that I would be his doctor. "Also, we can get you help and therapy," I added.

He seemed touched. "You've given me a chance to take my life back. Maybe if my brain still works, I can write again."

I smiled. "Well, this is a hell of a story—you can start with that!"

With our encouragement, he entered alcohol and drug rehabilitation and quit drinking. Last I heard, he was making a successful living as a writer. He was one of the lucky ones. It often takes several attempts for the practices and life changes required for true rehabilitation to fully sink in and become a sustainable change.

Trust is one of the most crucial elements in initiating the healing process and allowing the soul to unfold. The act of trust brings a greater sense of well-being and positive energy. It opens our hearts, minds and spirits, and enables us to give more fully of ourselves to our loved ones and the planet. Think of how you feel when you distrust someone, or something. Kind of closed, shutdown, maybe even a little dark, right? Now envision yourself living in full trust . . . doesn't it feel like exhaling into a pool of fresh, clear water?

Trust throws the doors of healing wide open and allows the energy to flow in.

Few dynamics or relationships in our lives require our trust like health care. Without trust, it is very difficult, even impossible to get well—or even allow needed treatment. This runs across many different levels and touches upon all aspects of health. We must trust not only our practitioners and treatments, but also our body's ability to heal. We must trust that the process our body is experiencing is perfect in some way, regardless of how imperfect we might judge it to be.

There is no question about the power of trust. The placebo effect of medications accounts for a 30 percent positive response rate from a simple sugar pill. Why is that? How can a drug with no tangible benefits work for 30 percent of the test group? Simple: Those patients *trust* that the pill will help them. By activating trust within their minds, their bodies open up to healing at a level far beyond the impact of a pill. Which gets to my biggest point: No matter how good the treatment or the practitioner, if there is no trust, healing will not occur. Trust opens the gates for healing energy.

Another major part of healing is love—and in particular, *loving thyself.* Let's say I rip my knee while running a marathon. I know myself well enough that, once I see my doctor to fix the physical damage, my trust in the doctor and healing process and my confidence in my body's ability to heal will enable me to recover far more quickly and fully than if I distrust. In order to love, though, we must feel and live in trust.

The place to start is *right now*, regardless of how you feel, the condition of your body, or whether or not you are facing disease or other health challenges. Loving our bodies exactly as they are opens up the channel of trust, which allows that inward flow of love to occur. With trust, your body is more likely to heal and for you to continue life's journey in a higher state of wellness. On a higher level, your growing degree of trust will lead to the wondrous flowering of your unfolding soul.

Asking for Help

For many, one of the hardest things to do is to ask for help. It is partly embedded into us by societal expectations. We may not have enough knowledge or skill. Or, we don't trust ourselves to handle the situation, whatever it might be. *I am weak for asking for help,* we sometimes think.

It would seem anyone who visits a doctor for more than a routine checkup is operating from a place of trust and asking for help. But you'd be surprised! Believe it or not, people often bring along their many self-imposed obstacles to asking for and receiving healing. They are often afraid to reveal how much help they really need, for fear of being "discovered" for whatever might have caused the ailment, perhaps deeper issues they don't want to expose or deal with. They keep their real wounds tightly covered and hidden. They feel embarrassed, or unwilling to take responsibility for the healing work that will follow.

One of my patients exemplified this. Celeste came to me while in her 70s, though she looked significantly younger. She came to see me after failing to reach her health goals with at least five previous doctors. She spoke quickly, trying to get out everything on her mind. "Dr. Randall . . . oh, I am afraid. My heart beats so fast, like this: *boom-boom-boom-boom-boom!*" She spoke as fast as an auctioneer running up the ante on a hot item. "I am afraid I am going to have a heart attack or die. Am I going to die?"

"No, Celeste, it will be OK," I said. "Let's talk a little more and figure this out."

She shook her head rapidly. "No, I already did this with five other doctors. They couldn't figure it out. What are you going to do?"

"I promise we can get to the root cause. The body is like an orchestra. We have to look at all the players and see how the whole system runs when we bring the whole thing together."

Celeste began nodding. "Yes, yes, that makes sense. But I can't sleep at all, maybe two hours, then I wake up panicked. I can't go out of the house at all. Maybe around four or five in the evening . . . *maybe*. I cry all day! All the other doctors wanted to do was give me drugs and antidepressants. I'm not depressed, Dr. Randall."

I sat still, absorbing her words, feeling her fear, pain and anxiety. I'd heard this type of patient story before. "I believe you," I said softly. "Now, what about your hormones?"

She sat bolt upright. "Oh no! I can't take those. I don't want to get cancer. My other doctor told me I'm too old, anyway."

Her concerns had some validity. The key word is *had*. She gave me the opportunity to fill her in on a solution that would help her, if she could open up and trust.

"Let me explain to you the new research," I said. "Bioidentical hormones not only do not cause cancer, but they *protect* you from cancer, cognitive decline, osteoporosis and heart disease. They also reduce anxiety and help you sleep."

I explained how the Women's Health Initiative Study, published in 2002, villainized estrogen.[5] Women that used Premarin (a conjugated form of all three forms of estrogen [E1, E2, E3] sourced from pregnant horse urine with synthetic medroxyprogesterone) had an increased risk for breast cancer, heart disease and stroke. When looked at more closely, the synthetic progesterone likely caused the cancer. "Natural progesterone and bioidentical estradiol are another story and have more benefit than risk," I concluded.

Celeste looked at me, dumbfounded. Obviously, I was the first to share the latest on bioidentical hormones and their hugely positive effects with her.

"Are you sure?" she asked.

"Yes. As long as you don't currently have an estrogen receptor-positive cancer, you are safe. Bioidentical hormones are protective and can help you."

"OK, but I'm on thyroid medication for a hypothyroid condition. Will hormones mess up my thyroid?"

My answer surprised her. "No . . . but they may help it. Perhaps we should check your thyroid is well."

"Yes, yes. Check everything," Celeste said, her eyes gleaming with light for the first time in our session.

I knew I had her trust. I *really* wanted to dig down to the root causes and define the big picture. "Let's also check your neurotransmitters, along with your hormones. You are out of balance," I said. "In the meantime, I want you to take a medicine for a short time to protect you from the irregular heartbeat."

She seized up, anxiety gripping her. "Oh no! See? All you doctors want to do is push pills."

"Not really. I don't prefer pharmaceuticals," I said calmly. "Until we get the lab results, though, let's be safe. I promise it is just until we get to the root cause."

Reluctantly, Celeste agreed. For her heartbeat, I prescribed Metoprolol, a well-tolerated beta blocker. It reduced her palpitations long enough for her to begin to trust me, her body and healing process.

Over the course of the next year, we balanced her hormones with estradiol progesterone creams, and found out she had a hyperthyroid condition from medication over-prescribed by another doctor. When we reduced that, her palpitations ceased completely. Her anxiety began to lessen with neurotransmitter and adaptogen support. Much to her delight, we were then able to withdraw the Metoprolol beta blocker.

About a year and a half after Celeste first came to see me, we met in my office. She was light and happy. "Oh my God, Dr. Randall, it is amazing!" she exclaimed. "I can sleep up to four hours now, and then wake up and sleep another two hours."

I smiled warmly. "That's great!"

"It's so much better. Why couldn't the other doctors figure this out? You've given me my life back. I am volunteering now at a hospital. I can go out!" Then she thanked me in a way that touched me deeply.

Celeste's biggest victory? She shifted her mindset. She learned to trust. She willed herself to receive help one more time—which made all the difference in her life.

We all need help at one time or another. The wise ones know when to ask, and how to apply the assistance they receive. I know as a doctor, the key is to foster trust by creating a calm, comfortable environment and being willing to listen and receive whatever the patient shares without judgment. This allows the patient to open up and reveal their weaknesses. We practitioners need to be there for our patients, so they know they are safe and can trust us with their secrets, no matter how dark. Another challenge is to coax the patient to let down their guard and ask for help. This takes constant guidance and an even stance.

My mother offers a good example. Years ago, when she underwent cancer surgery for an adenocarcinoma of the right upper lung, I took a medicine bag to use for her healing. We did this in addition to a multi-disciplinary approach with herbs, hands-on healing and prayer. I packed her medicine bag and filled it with key personal symbols for her, essential herbal medicine and nature-based healing energy. This is the same medicine bag I took to Joshua Tree for my vision quest. On the medicine wheel, bears are the guardians of the West—the physical plane. She needed physical protection for the surgery. The image of the bear at sunset, with water sourcing from her great paw, formed the essence of a continuing stream of life. The feminine energy of water is a flowing continuum for women from generation to generation.

During the days prior to surgery, I asked my mother to sleep with this medicine bag. She looked at the bag. "Oh, Honey, it is such a pretty purse . . . are you sure?"

It's such a pretty purse? Let's just say she was not familiar with medicine bags or bear medicine. However, she trusted me. "Yes, Mom, it's for your healing."

She loved and trusted me so much she dutifully slept with the medicine bag.

The day of her surgery arrived. Family members joined me in taking her to the hospital and sitting in the waiting room. (I was not part of the surgical team.) Some hours later, the doctor came out with a very surprised look on his face. He informed us that the adenocarcinoma tumor was gone—*gone!* Somehow, he added, it had necrosed. *Somehow . . .*

I knew what really happened. The bear did her job, the bear medicine followed suit, and it helped bring about my mother's physical healing. She faced an uncertain life span prior to surgery. Afterward, she lived for nearly 20 more years, until she died of natural causes at age 93.

The lesson learned? Trust your healing process, trust your body, trust your healers and trust those that love you. Also, allow the healing energy of love to flow fully, without any blocks.

Another trust-related issue I see often comes from patients who have been previously diagnosed or given a dark prognosis. Rather than viewing that as a doctor's learned opinion and setting out to heal, they often take it as the beginning of the end. I feel doctors and practitioners need to understand how diagnoses can act like sentences or spells and actually arrest the healing process. They need education on how to dispel these types of closed-ended diagnoses and prognoses. They need to assure patients that, for every problem, there is a solution. They can also reassure patients that official diagnoses are merely words used to code for billing reimbursement, or descriptions of a problem ready to be solved.

Imagine how different life would be for a cancer patient if we focused on living their life to the fullest while being treated. Or, if we made the most of a dementia patient's future by giving them natural medicines—and cognitive-strengthening exercises—instead of wallowing in the throes of a tough diagnosis that goes something like, "we all know how this is going to go . . ."

All people can heal, even if that healing isn't necessarily or completely physical. Some get cured, but all can heal and move forward.

Most of us know what it feels like in a doctor's office when a difficult diagnosis or prognosis is made—if not for us, then for a loved one. Now imagine what happens when a soul doctor like me sees that same diagnosis—and changes the game on the prognosis. When the anticipated dreadful medical prognosis *does not* come or proves to be otherwise, patients relax and slow down. The stress lines in their faces smoothen; already, the healing process has begun. Why? Because they are liberated from the fear that they will not be heard or treated in an uncaring way by doctors too concerned about economics or diagnosis codes or pressed for time to focus completely on them. Patients are astounded that a doctor such as me will actually sit and intently listen to everything they have to say. It returns them to a state of hope.

When people are given the attention they deserve, it fosters trust in the patient-doctor relationship. It also creates a sense of freedom crucial to healing. This trust begins the flow of healing energy between doctor and patient. The first step should always be to remove fear from patients . . . and their fear *of us*! Many patients are afraid of what we will do to them, what we might find out or how we may judge them for life choices or behaviors that led to their health challenge. Most of all, they are afraid that *we will not listen to them.*

I always strive to give my patients a feeling of being safe, free, empowered and listened to. When they do, I explain, "The new name for holistic medicine is integrative medicine and functional medicine. We make use of healing disciplines in addition to Western medicine . . . we keep our options open." All of that is well and good; who wouldn't want to know all available options for care and treatment? However, that's not what healing and a trusting rapport between doctor and patient comes down to. "Most important is that we (you and I) work as partners to design the most optimal health plan for you. A plan you help to create, understand, agree upon and feel like you can accomplish," I say.

Their faces light up. The seeds of our relationship and their healing sprout.

Part of returning to the road of health is also learning to trust our own inner teacher and the truth that comes from within. We need to become aware that we have access to inner guidance, and then learn to trust it. Often, we are not in touch with our own inner guides and do not know how to listen to ourselves.

A simple way to directly communicate with our body consciousness comes through guided meditation. Get into a quiet space and frame of mind, and tune into the part of the body causing trouble. You can do this on your own or with a professional, and perhaps record it in a journal later.

An Exercise to Build Self-Trust

Here's another way to use meditation to build self-trust and empower yourself: go to a quiet spot in the garden, or wherever you feel safe. Ask a simple "yes" or "no" question of your inner guide, something like, "Would exercise be good for me today?" The answer will either be a resounding "Yes" that feels like it's lifting our hearts, or a solid "No!" that causes them to sink in our chests. Trust the feeling. You will know. The right answer is usually the first we receive, before our thinking minds can interfere. If our minds flip back and forth, this is not what we are looking for. By clearing our minds through breathing deeply in and out, we can try again.

Look at these and see where you stand today—and see what you can do to better trust yourself, your *right* to have optimal health, and how by trusting yourself, the healing process and your doctor better, you can improve your health and well-being. The questions:

1. Do I trust certain kinds of therapy, and not others? (Think of Western medicine, traditional Chinese medicine, homeopathy, Ayurveda, American Indian, herbal, integrative medicine, micronutrient, nutritional or functional medicine. Answers to these

questions will help you to choose a healer, and/or appropriate therapy for yourself.)

2. Do I trust my healer?
3. Do I trust my *inner* healer?
4. Do I know the qualities I need in a healer?
5. Do I trust in the process of healing myself? Do I trust my body's ability to heal?
6. Am I having difficulty getting in touch with my feelings and expressing them properly?
7. Do I have emotions I am uncomfortable expressing?

In answering these questions, you will uncover ways in which you need to develop trust, which will help move you more quickly into complete healing.

CHAPTER 5
Love, the Cutting-Edge Tool

While speaking at a conference in New Mexico, I met Tim. His story was quite intriguing. At age 39, he'd met and fallen in love with a beautiful European woman. He poured his heart into the relationship, getting married, moving overseas and accepting a stepdaughter into his life. Two years later, they returned to the United States, where his wife always wanted to live. Much to Tim's bewilderment, eight weeks after that, on September 11 (yes, *the* September 11), he drove home from a business trip to a living room filled with shipping crates. His wife's first husband had flown to the US to whisk her and their daughter back to Europe. She took nearly all the money and possessions she and Tim shared, with no further explanation, and flew away.

Tim was shocked and devastated. He was a healthy, fit man who loved life, and also had a strong spiritual practice. None of that could stop his resulting emotional tailspin. For months, he willed himself to sleep by silently hoping he'd stay asleep—forever. Finally, he moved to New Mexico on the advice of a friend.

I met Tim almost a year later. His heart was still shattered. After we talked for a bit, he asked me for a healing. "I need to feel my heart again," he said. Those six words should alarm anyone in the health-care or emotional health world.

I felt his spirit desperately crying out, the urgency of getting an intervention so he could feel better. "Come and visit with me tomorrow around sundown and we'll see what comes up," I told him. "Also take note of your dreams. They are messages from your soul and I think yours has something to say."

The next day, we met in a quiet mountain lodge. I sensed a distrust for women at large, but a desire to trust me. "Tim, I am here to stand with you and help you find your way," I said. "I will never cross that line. I am your friend and healer. I will never be anything other than who I am." I put my right hand on his left shoulder.

"Thank you. I know that is true. I can see it in your eyes," he replied.

As he shared his story, his eyes glassed over with bitter tears. "When I'm out, and a woman comes up to me, the first thing I think is, 'What does she want from me?' I've never felt that way before."

Given Tim's penchant for trusting openly, and loving and serving others, I sensed two things: first, his heart needed to reconnect with life. *Fast.* And second, his soul was preparing for an even deeper healing than he could imagine. He was journeying through a dark night of the soul. His very essence could not stand any more darkness.

He asked for a shamanic healing. Two days later, it was time. Intuition and energies beyond myself guided me to build a unique medicine wheel for healing his emotional body and opening his locked-down heart to the love of others and himself again. I took Tim by the hand and led him around the medicine wheel, enclosing us within its spiraling transformative energy. Sitting in the center of the circle, I asked him to speak images from his recent dreams. Some pertained to falling in love with something or someone, and stopping short—before the person could get into his deep heart. This affected his work, everyday social interactions and existence. The pain was palpable. The darkness was deep.

We began to peel off an armor of self-protection that threatened to entomb his heart. We used crystals, cards, essential oils and meditation techniques to pierce it. These energetic interventions focused his attention away from his circumstances, in order to reveal the subtle energy pattern, storyline and vibration illuminating the path for his soul.

We also talked of the meaning of romantic love. "I believe it true of romantic love what Rumi said so many years ago, 'The minute I heard my first love story I started looking for you, not knowing how blind that was,'" I said, referencing one of his favorite poets. "Lovers don't finally meet somewhere; they are in one another all along."

As his emotions began to bubble to the surface, I continued. "When we love so deeply and intensely, we must remember to recognize that it is the love emanating from us that makes us so happy and elated," I explained. "True love is generous and kind and given without expectation. Your love for her was like that, for the most part, and when she returned your love with selfishness, it shattered your heart because you expected her to be someone different.

"Even in love, we can never expect another to change or be anything other than who and what they are. If you want to have a butterfly, choose a butterfly, not a caterpillar hoping it will become a butterfly. Find exactly who you want and give everything you have, expecting nothing except for them to be who they are. And if they love you for who you are and do not expect you to change, you begin to share the same dream.

"This is the divine dance of lovers in love, of couples who dream together over lifetimes of closeness. But if you love another like this, you must *love yourself completely*. You must make your half of the dream dance perfect and whole before you can give it away. You must own it before you can give it."

Recognition of this truth shone through his eyes.

Tim has an old powerful soul, and thus needed a powerful medicine pouch. I made him medicine with gifts of animal hair, feathers and crystals from the totems that came to me during the healing. They would speak to him and guide him toward the future. His medicine bag included hair from a black bear's chest, a cardinal feather, a kernel of white corn and a clear crystal. I explained that the black bear is a dreamer and teacher, and the hair from his chest is strong physical medicine to protect the heart and help it mend, while strengthening his own path as an inspired teacher. "The cardinal feather is beautiful, delicate love medicine," I continued. "It will attract love into your life and bring in the perfect mate. The white kernel of corn is a spirit-seed from the White Corn Maiden to help give birth to new things in life. The clear quartz crystal amplifies the medicine, a symbol of keeping things pure and clear."

I placed sage in the bag to help Tim release the past and protect him from it, and also to clear his heart for love of self and others.

Then I listened as he spoke, cradling his words and feelings with the detached, unconditional love and support he so badly needed. Not only did he need a medicine woman, but a friend *he could trust*.

Toward the end of our session, after we had cleared a great deal of obstructive energy from his heart, Tim pulled a card that pointed to meeting someone. I saw an image of a fork in the road, next to a beautiful flowing river. The couple held hands on the road, while on the other side, another woman waved. "You will be with this woman and it will be rewarding," I said, "but she is most likely not the one who you will stay with and let into your deepest heart. However, your deepest heart will heal and be free to open again."

Eight months after this session, Tim contacted me. "You won't believe what happened," he said, "or maybe you will. I played a *kirtan* [sacred Sanskrit music] in New York. A couple of hours later, I checked my e-mail and there was a note from my ex; I hadn't communicated with her for six months."

"What did it say?"

He quoted the e-mail: "I am so very sorry for what I did to you, and I tell you this because I know I was wrong and I want you to one day be able to love someone else."

A pair of simultaneous healings resulted from our work: divine forgiveness between Tim and his ex; and Tim's heart again swinging open at its deepest point. The following spring, he came to Rancho La Puerta, the fitness and spiritual retreat in Tecate, Mexico, where I served as executive director and integrated medicine teacher. He looked like a different person. His face was relaxed, his green eyes sparkled and his self-confidence exceeded what I'd seen before. I stood before a healing heart and soul.

I gave Tim unconditional love and sense of trust (plus my skills as a medicine woman) at the precise moment his heart was ready to start healing. Timing is everything in health—no matter if it's mental, emotional, physical or spiritual. Even more so when love, or broken love, is involved. Any doctor or healer must understand this loving attention to *all* levels of a patient. It is the most vital tool in our bag.

The Most Powerful Healing Elixir

Love is the most powerful healing elixir in the universe, the medicine of true healing. Love not only heals, but also holds the atoms and the solar systems and universe in place. *God is love.* It opens the closed heart, parts the waters, mends the sick and wounded, and heals us and the world. It is the vital foundation for the relationship with self, community and earth. Put your hands together each morning and give thanks to the power that is greater than us.

For this reason, practitioners must listen to their patients and look at them with the eyes and ears of a lover. And every patient must realize that love of self and others fuels all of the medicines, treatments, care and maintenance they receive. When we doctors work from this place, we become interested in everything a patient has to say. I can find something I adore about each person who sees me. This does not imply a sexual relationship. On the contrary, any breach of the healer-client relationship would irreparably damage the healing process and shatter the healer's integrity.

I have found that if doctors and healers can focus authentic loving energy on their patients, they become empowered in many ways. *Regarding patients with the ears and eyes of the lover.* It's a level of active listening that would well serve humankind in general. It is vital for *true medicine*. When you get down to it, despite our advanced technology, the difference between treating a problem superficially and true healing boils down to *caring*.

Holding a love for patients and respecting their uniqueness empowers people to take responsibility for their own well-being. When patients feel safe and loved, they develop a greater capacity for loving themselves. Levels of endorphins and neurotransmitters test higher in happy people who express love and feel it in themselves.

Years ago, studies by David McClellen at Harvard showed that medical students who watched three different movies before exams had three different immune system readings.[6] He showed a war movie, a documentary on organic gardening, and a biopic of Mother Teresa. He found the war movie suppressed the immune system, the organic gardening film left the immune system as-is, and the Mother Teresa movie increased immunity. In other words, an expression of love increased immunity.

No Separation Between Healer and Patient

A true healer knows there is no separation between the patient and herself or himself. When love fills that space in between, healing occurs. In his book *Love and Survival*, Dr. Dean Ornish writes, "Our survival depends upon the healing power of love, intimacy, and relationships. Physically, emotionally, spiritually. As individuals. As communities. As a country. As a culture. Perhaps even as a species."[7] And, I would add, as a planet!

Let's look at this. In one study, researchers found that people without friends increased their risk of death over a six-month period. In another, those who enjoyed many friends over a nine-year period cut their risk of death by more than 60 percent. The famous Nurses' Health Study from Harvard Medical School, an annual tradition started in 1976, found that the more friends women had, the less likely they were to develop debilitating physical problems later in life. Instead, they would lead joyful, fulfilling lives. Researchers concluded that not having close friends or confidantes is as detrimental to your health *as smoking or obesity*. They also examined the reaction of women to the deaths of their spouses, finding that those who confided in close friends as "sounding boards" were more likely to survive the experience without any new physical problems or loss of vitality.[8] Similarly, in July 2016, a Harvard Men's Health Watch survey of 127,545 men on marriage and health found that married men were far healthier than unmarried men.[9]

On that subject, Dr. Ornish and his wife, Anne, wrote a breakthrough book, *Love and Survival: 8 Pathways to Intimacy and Health*, which proves that not only lifestyle, but intimate, loving relationships are the next step to transforming our lives in every way—physically, mentally, spiritually and emotionally.

Simply put, the love of our friends and our partners helps us to enjoy longer, better quality lives.

Quantum Physics and the Existence of Love

Before quantum physics broke onto the scene in the 1970s, we thought of life processes in a Newtonian, or linear fashion—first, process X occurs, which leads to process Y. The birth of quantum physics came from attempts to understand the smallest particle of light. It brought a whole new way of thinking into physical science.

Quantum refers to the largest leaps in evolution science and growth. It also is a very important word in healing. The word *quantum* is Latin for "how much," or quantity, and describes the smallest unit that can be called a particle in form. Quantum physics arose out of an intense desire to understand the physical nature of light. One group of scientists, who believed light emanated as waves, invented an instrument that unequivocally proved their theory. Another group, hypothesizing that light was particulate in nature, conclusively confirmed it as a particle form. This suggested a nonlinear conversion of light from one form to another, from particles to waves. Since light cannot exist as both simultaneously, the way in which it behaves could depend upon the intention of the observer.

In order for a particle of light to become a wave, it must undergo a vibratory transformation. Some advanced quantum physicists argue that the vibratory force that holds atoms together is *unconditional love*, and that this force permeates the universe. Today, astronomers and physicists know this force as "anti-matter" or "dark matter."

Let's explore this force further. During the past decade, quantum theorists and astrophysicists have ventured beyond the atomic level, past protons, neutrons and electrons, and discovered that in this vast universe with its billions of galaxies, there is more space than mass. A lot more. Atomic structure better resembles dancing particles separated by enormous gaps; a typical atom is 99.999 percent empty space. This holds true for every kind of matter, whether gaseous, fluid or solid; diamonds are just as "spacious" as iron. Thus, everything in matter, including our bodies, is as void as intergalactic space.

I submit that it is love that fixes that void. The particle or wave is determined by the energetics of the observer.

What holds it all together? My teacher, Joseph Rael, often recounts his grandfather's early teachings: the basis of life is vibration. He is not alone. It is common among shamans and physicists to attribute the pillars of universal life and matter to vibration. When Joseph was a young boy, his grandfather took him into the kiva (a sacred circular chamber for ceremonial work and prayer). During a ceremony, he told Joseph to watch as he walked through a wall, and across a beautiful field to gather herbs. He returned through the wall, carrying the herbs, and made medicine. "All things are possible when we are truly in tune with the vibration of life," Joseph told me. "It's all love. The universe loves us so much that it becomes what we want it to be."

The late Dr. Candice Pert's turn-of-the-21st-century work with informational molecules (neuropeptides, hormones and neurotransmitters that transmit biochemical messages) unfolded the secrets of vibrational energy in the human body by scientifically documenting their rapid change in form over time. She showed that each of these informational molecules may possess thousands of different forms, constantly morphing from one to another (vibrating, like light morphing from particle to wave). The role they play in emotions and feelings fills in the missing link between matter, emotion and spirit. She showed how high concentrations of informational molecules seem to pool in physical locations corresponding to the seven cerebrospinal chakras (root, sacral, solar plexus, heart, throat, point between the eyes, crown of head). There are at least as many of these substances and their receptors in the heart (center of love) or gut (solar plexus; center of intuition and immune system) as there are in the brain.

This also lays a firm scientific notion for why chakra meditation may be useful in balancing our energy and why people have been doing it for over 5,000 years. The informational molecules are not thought; rather, they move *before* thought can be attributed to them. They serve as split-second points of transformation within the body. First, we have the "A-ha!" moment. *Then* we decide what we think about it.

In the brain, where the crown chakra is located, health and thoughts of love are dependent upon neurotransmitter function. In the 1990s, I began using Sanesco neurotransmitter hormonal testing and therapy intensely when I was one of the first physicians to take holistic functional integrative medicine into the inpatient addiction recovery world, which helped change the conversation in addiction therapy.[10] We showed that holistic testing and treatments improved patient outcomes and outlooks, reduced their symptoms like insomnia, cravings, anxiety, depression and fatigue, and lowered the relapse rate. By the time I finished, we had over 5,000 different patient data points and half as many retests. We looked at levels of neurotransmitters (serotonin, GABA, dopamine, norepinephrine, epinephrine, glutamate, cortisol, DHEA).

I continue to use this system. Recently, I worked with a British physician who was born without adrenal glands. I wasn't sure it would be effective but I told her we might as well try. She was open to anything. After finding extremely low levels of her neurotransmitters and adrenal hormones, we went to work, treating her with targeted amino acid therapy. Her numbers reflecting total body neurotransmitters levels were markedly increased. She now feels better than she has in her entire life. "What have you done?" her friends asked afterward. "You look amazing. You are so different and happy! Even your hair is thicker."

Now she wants me to come to the United Kingdom and set up a clinic!

Once I find out the pattern of imbalance through Sanesco neurotransmitter and adrenal testing, my staff and I treat imbalances using biomimicry—yet another way to express love by mimicking the flow of nature. In this case, it involves targeted amino acid therapy. Nutrients and amino acids feed the chemical pathways. With that in mind, we correlate the patient's symptoms and history with the pattern on their tests. When we relieve a patient's symptoms and restore long-term health, annual or semi-annual testing can be done to maintain that health and prevent recurrences.

Quantum physics is similar to Sanesco, except that the "body" reflects the universe or totality of nature. We have that 99.999 percent of open space in every atom, and in the space between atoms. What holds our bodies and all matter together? According to seers from Dr. Pert to Joseph Rael to leaders of indigenous religions, it is the loving energy of the universe—unconditional love.

Exercise: Opening to Unconditional Love

Try the following meditation to put into practice the modern principles of quantum physics, to perceive the unconditional love beyond, behind and within everything.

1. Go to your power place and use your breath to quiet your mind.
2. Visualize a brilliant white light at the top of your crown, taking the shape of a beautiful lotus flower. As you breathe deeply in and out, the flower begins to open. It receives the divine white light energy pouring down for all of us to receive. Feel yourself being

washed completely clean by that brilliant light as it floods into your crown chakra like a waterfall, lighting up your crown, brain stem and heart as it cascades through your entire body.

3. Imagine that light passing down and through your body and lighting up your third eye (forehead area) and throat chakras.

4. Visualize a beautiful deep pink rose opening in the center of your chest. Feel the warmth as you begin to receive all the love that is there for you. Open yourself to all of the love from your family members and friends. Open to all of the love ever given to you, in this or any other lifetime.

5. Breathe in deeply and slowly. Allow yourself to receive the love that you may not have given yourself permission to receive before. Open yourself to unconditional love from the higher realms and from the earth herself.

6. Breathe out slowly and completely. Give love to your friends, family, community, Mother Earth and your God. Now give love to yourself.

7. Breathe in again. The love you transmitted will be sent back to you, multiplied and blessed by your act of giving. A verse from the Moody Blues song "Question" speaks to us receiving all the love back that we have given to others.

8. Focus on your breath, the vehicle of giving and receiving love. Inhale for five counts, exhale for six counts. Continue breathing in this pattern for 10 to 20 minutes, giving and receiving love throughout.

CHAPTER 6
Attitude Is Everything

Pray for change
Make the change
Fight for change
Be the change

—G. M. R.

In 2002, I experienced attitude in a healing situation from both sides of Alice's looking glass.

The prior year had been full of crushing disappointments. After my divorce in 1998, I moved from Malibu to Tucson to begin a new life as director of integrative health at Miraval, a top-10 destination health spa. They recruited me from my successful integrative medical practice to head up a new healing center adjacent to the existing spa. We designed buildings, interviewed staff and brought in new talent and services. I also wrote programming to create a new holistic health adjacent to Miraval; it was to include holistic medical and spiritual therapies and classes of all types. So I began teaching some of the classes. There was great excitement for this groundbreaking health center.

I also met someone, Jason, a deeply emotional and expressive Greek man introduced by my good friend Mathew. The three of us went out to dinner, and I could tell Jason liked me, in the way a woman *knows* a man is interested. His dark attractiveness drew me to him, though I was well aware such an attraction had always led me into trouble in the past. Still, he called, and we developed a friendship. We met for coffee and made a habit of talking until the wee hours of the morning about life, our experiences, philosophies and transformation. We loved hiking, working out in the gym and movies. Jason shared the life stories of his rise and fall financially, his survival from alcoholism and his own marital breakup. His heart had just been shattered again, by his longtime love.

At that point, perhaps I should have turned and run, but I felt like we had something in common. Something we needed to overcome together. Besides, I liked him. Spirit brings people together for a reason, and Jason and I were good for each other's souls.

One day, Jason asked me to go camping with Betty and Tim, his long-time friends from the East Coast, who also lived in Tucson. When he picked me up, he stood in the doorway in his jaunty way, left hip sticking out, leaning on the doorjamb—with a .357 Magnum pistol strapped to his right leg.

I looked him up and down, my eyes falling on the pistol. "I thought we were going camping, not on an espionage mission," I said.

"Yeah, bears . . . you know . . . can't be too careful."

"OK, should I bring my forty-five?"

"No, I think one gun in the family is enough."

We laughed. Actually, we laughed a lot, one reason why we liked spending time together. We were so involved in our banter that we forgot to get half the things on the camping grocery list. Finally, we fueled up before heading into the mountain forest toward Mt. Lemmon, the highest point in the Santa Catalina Range of southeastern Arizona at almost 10,000 feet.

After Jason pumped the gas, he popped back in the car and picked up our conversation. "So anyhow," he said, "there was this guy and he—"

Thump!

The huge sound came from the back of the car, cutting off his words abruptly. "Someone hit us with a bat or something? What was that?" I asked.

We pulled over and got out. The pump nozzle still hung out of the gas tank. A gas station attendant sauntered in our direction. "We're so very sorry," Jason said.

The attendant calmly smirked. "It happens all the time. Almost once a week. At least you weren't drunk." He sized us up. "Just otherwise occupied, I figure." He returned the nozzle to the gas pump and returned to his retail area.

We slid back into the car, laughing so hard we had to pull over again. We hugged each other while shedding tears of laughter. "Wait until we tell Betty and Tim," I said.

Every time we mentioned our gas station moment that night, we laughed until I almost wet my pants. Camping was a blast. We cooked steaks and corn, giggled and told scary stories about extraterrestrials around the campfire. Jason's people were so fun and warm hearted; they became some of my dearest friends.

Everything remained great until a recession hit the economy in March 2001, followed by the burst of the dot-com bubble, which crashed a lot of businesses. The company that owned Miraval sold out to go private, in order to balance their debt. I realized the healing center was not going to happen anytime soon. It was very difficult to part from something I believed in so strongly. *It's not the initiative itself,* I thought. *Just about money. Everything in its own time and rhyme.*

Jason dropped the next bombshell, deciding to reunite with his old girlfriend. "Bad timing," I said, plenty of sadness in my voice.

"No, the timing was perfect. We needed each other," he said.

He was right.

I couldn't help but take some of this personally. Furthermore, Jason's decision added to a feeling of mounting, impending doom from which I had been distracting myself. My intellect told me that the economy was responsible for my dreams at Miraval falling through, and that Jason needed to work out his own issues. Unfortunately, though, my attitude headed south. Thoughts of inadequacy allowed the dark clouds of doubt, unworthiness and self-judgment to creep into my heart. I dipped into a dark night of the soul.

A Dark Night

It turned out to be a very dark night, and my attitude was not helping. I was forced to sell my beautiful house on 10 acres in the Tortolitas of Arizona, complete with organic gardens and orchard. It was awash in saguaros, cacti and fauna, more beautiful than the nearby Desert Museum. A beautiful mountain lion would share the backyard with my dog, Ruffy; the mountain lion's tail would wag up and down lazily like a snake as she rested in the soft grass. It was her home before ours. Not 12 feet away over a short garden fence, Ruffy sniffed around the yard. We were in harmony with each other, and with the surrounding nature.

The worst, though, was that a woman I thought was my friend and teacher betrayed me in every way one can be betrayed. She was a shaman and medium who attempted to injure me mentally, emotionally, physically and spiritually. She tried to take my soul. Eventually, my strength, attitude and spirit pulled me through.

It was very disconcerting. And noticeable. My friend Harold Greene said, "You are amazing the way you go through all these changes and rise like the phoenix from the ashes . . . but I'm worried about you."

Even though I felt dashed and a little worse for wear, I asked, "Why do you say that, Harold? I'm a survivor."

"Well you know better than me, doctor, when people undergo repeated severe stresses, something bad happens to them . . . like cancer or a heart attack. A person can only take so much."

He was right. However, my teachers had given me the tools and knowledge to heal, and a spiritual practice to keep my soul strong. There was one thing I could do, one change I could make, a change I desperately needed to move forward: my attitude.

A colleague at Miraval, Diane, asked me repeatedly to see her shaman. I didn't feel I had the room or energy for another shaman or teacher in my life, but eventually I acquiesced and called her to set up the appointment.

I became proactive, designing a program for myself as if I were my client. It combined immune system enhancers, adrenal support, exercise and prayer. When you suffer repeated stress events in a cascading way, your spirit and attitude tumble and the body begins to suffer as well. The immune and adrenal systems become dangerously depleted. So I needed to bolster myself physically. The additional supplements I self-prescribed brought my pill count up to 20 a day, not counting elixirs, powders and teas. It seemed like a part-time profession, taking supplements three times a day. Using the tools I gave to my patients, I put them on the kitchen table to take with my meals, and took the opportunity to say *thank you* to the plant spirits within the supplements and visualize my body as healthy and strong.

I felt so weak that the next piece of my program, exercise, became the hardest part. I rented a sweet little Santa Fe style house in the Catalina Range foothills above Tucson, complete with a swimming pool. The owner lived on the property and kept up the pool, but didn't like to swim. Well, I was a swim champion as a kid, so I knew what to do in that pool! I built up my endurance and flexibility, and soothed my emotions in the cool, blue water. I made a daily practice of sunrise meditation and prayer, followed by swimming and water aerobics. I needed the yin of the water to cool my heated adrenals and emotions. I felt my strength gradually return.

Visit with a Shaman

About two months after I moved in, Diane picked me up for my healing with the shaman. "You know, he is impossible to get in to see, but he is making this exception because when I called, he got some kind of intuition," Diane said.

"What did you tell him about me?"

"Nothing really. Just that you had been through a series of difficult events, including losing your husband, job, boyfriend, house, and a girlfriend that betrayed you."

I grimaced. "Well, when you put it like that . . . it does sound bad."

"I didn't mean it like that," she said.

"I know. Just my stuff. How much does he charge?"

"Not much. By donation only."

We drove to a remote location outside Tucson, bouncing on a washboard dirt road the last third of the trip before arriving at a small brick house in obvious disrepair. Two large Labrador mix dogs, one black and one yellow, barked and wagged their big bushy tails. We walked into the house through the kitchen, where the shaman's wife asked us to have a seat. I was used to healings in the kitchen from early experiences with my Lakota grandfather and grandmother, so this felt good to me. She was thin and wrinkled, her hair the color of old wheat straw. Her clear blue eyes shone and beheld a kindness that broadcast her strong spirit. "I'll go get him," she said.

These are no-nonsense people, I thought. *I like this.* My attitude was right where it needed to be.

An unassuming thin man with yellow-white hair, a flannel blue plaid shirt and blue jeans sat down at the table next to me. He looked me up and down, took a pad of yellow lined paper his wife laid in front of him, and began to write and draw. "Yep," he said as he drew. "It looks like this. You got some blockages down here." He was drawing a likeness of a body. He made a marking down by the knees. "Did ya have surgery there or something?"

He'd picked up on my worn knees and previous arthroscopic surgeries! I nodded. "Yes."

"Thought so, we can fix that, no big deal . . . also a little problem here in the neck . . . probably just stress." He drew some more, and then stopped. "This is the biggest problem I see," he said, confirming my pain. "I've seen this before. It's the work of a woman I know. She splits open your base chakra and slices ya all the way up, like this"—he drew on his yellow pad of paper—"so she can tap your energy. You gave it to her, whether you know it or not. But you did try to cut her off, didn't ya?"

"Thought I did." I really did think so, though sometimes, it takes a while for your heart to catch up with what your mind really knows.

I was so relieved to hear him confirm what I'd suspected. This is why even healers need healers. Still, he shook his head. "Well, not completely," he said, addressing my comment. "We can fix that, though. Although you gotta continue to do your work and take your energy back. That's part of it."

"Yes, I will," I said affirmatively; that's what I'd been doing the past two months. Slowly getting my energy back, then working on taking my power back.

He wasn't done evaluating. "Also, you got a block in your mouth. We can fix it, but you have to start speaking your truth. That's why God put you here. It don't matter if some people don't get what you say or don't agree with you—the right people are gonna get it. Understand?"

"Yes, I understand."

"OK, then let's get started."

The shaman took his pencil-sized feather and used sage smoke and worked on my chakras. It was simple, no-nonsense. Just like him. In that reading and healing, he helped strengthen a change in perspective and attitude I so badly needed. In describing the drawing and what he saw in me, he also reminded me of how our attitudes not only can take us down mentally and emotionally, but also physically and spiritually—*especially* when coupled with traumatic, stressful events and when you give your power away.

Our Attitudes Control Our Lives

Like everyone, I have endured a number of roadblocks and obstacles. Life is like that. I attribute my ability to keep healing and returning to full strength to a positive attitude. That includes always looking back and finding the gifts I have learned through those difficulties, which was certainly the case as I worked with the shaman. Then I pass it forward, teaching that wisdom to others so maybe it's not quite so hard for them as they take their healing journeys.

Our attitudes control our lives. Attitude is our secret power. It is of paramount importance that we know how to harness and control its great force.

Our intentions and attitudes create the types of experiences we will move through, health and otherwise. We attract to us what we emanate most strongly. When you're not well and your energy is low, then your life vibration is likely low as well. The key is shifting low-vibration energies to high-vibration. Low-vibration energies (fear, anger, hate) slow or stop our overall energy flow by externalizing or giving away our own power. When we can understand this, we become more willing to draw our energy back. Also, when we comprehend that projecting low-vibration energies draws more of the same to us, we are more willing to shift our perspective and begin attracting what we truly want: love, joy and happiness.

One of my heroes, Dr. Norm Shealy, has promoted positive attitude from day one. Norm is the grandfather of holistic medicine, who pioneered pain medicine by inventing electrical nerve and spinal cord stimulators, among other works. Now 90, his new book *Life Beyond 100* speaks of attitude being the key to longevity. As well as making it through hard times.

After I returned home to Tucson, my attitude was really good. The shaman's healing strengthened me big-time. It explained what was draining me and how to stop giving my energy away. Between that and a continued daily practice of meditation, prayer, swimming, and adrenal and immune system support, my energy elevated enough to form a new consulting firm, GM Randall Corporation. My good friend and consultant, Michael Figueroa, was instrumental in teaching me how to form and run such a firm. I am eternally grateful to him. This firm became the safety net for my financial stability, and the cornerstone for all Randall Wellness Network endeavors to follow.

New Challenges

One day, just when I was feeling strong and healthy again, I looked into the mirror and noticed a peeling bumpy place on my lower lip. I scratched it off and carried on, doing well on the lecture circuit, and interviewing for a job at the prestigious Canyon Ranch in Tucson.

Soon, I began to notice strands of my beautiful flaxen hair everywhere. It covered my office chair and pillow. Whenever I shampooed or brushed it, my hair would come out in handfuls that clogged up the drain. Bouts of diarrhea, nausea and weight loss followed. I called my friend Donna. "If I didn't know better, I would think I was on chemotherapy," I told her. "I can't eat. I have no energy. I'm losing weight and my hair is everywhere—it's scary!"

Coincidentally, I was consulting for six patients with late-stage cancer—one with aggressive thyroid cancer, another with lung cancer wrapped around his aorta, plus patients with colon cancer, breast cancer, melanoma and uterine cancer. In each case, I suggested heavy regimens of herbal and mushroom immuno-modulators, adaptogens, antioxidants, organic vegetarian diets, prayer and spiritual practice, along with exercise very similar to what I was doing.

Meanwhile, my hair kept falling like snow. During the July 2002 solar eclipse, I decided to visit the only wig shop in Tucson. My comb-over hairstyle rivaled some of my old medical school professors; it was becoming obvious. I walked into the wig store, largely ignored by the indifferent Korean ladies that tended the shop. I eventually asked to be shown the natural hair wigs, thinking they would be better than synthetic. One of the ladies showed me some over-teased champagne-blonde options, not exactly my idea of the way to mask the loss of my pure white, naturally silky hair. I looked around the store a little longer and found a synthetic wig close to the right color, with a natural-looking pink-colored part instead of the "woven look." I took it to the mirrors and waited to be assisted. The ladies walked by me on several occasions without offering help.

While sitting and waiting, I watched some of the other shoppers through the mirror. I noticed something: many were already wearing wigs. *Of course!* I thought. *This store is right across from the University of Arizona Medical Center.* They slipped into the corners very self-consciously, taking off their wigs, trying on new styles, covering heads as bald as bowling balls.

One of the shop attendants came up behind me. "Are you going to just sit there?"

"Well, no . . . I mean *yes.* I haven't done this before," I replied. "How do you put it on?"

"Like dis." She took the wig off the mannequin, her hands on each side, and shoved it onto my head in one swoop. The bangs hung down below my nose. I peeked out from the mess of Marilyn Monroe–colored locks and saw how pathetic I looked with little wisps of my remaining hair sticking out on the sides. I plucked it off and ran tearfully to the back of the store. There, a heavy woman tried on large wigs to compensate for her size, I suppose, not to mention her baldness. She looked at me through thick glasses, her head shining beneath the harsh store lights. "It's not easy, is it?" she said.

"No."

We cried and held each other for a long time. I understood how she felt as she comforted me. I left the store, never to return.

I felt the need to grow, in skills and attitude. I put more energy into my private consulting, in addition to taking a job in an ER. This was a fascinating way to upgrade my Western medical knowledge at the same time as testing out whether holistic medical skills had any place there. Plus, it gave me a paycheck and another way to be of service, which always helps my attitude.

One night, I had a dream. I was at the doctor's office, and he was very gently looking at my hair. He picked up little strands between his fingers. When pieces fell out, he studied them with a magnifying glass, then held them to the light. I could see my scalp was bright red, as if burnt.

"You have cancer," he said . . .

The next day, I told the dream to one of my dreaming women. We convinced ourselves it was a metaphor and a reflection of my recent experience, not actual cancer. My hair continued to fall out, though, and I continued to feel ill, so I made an appointment.

My doctor examined me carefully and suggested we take blood tests before he sent me to the dermatologist. All of my tests returned with normal results, to my great relief. Still, he referred me. Then the dermatologist offered up a surprise. After listening to my story, he carefully and gently began to look through my hair and examine the pieces that fell out, just as in my dream. "Your hair loss is from stress," he concluded.

"Stress?"

"When you are severely stressed, your body gets rid of what it doesn't really need to survive. What you thought were the roots are actually the cuticles. It will grow back." That issue solved, he looked at my mouth. "What is that on your lip?" He began to examine my lip and inside of my mouth. He was not pleased. "We had better biopsy that."

"Can you take the whole thing out?" I felt like I was already falling into the bargaining stage.

He paused for a moment. "Well, I hope so . . . the thing is, it goes through to the inside of your mouth. We'll see."

"What do you think it is?" *Please don't say cancer.*

"I can't be sure. Don't worry now. We'll find out soon. I'll put a rush on it."

I convinced myself it was going to be fine.

I woke up two days after the biopsy with the feeling someone had run a stake of fear through my heart. Usually courageous, I was taken back by these unfamiliar feelings. I ran to the phone and called my dermatologist, intending to leave a message. Much to my dismay, he answered. "I'm so sorry to bother you on Sunday . . . I . . ."

"Madeleine?"

"Yes."

"It's so funny you called. I just came into the office to see if your biopsy report was finished."

My heart started pounding. Hard. "What is it?"

"Positive for invasive squamous cell carcinoma."

Cancer.

My stomach rumbled into somersaults before sinking into my pelvis. Cold sweat dripped from my armpits. My mind began to race a thousand miles a minute. Why me? I'm so healthy and careful. Did they mix up the biopsies? It's not fair! How can I do my work without a mouth to speak and teach through? What did I do wrong to deserve this?

Then, I thought of all my patients that had experienced this same feeling, the feeling of finding out for sure. My next thought: how do I turn this around? Thankfully, my attitude was far better than after I lost Miraval, Jacob and my house.

First things first. "What do I need to do?"

"I know a great plastic surgeon," the doctor replied. "I'll get you in next week and you can see him and set up your surgery. You'll have to let him assess to see if it can be locally excised, or if it has spread too far inside your mouth or lymph nodes. If so, your jaw and tongue may need to be resected."

I felt like a huge club had struck me down. "Oh, God."

"Don't worry—he's the best." The doctor's voice was reassuring.

Immediately, I began preparing for the surgery. I asked a few choice friends and fellow healers to pray for me and send healing energy. Amazingly, all knew that something wasn't right; whether in person or long-distance, they felt a waning, inward flow of my energy, which happens when we're fighting disease, especially something as invasive as cancer. Among those was my friend Dale. We corresponded back and forth, at one point bringing in one of my biggest life influences, Deborah Szekely. I'd like to share some of our correspondence:

Dale: *This is really a bittersweet message and I feel moved to comment rather at some length.*

I had felt something about your health, for a month or two, but I don't believe you had told me anything was wrong. I did not pick up about your hair.

Me: *Remember about my medicine—I do things before they happen to soften the situation in this plane of existence. I don't think I will need chemotherapy or radiation, and I am following my own program for cancer patients. I believe it was a practicing for the letting go of my lip—the letting go of my hair. Also, this is the one-year anniversary of my moving to this house and letting go of Miraval. I needed to shed it all so I could move forward with the work I have to do.*

Dale: *The hair loss is the least of it, but you're right, as it would affect your appearance temporarily. There is a solution.*

Me: *My hair actually has come back so fast it looks kind of cute now. My hairdresser cut it in a long layered look and it's curly. I had forgotten it was wavy. Looks good. I keep visualizing it growing and thick.*

Dale: *Of course, there are wigs.*

I then told Dale about my lousy visit to the wig shop, and the experience with the woman who had cancer.

Dale: *How bad does the lesion look after the biopsy?*

Me: *It looks fine. No one can even see it. It's about five millimeters, but may be larger underneath, as the whole lip on the bottom is peeling and there is a lump inside my mouth. We won't know until the surgeon gets in there, and he and I both want to do it in one step if possible, with a pathologist standing by. The idea is that he keeps cutting until he gets a clean margin. Then he figures out how he's going to fix it.*

Dale: *Madeleine, your brilliant mind and sweet spirit should absolutely shine through. And you know there are times that God shows people what He wants them to see. So I would suggest that you carry yourself as a beautiful woman in the way that you have always seen yourself.*

Me: *Thank you. I will remember this and do my best.*

Dale: *You have my prayers in abundance. God will see to it that you are where you are meant to be! And I know that is helping others. You are humble, Madeleine, and also under a lot of stress right now, but this woman, Deborah Szekely, has seen something in you that needs to be developed even further. And the very brilliance you mention in her, I think, will make her encourage you even more to eventually work by her side. Remember ALL THINGS ARE POSSIBLE!*

The Surgery

Later that same day, my mind and heart already filled from the conversation with Dale, my very good friend Victor the Yaqui Deer Dancer took me in for my surgery. Before we left the car, I asked him, "Victor, will you do me a favor?"

"Sure, that's what I'm here for," he said cheerfully.

"I want you to kiss me . . . for real. So I can remember what it feels like. I want to have the touch of someone who cares for me on my lips."

We'd always been like brother and sister, but our kiss is one I will always remember.

We entered the clinic, and they took me straight back to prep for surgery. I did not want a general anesthetic, or semi-conscious sedation; we were going with local anesthetic, if possible. I began to place myself into a deep meditative state. While the doctor worked, I felt in two places at once—on the operating table, and in the center of a circle of people, elevated and full of love. The sound of chanting rose and fell through my mind and soul.

The doctor left the room to wait for the frozen section. When he came back, my body tightened up like a drum in the heat. "The margins are far from clear. We need to keep going," he reported.

It took me a while to get back to my "other place." But eventually, I calmed my fears and again heard chanting. The doctor again left to wait for the result. It seemed to take an eternity. Finally, he burst back into the room. This pattern of cutting and waiting repeated at least three times. I could feel the tension building in the surgeon. When he again reentered the room, he said, "I don't know if we should be doing this here. We should be in the hospital in case we have to go deeper. What do you think?"

I was taken aback, totally vulnerable, split open figuratively and literally. *Why is he asking me?* I sat up and felt warm blood running down my neck. The tray tipped over, spilling surgical instruments onto the floor.

It was time to speak my truth. "Look, I'm in no place to decide," I said. "You already have me opened up. Why don't you give it one more try, and if it is positive, we can reschedule and go to the hospital with a new plan?"

"Yeah, that's what we'll do." He turned to the nurse. "Jenny, re-prep her. She just broke sterile field."

I lay there wondering where I got the energy to sit up and speak out, but I was glad it was decided. Somehow I felt good, like everything was going to be alright. All the tension left my body with the last chunk of tissue that left the room. It was gone. I felt and intuited the cancer was gone.

The Power of Distance Healing in Action

As for the chanting that moved through my mind and soul? During the surgery, I also received some major help from 400 miles away. My friends Jozef and Julia, both powerful healers and directors of Sierra Dove Center for Healing in New Mexico, engaged in a concerted long-distance process that tuned into my energetic body and worked with it. At the same time, 150 miles north of Sierra Dove, my name was placed in a powerful healing circle outside Albuquerque during a kirtan (ancient Sanskrit chanting, each seed syllable that is sung resonating with spirit). The group chanted for two hours, then chanted the Sound of Creation, "Aummmm . . . Aummmm . . ." for 10 minutes while focusing specifically on me. The energy and effort spread far beyond myself or my own actions.

After the surgery, Victor drove me home. He stayed with me, and we watched funny movies. My lip was the size of a small banana. I used ice and took Arnica Montana, as well as pantothenic acid and vitamin C, to promote healing. Less than two hours after the first movie, Victor said, "Hey girl, you're getting better already."

I looked at him. *Sure.* "No, really," he insisted. "Look in the mirror."

He was right. My lip was half its previous size.

One week later, I met the surgeon to hear the final pathology report and to have my stitches removed. He was unsure about my prognosis when he discharged me after my surgery, taken aback by the size of the tumor. I waited in the room, this time with none of the sense of dread I had previously experienced. Then I heard the doctor rustling my chart outside the door.

He walked into the room. "Good news! The final pathology was all clear."

I sighed deeply. "Thank God!"

He looked at me, his eyes widening. He adjusted his glasses to be sure he was seeing correctly. "I don't think I've ever seen anyone heal that well and that fast after that much work. I took out a piece of your lip equivalent to the size of my little finger, and there is no visible distortion whatsoever!"

"Yes. You did a great job."

I silently said another prayer of gratitude to God, my beautiful friends and angels that helped me through this so quickly, all the vitamins and herbs and tinctures and potions. Everything. I was so grateful to be healthy again.

I wasn't alone in healing. At that same kirtan in New Mexico, the devotional chanting also focused on two other people. One, a stroke victim, made an amazing recovery, walking again with the aid of a walker, regaining 80 percent of her strength and the use of her left (formerly paralyzed) arm. The others were a father and son long-estranged due to the son's alcoholism. On the following Christmas Eve, the son traveled to the father's Nebraska home and reconciled their relationship. He also quit drinking after a five-year tailspin and brought his life back into alignment.

The common thread in these healings and transformations? Positive, "I can heal" attitudes on the part of the person—and the willingness to open to help from others.

Stop Blaming Yourself

Unfortunately, when we fall ill or are diagnosed with a disease, we tend to judge and blame ourselves. We automatically assume all illness is unnatural and undesirable; sometimes, we feel it's the result of some wrongdoing on *our* part. Even spiritually developed people can fall into this pit. They blame themselves for not having appropriately completed their inner work, thus creating their disease. This type of thinking drains our power and strengthens the grip of the illness. Our soul will use whatever means necessary to enlighten and educate us. The trick is to take back our power by removing the judgment and finding the gift in the illness.

Also, it is the healer's job to remove our self-judgment and help us return to our power.

Illness is not necessarily a bad occurrence, even though it feels that way. It is more often an enormous opportunity to learn and evolve into wisdom. Meet Karen, a 28-year-old who saw me for a symptom complex that involved her reproductive system. Her symptoms included recurrent urinary tract infections, uterine bleeding from fibroids and pain from endometriosis. She had seen many different types of doctors. Most recently, despite her young age, her gynecologist suggested a hysterectomy. I took a Western medical history and reviewed the data she brought from her other physicians. It lined up with the diagnoses. However, when I took her spiritual and emotional history, I learned something more than paper and lab results could explain. "I've had a poor opinion of myself since I was a little girl," Karen admitted.

"What do you mean?" I asked. "That was a long time ago and you were so young. What could you have possibly done to make you so hard on yourself to this day?"

"It's so awful. I don't know if I can talk about it. I've never been able to talk about it."

I looked steadily into her trembling eyes. "You don't have to talk, but I'm here for you if you ever want to."

We worked on her physical symptoms with natural remedies, including cranberry extract, berberine and D-mannose to prevent recurrent urinary tract infections, and natural progesterone cream, chaste tree and cramp bark to reduce her fibroids and pain from endometriosis. After about four months of therapy, she felt physically better and began to trust me.

One day, she confided in me. "I was raped by my brother. I didn't even know what we were doing. I thought it was a game," she said.

No wonder her reproductive system was shutting down; it was the center of the injury to her entire being, depriving her of new life—and the ability to live her own fully.

I reached out and held her tight. "This is not something you chose. It's not fair to judge yourself like that. What if the same thing happened to your best friend and she told you? What would you say?"

She looked up at me, her eyes wide. "I'd say, 'It's not your fault.'"

"Of course you would. Would you like to learn how to let it go? It's ancient history and not serving you anymore."

Since her rape, she'd held a harsh judgment about herself: *I am impure.* "Yes, I would. Very much so."

I guided her through a meditation to remove the traumatic vibration of her brother's act from her auric field. I also recommended the "I Am" meditation (which appears at the bottom of this chapter). She changed her daily mantra to "I Am Pure."

Between this work and the natural medicines, her pain, bleeding and urinary symptoms ceased completely within three months. She took back her power by releasing the judgment she'd laid upon herself, and her body moved back into balance. When I last heard from Karen, she was married with two little girls and was healthy and very happy.

Give Yourself Permission to Heal

What have these stories illustrated? Quite a few things, but above all, we must adopt a positive "I am healthy" attitude when dealing with our health, whether it is good or challenging. That starts before the healing process can even begin. *We must give ourselves permission to heal.*

If we are working with a healer, we must give the healer permission to show us the return path to wholeness. The doctor, or healer, must also respect our state of readiness to release the illness. Even if the healer is convinced she or he has the tools and "know-how" to help the patient, a good outcome is not likely unless we're ready for it. The following words, when spoken aloud, set the stage for healing to occur: "I give myself permission to heal, and I let go of anything that no longer serves me."

While an intern in the Cardiac Care Unit at UCLA, I took care of the 85-year-old mother of famed photographer Richard Avedon. She was admitted for an irregular heart rhythm and congestive heart failure so severe that she required a ventilator to breathe on three different occasions during her hospital stay. After the third time, I removed the tube from her lungs. She told me, "If you put that tube back in my lungs again, I'll die!

Please, I'd rather die than have that tube and be back on that machine. Promise me, Dr. Randall, that you will not let that happen."

"I understand. I promise I won't let that happen."

I told the resident of her request and went downstairs for lunch—my first meal since breakfast the day before. As I stood in line to pay, my beeper went off. The voice on the overhead page announced, "Code Ninety-Nine CCU, Code Ninety-Nine CCU." I ran up five flights of stairs and arrived before the Code Blue team could intubate her.

"Stop!" I said. "No tube!"

"Any better ideas? Her oxygen is falling," the resident snapped back.

"How about a positive pressure mask? Just give it a shot. It's what she wants."

"OK," the resident replied. "Her blood pressure is stable. Respiratory, get an IPPB machine. Stat!"

My patient's oxygen level rose and stabilized, as did her heart rate. She recovered fully and was discharged from the hospital. After a few months of rehab and recovery, she took a trip around the world. She sent me a postcard from every country she visited to remind me how grateful she was that someone listened to her wishes. "Respect is love in plain clothes," said Frank Byrnes, the President of Human Potential Consultants.[11]

How true.

Attitude of Your Support System

People who are ill unknowingly give their power away, not only to their illness, but also to a health-care system that creates dependency by treating every patient the same, not listening to them and not taking enough time to find out what is really going on. As a medical doctor, this distresses me to no end. It is so *wrong* and counterproductive to healing.

But I'm also a healer, so I can do something about it. And I do. As healers, we must return the power to patients by teaching them how to reclaim their own power, which changes their attitude in a way that elevates their health and wellness. I tell my patients, "We (doctors) work for you. Tell me what you need, and I'll help you get there."

Another way in which we relinquish our power, as mentioned earlier, is by projecting lower-vibration attitudes and emotions—anger, fear, resentment, guilt and sorrow. These attitudes produce feelings of weakness, exhaustion and physical depletion. Did you know that six minutes of sustained anger causes a measurable depression in the immune system that can last for up to *six hours*? On the other hand, high-vibration attitudes and emotions such as love, joy and happiness augment the healing process. If we turn six minutes of sustained anger into the same amount of sustained happiness or appreciation, our immunity *improves* for up to six hours! Scientists at the HeartMath Institute have performed studies that have shown this technique effective in reducing work-related stress, improving job satisfaction and work performance, enhancing well-being, and reducing body pain.

This brings me to Perry, a 55-year-old man who suffered from recurrent viral infections, exhaustion and depression. Blood chemistries revealed his cholesterol and triglyceride levels to be dangerously high. He also had borderline diabetes. "Perry, this is not acceptable and could be dangerous," I said. "It's crucial we act quickly."

We got to work by addressing the immediate threat to physical health with medications and dietary change. Normally, I like to control lipids with diet, exercise and herbs, but he was at serious risk for stroke. In this case, I prescribed pharmaceuticals and fish oil to lower his cholesterol and triglyceride levels, and daily aspirin to reduce the risk of stroke. I advised him to refrain from eating animal fats and refined carbohydrates for the diabetes, and suggested he begin a reasonable exercise plan. This protocol restored his blood tests to less dangerous (but still elevated) levels within six weeks. Unfortunately, though, his levels of exhaustion and depression had not improved.

Early on, I learned from Perry's wife that he was an extremely negative person who stayed up every night listening to late-night "shock talk" radio about governmental conspiracies and impending planetary disasters. He carried this negativity throughout his daily activities. Even though he enjoyed financial security and a wonderful marriage, he always saw the cup as half empty, not half full.

I came up with an idea. "Perry, maybe you need a change in scenery. Why don't you and Jenny take some trips away from home?"

Perry agreed, and became a changed man on these trips. He was much more positive, and returned home healthier, happier and more energized. However, when he returned home and relapsed into his old patterns, the negativity, exhaustion and depression returned.

We needed to balance his ingrained negativity at home. After thinking of their strong financial situation, I recommended that Jenny figure out how to get Perry to travel several months a year. They created a good solution: keeping homes in several different parts of the country. This resulted in the feeling of always traveling; consequently, Perry is a healthier, more balanced man.

As this example illustrates, people close to us can participate in creating our health reality as well. In fact, a positive support person is crucial. The support and non-judgment of family and friends are important for reestablishing health and balance. I think of Susan, a woman in her early 50s who came to see me with multiple physical complaints, chest pain and insomnia. We performed a battery of tests, including a chest X-ray, echocardiogram, and stress and blood tests. They did not reveal any threatening heart or lung problems. While relieved, she said, "Dr. Randall, you've got to give me some Dalmane. I can't sleep; I'm too nervous. If I don't have pills, I just drink more, and it's hard on me."

Her comment alerted me. I needed to be careful. "Susan, we have got to find a better way. This is dangerous. I will only give you a few Dalmane and you must stop drinking with them, or I won't give you more."

"Honestly, I don't even want to drink. I don't drink during the day, but only to sleep."

I nodded. "I also want you to go to AA."

She agreed. While listening to her, and reading her facial expressions and body language, I intuited her anxiety resulted from her home life, although the cause was not clear to either of us. Her husband, a seaman, was away for three months or more at a time.

I began by teaching Susan how to meditate. "You know, Susan, meditation has been shown to help combat insomnia and an hour of meditation is equivalent to six hours of sleep," I said, then asked her to come back in three weeks.

When she returned, she had improved remarkably and stopped drinking. She described how much she enjoyed her newfound skills. "When I meditate, I feel so peaceful and all the tension just pours out of my body. I'm not afraid anymore and the people at AA helped me, too," she said, her voice noticeably lighter than our last visit.

When I saw her again two weeks after that, she told me she no longer needed pills to sleep. She was well on her way to full recovery, health and wellness, led by her attitude and newfound meditation practice . . .

Then she hit an obstacle. Three months later, she came into my office looking haggard, 20 pounds lighter than her previous visit. She'd suffered a relapse, a "backslide" as it's known in AA. I asked if she was meditating. "No, because my husband was home and I'm too busy caring for him," she said.

Not a valid excuse. "I'm asking you to give yourself 30 to 40 minutes a day. You can find that time. If you break down, who will be there to care for your husband then?"

What she said next really saddened me: "My husband does not believe in meditation or AA. He says it's all in my head."

Susan completely lost her tool for making her well because of a judgment her husband held about meditation and AA. In giving away her power, she gave away her health and returned to alcohol and sleeping pills. Her situation starkly emphasizes the need for positive support from our family and community in our recovery and for maintaining our balance and positive attitude.

Try the "I Am" Meditation

In working with healing, you may find areas in which your progress is obstructed. For example, you may find that after experiencing an illness, you cannot move beyond it into introspection to bring back your power. Your personal power may still feel low or tapped out. Making a conscious attitude change might not be enough. It requires a deeper solution. Using the "I Am" meditation is one method of moving through this obstruction deeply. Here's how it works:

1. Go to your power spot where you feel safe, comfortable and won't be disturbed.
2. Clear your mind of chatter and all other thoughts.
3. Begin to visualize Your Perfect Self. *Who am I in my most perfect state?* Chant the mantra "I am power, I am whole, I am healed." Continue for 10 to 15 minutes or until you feel complete.
4. Observe any concepts or images coming to you. Send energy to areas of your body that may be in need.
5. Make a note of the images after your meditation is complete. These may help you in reclaiming your personal power.

This same process can be used for any beneficial action to help you improve and strengthen your positive attitude on your healing path—or toward any other high-vibration goal, such as abundance, compassion, strength, patience and wisdom.

CHAPTER 7
The Science of Intuition

"Let us very carefully examine the wisdom of the day and nourish those ideas and inventions whose roots are deep in the soil of harmony. Let us recall that what each of us does will come around the sacred wheel and touch us again. As the pebble in the stream makes many ripples, so does each word and thought we hold in our minds."

—Dhyani Ywahoo, Cherokee Teacher

Why do many Western doctors close off to information that comes from outside the mechanistic, scientific physical realm? Why do they deny our inner wisdom, our intuition? Especially when we have the power to prove its existence within the physical realm with modern technology and tests? Not to mention the right guidance it provides in our health and our lives?

Intuitions are perceptions from beyond the physical senses; they serve our highest and best good. They are innate to who we are, as vital to our walk as our skin and feet and minds. They are the guiding forces of "things not yet seen," whispering silently from our inner wisdom, gifts from the source of all knowledge. We can and should regularly turn to our intuition. Some intuitive messages are soft nudges toward decisions that result in more joy, happiness or clarity, like "gut feelings," "hunches," "sudden inspirations" and "inner guidance." Others are full-fledged warnings we would do well to heed, such as "gut punches" or "bricks on the head." Each piece of information comes to us through a non-logical, more spiritual realm.

An intuition might be a communication to guard the safety of our loved ones or ourselves from a dangerous situation. Or, it could lead us into the right situation at the right time for a life-altering event. Once in a while, if we're not listening, and ignoring inner signals and warnings, our intuition will message us in uncomfortable ways that demand our response.

Sadly, in our busy adult lives, we tend to veer away from listening to our intuition while focusing on everyday concerns. As children, intuition was as firmly wired into our beings as our next breath. However, our social obsession with "just the facts" and "if you can't see it, it doesn't exist"—the physical life—clouded our inner perception as teens and adults, until many of us disconnected. When that happens, we lose our most powerful ally in life. As medical intuitive and author Dr. Caroline Myss wrote in *The Creation of Health*,

> *Intuition is so natural, so ever-present, that it is accepted without question when it comes in the form of a symphony or a great painting; it is, however, often somewhat grudgingly acknowledged by non-intuitives when a great scientific invention or theory is the result of intuition.*[12]

In her book, *Dr. Judith Orloff's Guide to Intuitive Healing*, Dr. Orloff defines intuition as:

> *A potent form of inner wisdom not mediated by the rational mind. Accessible to us all, it's a still, small voice inside—an unflinching truth-teller committed to our well-being. You may experience intuition as a gut feeling, a hunch, a physical sensation, a snapshot-like flash, or a dream. Always a friend, it keeps a vigilant eye on our bodies, letting us know if something is out of sync.*[13]

I practice medicine by using an integrative, intuitive approach. A merger of science *and* spirit greets everyone who walks into my clinic. Science and spirit are not mutually exclusive nor, in the spiritual view, separable. Only creative categorization pulls them apart, which the Cartesian and Newtonian philosophies did to create what we know today as Western medicine. Along those lines, the late Malidoma Patrice Somé, a well-known African shaman, said that computer technology and the internet offer the closest thing to the mind of God of any tangible item on our planet. Problem is, some treat the internet *as* God. Joseph Rael explained to me that, in honoring technology, we have become so wrapped up in the material aspect that we lost our sense of spirit and connection to our earth and our soul. Within the technology, however, is precisely the gift that can return us to the infinite vastness (the Great Spirit).

Men and women of spirit understand that science is part of the answer. Why can't they also understand that *spirit* is part of it, too? Every spoke in the wheel is of equal importance (physical, emotional, mental, spiritual). If one spoke is missing, there is imbalance. Without that balance, our intuition can also become cloudy and the guidance we receive off-kilter.

The greatest advice I can give you as a medical and soul doctor is to reconnect with your inner wisdom. *Now.* When we listen to our inner wisdom, we gain information to heal ourselves, and make it possible for those who follow us to do the same. Joseph Rael also taught me that if we do something new on the planet, we make it possible for all who follow us to have that gift. Spontaneous healing and cures for terminal illness have occurred as a result of remembering the wisdom of the body, seeing it for what it is and *acting upon the guidance.*

There are no limits to what we may discover when we connect with our inner wisdom. People have actually spun new threads on a DNA spiral within one lifetime. We've come up with miraculous treatments for cancer and HIV, which leads to AIDS; the death rate from the once impregnable HIV virus has been sharply reduced since it first appeared in the early 80s. In 1990, the death rate was nearly 100 percent, according to the Centers for Disease Control and Prevention.[14] In 2020, according to UNAIDS, the death rate was less than 6 percent of all HIV cases worldwide.[15] Likewise, many of the tech toys, most memorable books and songs, great inventions and causes of our time began with a hunch, a dream or a vision—all forms of intuition.

Intuitive Medicine and Inner Wisdom

How far back does this "new" practice of intuitive medicine go? The Greek physician Hippocrates, considered the founder of Western medicine, learned about intuitive medicine from Eastern practitioners. Healers of all stripes have practiced with the knowledge of their training and counsel of their inner wisdom for thousands of years. In fact, medicine used to be a primarily intuitive art. However, most modern Western scientists have closed themselves off from intangible sources of information because they do not comply with the current requirements for scientific proof (data from randomized double-blind studies).

Not until the breakthrough work of Dr. Norman Shealy and Dr. Caroline Myss in the 1990s did intuitive diagnosis in the Western world rise above crystal ball reading status. There is still a long journey ahead of us, but pioneers like Gladys McGarey, Dr. Shealy, Dr. Myss, Dr. Larry Dossey, Dr. Judith Orloff and Dr. Valerie Hunt have opened the doors and affirmed our right to use intuition as a tool on our path of healing—as doctors, patients and in our healing of self. For my part, I taught intuitive medicine as a UCLA Medical School professor in the 1980s and 1990s, one of the first physician-teachers in the US to educate medical students on how intuition is useful to their practices.

Dr. Orloff makes a comment in her guide to intuitive healing that speaks to both the awesomeness and subtlety of our intuitive power:

> *We all possess within us an intuitive healing code that contains the blueprints for health and happiness, and for the survival of everything that is good here on earth. This code is written in the language of silence, metaphor, imagery, energy, and [a] knowing that may seem alien until we are taught to decipher it.*[16]

We need to learn to decode the metaphors that our body and the planet utilize to communicate with us via signs or symptoms, or how our soul speaks to us through intuition and dreams. If this seems distant, unattainable or just "out there," consider how one of the greatest pieces of music, Handel's *Messiah*, evolved. Handel received a few notes in a dream. That lit his mind afire. He locked himself in his room, ignored all meals sent up to him and wrote the draft of his timeless masterpiece in *three days*. Three weeks later, he was finished with the final version. Less than a month! He listened to the metaphors his body that spoke to him, acted in *complete trust* and blessed the planet with what moved through him.

Two of rock music's greatest and most romantic ballads ever, the Moody Blues' "Nights in White Satin" and Jefferson Starship's "Miracles," were written in much the same way. Feeling great adoration for all women while between relationships, 20-year-old Justin Hayward sat down—and out poured "Nights" in an hour. A few years later in southern India, Jefferson Starship's Marty Balin finished a devotional sitting with famed guru Satya Sai Baba, felt his girlfriend's energy pour through his heart and scribbled the lyrics to "Miracles" in 30 minutes on a yellow legal pad. Each ballad was among the 25 most-played radio rock tunes of the 20th century. A half-century later, they still pop up regularly on classic rock stations. They are timeless, universal songs—what happens when intuition is given a voice.

This unseen communication helps to govern our health and balance. We learn to be aware that these things are occurring, and then we begin to understand what the metaphors mean.

We're still reawakening to doctors and scientists recognizing the validity of intuitive diagnosis (though its practice is slowly increasing). I maintain that medicine can be scientific while allowing the artful, spiritual and magical aspects of its true nature to be expressed and utilized in a beneficial way.

Why so much controversy and problem accepting the value of intuitive diagnosis? And intuition itself? Why would we turn our backs on our inner guidance, one of the most powerful guiding lights and forces we carry as humans? In the most general sense, scientists make observations about the phenomenal world. They find patterns to help make predictions for greater control over these natural phenomena, generating knowledge to seemingly direct the powers of the natural world. This comforts our society because it counteracts the fear of the unknown, which troubles us most. It is useful for doctors to align themselves with science, because of the treatment and healing benefits that instruments, technology and scientific findings bring—along with our widespread belief in the power of technology.

Descartes, Newton and the Start of Western Medicine

Let's return to the history of medicine. Medicine evolved by bringing intuition and scientific treatment together to help treat ailing men and women. Consider these three statements: "In nothing do men nearly approach the gods, than in giving health to other men"; "A doctor is consolation for the spirit"; "Conscientious and careful physicians allocate causes of disease to natural laws or disturbances of the inside man, disconnected from Nature." All came from the Greek philosopher Aristotle some 2,500 years ago.

In the 16th century following the Renaissance, the emergence of science created a gap in this science-intuition unity. The thinking minds and doctors of the day began separating the two. There was no place for spiritualism in the theories of French mathematician René Descartes (1596–1650), who separated mind and matter as independently functioning entities. Descartes summed up his idealistic philosophy, Cartesianism, by the words *cogito, ergo sum* (I think, therefore I am). His philosophy of dualism became the basis of scientific and medical theories accepting the separation of mind and body; the world has not been the same since.

Sir Isaac Newton's theories also sought to demystify much of the observable world. They increased the power of Western science and helped influence the separation of modern medicine from the mysteries of the universe. Newton invented a scientific method that became universal in scope, a set of four rules for scientific reasoning, stated in the *Principia*:

1. We are to admit no more causes of natural things such as are both true and sufficient to explain their appearances;
2. The same natural effects must be assigned to the same causes;

3. Qualities of bodies are to be esteemed as universal; and
4. Propositions deduced from observation of phenomena should be viewed as accurate until other phenomena contradict them.

While these concise rules for investigation were revolutionary, this "cause and effect" method virtually eliminated the contribution from mysteries of the unseen or intangible world. Independent emotions or thoughts cannot exist under these rules. Nor can feelings. This analytic method far exceeded the more philosophical and less scientifically rigorous approaches of Aristotle and Aquinas. Newton used his rules to refine Galileo's experimental method, creating the compositional method of experimentation still practiced today.

Newton gifted us with a great legacy for scientific development, but he dealt a serious blow to the use of spirit and holism in medicine. Perhaps this was a sacred, necessary journey, leading us down the path of scientific knowledge and tools in order to return us to the whole-person approach, which we've finally begun to see in the last three decades with integrative and functional medicine.

Let's fast-forward four centuries. Western medicine has subdivided into multiple myopic specialties (the cardiologist for heart problems, the nephrologist for kidney problems, the gastroenterologist for stomach problems, the neurologist for brain and neurological disorders, and so on). It is not uncommon to see pharmaceuticals adversely interact with each other, sometimes fatally, in people prescribed so many different medications for their different body parts. Diseases caused by medicine or the medical system, known as iatrogenic diseases, are a frequent cause of ICU hospital admissions today. The current model of medical specialization by design leads physician specialists to ignore the whole person, the whole physiology—not to mention the patient's emotional, psychological or spiritual condition. In today's sprawls of medical offices, clinics and hospitals, it is saddest to realize few doctors are truly looking after the whole person. Often, one specialist does not know what the other is doing.

Now it's time to reconsider the spiritual and return balance to our medicine, ourselves and our planet.

Physicians and healers of all types need to develop sound practical and technical skills and master specific healing and diagnostic techniques. In *The Creation of Health*, Caroline Myss writes:

> *Traditional medicine and holistic health represent more than just two different approaches to healing disease. They illustrate two essentially different paradigms of reality.*[17]

I agree with her in one sense, but I would submit that, no matter the technology, mastery always includes a certain intuitive process that separates the true master from the skilled clinician. I also suggest the birth of a third paradigm that encompasses its two predecessors—traditional medicine and holistic health. This includes and recognizes intuition, as well as knowledge and technical skill.

In my years as an endoscopic surgeon and teacher, I noticed certain students were naturally sensitive to the differences between patients and their anatomies. Those students showed a real talent for diagnosing problems, performing endoscopic procedures, and communicating and connecting with their patients. This same quality can be applied to the sensitivity we feel for the energy fields of a person or the flow of energy in our own bodies. Beyond recognizing that these energy fields exist, true healers become aware of the precise nature of energy flow in their own bodies. Healers then begin to sense themselves as radiant beings capable of giving and receiving the healing light of unconditional love.

At the same time, people are awakening to the assistance continually available to us from beyond our sensory level of awareness. While most people still work primarily through their physical senses, millions now meditate, visualize, pray or otherwise tune into their inner guidance, viewing life from the "inside out," the flow of the power that creates, manifests and heals. The flow of optimal health.

Merging with Patients' Energies

In the 1980s, I had the great fortune to work with Valerie Hunt, a professor of psychological sciences at UCLA and the founding mother of intuitive and vibrational sciences. I assisted her in measuring the energies of healers as they merged with the energies of their patients. She was probably the first to electrophysiologically measure peoples' energies and chakras. In her book *Infinite Mind: Science of the Human Vibrations of Consciousness*, she describes how we all have intuitive ability and a vibration.[18] I always say it's like a muscle you haven't used before and have to build it up. Once it gets strong, so will your intuition. As doctors, we can follow our intuition, conduct a test on a patient and measure if our intuition was correct. The vast majority of the time, it is.

One morning, I welcomed to my clinic Kathryn, a 57-year-old counseling psychologist who experienced abdominal pain for 15 years due to recurrent acute pancreatitis. Ten years prior to our first visit, she underwent a surgical procedure to drain her pancreas and alleviate the problem.

Although she had once been able to control her symptoms with extreme dietary restriction, nutrient therapy and enzyme replacement, her symptoms had progressed beyond control. On her third visit to my office, she exclaimed, "I need an intuitive body detective; I can't take it anymore!"

What a significant and passionate statement, considering it came from a very quiet, even-tempered person. Through it, Kathryn gave me permission to look into her energetic field, opening herself completely to me on every level. I closed my eyes and asked for an answer; it was given to me in a split second. I informed her of the visual I received: "I see an image of your pancreas struggling to empty its secretions through a narrowed passage. I know this sounds odd, but I also see many distraught human faces in your pancreas."

Specifically, I intuited that she, as a psychologist, was absorbing the troubled awareness of her clients, and not allowing it to pass out of her body. "Kathryn, I don't know how to ask you this any other way but directly," I said. "Are you taking on the suffering for your clients?"

Kathryn was herself intuitive, an empath. My question moved right into her eyes. "Letting go of *their* pain has been my challenge in working with clients for a long time," she said. "I'm so used to it, I don't think anything of it. But I believe you pegged it . . . what can we do?"

We agreed that a Western medical solution needed to be complemented with some sort of energy work. "You know the success of this therapy is riding on your willingness to empty yourself of pain that does not belong to you," I said.

"Yes, I'm ready. I should have done it a long time ago. I just didn't realize . . ."

I stopped her in mid-sentence. "It's important not to take this in the form of guilt. Just learn to let it go. The time is now and that's perfect. We'll work on the techniques to keep it from building up in you again."

"OK," she agreed.

We scheduled Kathryn for an ERCP (endoscopic retrograde cholangio-pancreaticogram) and sphincterotomy. This procedure is used to image the pancreatic drainage tubes (ducts) and create a larger opening to empty into the bowel, in order to relieve the scarred and abnormally narrowed area. Kathryn had undergone numerous ERCPs in the past, but each time, the injection of dye into her ducts caused a severe episode of pancreatitis (inflammation of the pancreas), resulting in worsened pain and prolonged hospitalization. I thought the combination of this chronic process and scarring from a previous surgery narrowed the passage of her pancreas drainage. The UCLA doctor who performed her procedure is also a proponent of integrative medicine; she practices traditional Chinese medicine and acupuncture as well. Her Western medical management was complemented with Eastern, energy and spiritual medicine.

The night before the procedure, I performed a combination of color and pranic healing (a powerful technique through which universal energy passes to specific areas that need healing). We also performed acupuncture and prayer to strengthen her Chi and help prevent damage suffered from her previous procedures.

This time, the procedure succeeded. Unlike her previous surgeries, she showed no signs of complications or pancreatitis afterward. On the following day, when her second set of laboratory studies showed everything was OK, she was released.

After she recovered, we celebrated! We designed a guided meditation to allow the energy of her patients to pass through her without her absorbing any of their suffering. I reminded Kathryn of the Buddhist approach: "Breathe in suffering, breathe out compassion." I also taught her simple energy clearing techniques like sage smoke, a salt lamp in her office and sea salt baths. All have the potential to clear attachments and negative energy. Most importantly, I reminded her to always hold the intention and willingness to release the negative energy and allow it to pass through her.

Within two weeks of her integrative treatment, Kathryn was eating caviar. She'd dreamt about caviar for years, but could not eat it because of the delicate nature of her pancreas, in particular its inability to tolerate fat. Eating caviar was her one-time celebration of a healthier life moving into the future.

Today, Kathryn knows that the power of intuitive diagnosis and the combination of medicines from seemingly different paradigms made her pain-free for the first time in 10 years. When she feels tension building inside, she knows her body and intuition are giving her messages to release the suffering and cleanse her energy before it manifests in her physical body as disease. She remains disease-free to this day.

Become Your Own Intuitive Healer

We can participate fully in our own healing by listening to our intuition. In order to hear what our souls are trying to communicate to us, we need to learn to quiet the mind and to trust the information we are being given. This is not to say that we should forego formal medical evaluation or treatments. It is, however, a wonderful technique for learning to listen to our own bodies and tune into what they need, which can be used as an adjunct to traditional methods.

There is constant communication between our souls and higher minds. This communication from spirit transmits through our soul, the bridge between spirit, mind and body. Our awareness of this information flow depends on our focus level and practices to remove obstructions from the soul. For example, doubt or lack of trust, and interference from external energies, obstruct the energy flow of intuition.

How do you gain greater access to intuition? First, accept that it exists. Then open yourself to revealing it. Become receptive to a greater sense of awareness. It may come as a body sensation, an emotional or "gut" feeling, or a dream. Once you accept the flow of intuition and receive it, you need to trust it. "Don't think so much," Joseph Rael says. Open yourself to the content of the information. Do not try and control the flow. If you think too much about it, you will cut it off or end the transmission. Just allow and accept it, however unusual it may seem.

After years of practice, you might find what I do: intuitive flow comes innately, part of my natural thought process, integrating as it flows.

Once you become proficient at these steps of acceptance, receptivity, awareness and trust, you are ready to engage in the intuitive process. Dr. Orloff offers a five-step framework:

1. Notice your beliefs
2. Be in your body
3. Sense your body's subtle energy
4. Ask for inner guidance
5. Listen to your dreams

As a doctor-healer, I might add, do check it out! See an expert; do a test. Verify it. Most of all, stay open and listen. I always "get the mail" when I'm in the shower. I suppose when my mind isn't tightly focused on a problem at hand it is more open to receive. Dreams and meditation are other times we are more open to receive.

CHAPTER 8
Shift Happens

"When humans participate in a ceremony, they enter a sacred space. Everything outside of that space shrivels in importance. Time takes on a different dimension. Emotions flow more freely. The bodies of the participants become filled with the energy of life, and this energy reaches out and blesses the creation around them. All is made new; everything becomes sacred."

—Sun Bear[19]

The role of the healer is to shed a different light or perspective on a problem or illness facing the client. By changing our perspective, our relationship to an illness or disease changes as well. This change in consciousness allows the opportunity for wholeness and well-being to return to our bodies, minds and souls.

Such a transformative shift happened for Melanie, changing her life forever. When she was 49, Melanie came to me in a major depression, requiring antidepressant therapy to function. Eventually, even that stopped working; her depression deepened, taking her energy lower and darkening her moods, thoughts and state of mind. She was scared to death. The root of it? A sincere and unfulfilled desire to have a meaningful lifelong relationship. Although married for a short time earlier, Melanie had spent most of her adult life single.

Melanie had known and trusted me as a friend and healer for a long time prior to her visit. She promptly requested a ritual. "Are you convinced that finding a partner in life is what you want?" I asked.

"Yes!" she replied without hesitation.

"Are you ready to let go of the old emotional attachments holding you back, even if it's hard and doesn't make sense—and even it if doesn't turn out like what you expected?"

"Yes, I'm ready, and I release all expectations."

Melanie's power spot lay under a huge mother oak tree near a stream in the Santa Monica Mountains. We headed there to perform her ceremony.

We set a sacred space, using smooth river stones we gathered from a nearby stream to build a medicine circle. We cleansed the inside of the circle and stones with sage smoke and used sweetgrass to encourage the entry of sweet things into Melanie's life. After we placed the stones and set the circle in a clockwise fashion, we sang them awake and danced in a counterclockwise direction, the feminine direction. I waved the night eagle (owl) feather over Melanie and around the circle of stones, and a sweet breeze caressed us with a tangible opening of the energy vortex. The energy whirled around us, assisted by humming from the stone beings, the swaying mother oak and other forces of nature.

Melanie lay in the newly created medicine wheel with her head pointing south toward the emotional plane, where her healing needed to take place. The stones she chose for this healing glistened and vibrated in the light of the setting sun. She declared her readiness to let go of her old emotional attachments and blocks and make space for her partner to step forward and join her in a new life together.

We prayed and sang until the sun went down. I began to sing a beautiful Lakota song to the first star in the heavens . . .

> *Oh la wah luaho luaho luaho . . .*
> *Oh la wah luaho luaho luaho . . .*
> *Oh la wah luaho luaho luaho . . .*
> *Oh la wah luaho luaho luaho . . .*

Just then, the Hale–Bopp Comet flaunted its glorious tail over the mountain tops. A lone coyote came out of the forest and sat just outside the south portal of the medicine wheel, only about 15 feet from Melanie's head. As I sang to the tailed star, the coyote guardian, totem of the south, joined me in high, harmonic howls. When the song was finished, she stopped singing and returned to the southern brush. It was a moving and enchanting omen for Melanie's recovery and realization of her prayers.

During the course of the next year, Melanie lost her beloved home of six years on a horse ranch and changed her profession. At first, this was sad and devastating. "Remember, you promised to let go of the old in order to open up to the new," I reminded her. "You don't know what the Universe has in store for you. I know it's hard, but trust spirit. You asked and the signs are strong."

Sure enough, shortly after her move, she met the man of her dreams. He was the widower of one of our dream sisters, who had died suddenly from a respiratory illness. They fell rapidly and passionately in love, and within months, she was very happily married to the man for whom she prayed during our ceremony under the comet-lit sky, accompanied by the song of the coyote.

Shifting Consciousness and Changing Perspective

Throughout the centuries, shamanic healers have used various techniques to shift consciousness in order to heal themselves and others. Changing perspective is a simple and central form of this healing. That's also the case for neuro-linguistic programming (NLP), developed in the mid-70s by John Grinder, a professor at UC Santa Cruz, and Richard Bandler, a graduate student. NLP is a set of models of how subjective experiences impact communication—and vice-versa.

NLP uses a technique called "reframing" to shift consciousness and effect beneficial change in behavior. It is an elemental part of shamanism, perhaps more acceptable for some because of the modern scientific name assigned to it. Referring to it as "NLP" is reframing, too. Consider a person who says, "I'm afraid I have cancer." If that person can shift, or reframe, their perspective to state, "I have something out of balance," then they have affected a positive shift in their energy. Love and healing can now take hold. Anything that can be used to create a radical discontinuity in the way an unwell person's reality is assembled, without causing harm, opens an opportunity to restore balance between the physical, emotional, mental and spiritual bodies. This ultimately results in healing of the immediate disease and forges a big step toward greater health.

Shift can also happen when people feel blocked from moving from allopathic to holistic medical care. They may be fearful if they have no experience with this type of medicine. The most common thing I hear is, "My insurance won't pay for it." However, it is interesting how much their willingness increases when they become very ill and/or desperate. There are also those who learned of me from others, or patients who wanted to experience the extra measure of healing. With my practice, they feel safer because I am a highly trained allopathic physician who has a foot in both worlds. Once they experience the gentle touch of holism, they can mentally make that shift while being further educated through their own experience and success. More recently, people come to me because they want the holistic approach. That is very refreshing as it means it is spreading and taking hold in our medical system, even without third-party carrier support. Although there are institutions like Mimi Guarneri's Pacific Pearl in San

Diego and others, I see the majority of future medicine covering all kinds of holistic medicine and a time where it is commonplace for us all to work together. That is the real power of medicine at its best.

When you're looking at your own mortality, and want to keep on living, then shifts can and often do happen quickly. I'm reminded of a friend whose mother, a lifelong smoker, was diagnosed with metastatic lung cancer that first appeared in her lower spine. A 67-year-old former nursing school student and firm adherent to allopathic medicine, she was initially given six months to live. She did a round of chemo, but also turned to my friend and said, "Call everyone you know about all these different types of healing you're into; I want to look into it."

She was not done living. The terminal diagnosis shifted her perspective suddenly and quickly—and so did her decision to consider other treatment options. Soon, she was visualizing trips abroad, receiving pranic healing, taking a few supplements, exercising when she could and receiving healing prayers from a 3,000-member prayer group. Close to "D-Day," the six-month mark following her diagnosis, she got the golden "you're in remission" call from her oncologist while spending a week in the Holy Land with her cousin, a nun.

After two years of traveling extensively, her cancer returned and assaulted her vital organs; she knew what that meant. Her time on earth was coming to a close. She went to her oncologist, who recommended a month of bed rest followed by a round of intense chemo. Her response? "In a month, I'll be taking a cruise down the Danube River." Off she went to Central Europe. She lived five more months before slipping into a coma on Easter Sunday, a most auspicious day for any devout Catholic. She passed a couple hours after midnight.

Her goodbye present to the world, besides all the love she poured into it? When the hundreds who attended her celebration of life service filed out, the first thing they saw was a poster of her, smiling while sitting atop a camel in Egypt. What a send-off!

How do we shift our perspectives? Are there activities or steps we can take to shift our consciousness and train it on what ails us?

It begins with creating an altered focus of attention. One method is through ritual or ceremony. This moves us out of the personal realm and into the transpersonal realm, which is where consciousness transforms. We begin by establishing a sacred space, removed from ordinary reality, which generates an energy that opens the window of opportunity for change. In days of old, our ancestors would go to a place of power atop a mountain or high desert mesa, near a river, to the ocean's edge, or within a forest. Today, our busy culture and vast property development has cut us off from many of those sacred spots. Even so, we can still create that sacredness within our own spaces and ourselves, the sacredness that feeds and blesses our shifting, changing perspectives. As Joseph Campbell once said, "Your sacred space is where you can find yourself again and again."[20]

Simply put, I ask my patients to look through the other end of the binoculars, to change their focus from fear-based to love-based. This way, we can find the gift, the metaphor of the illness. Metaphor allows us to transcend out of our present state, and release the physical, emotional, mental and/or spiritual grip a disease might hold on us.

Setting the Sacred Space

In the first year of my studies with Joseph Rael, he gifted me with an eagle feather. He intuitively knew I wanted an eagle feather to use in my healing. He gave me the feather after a ceremony in the kiva. It was wrapped in a red cloth, customary for sacred items. His mate beaded the stem in swirling iridescent blue beads. They stood together and handed it to me. I was thrilled. "Thank you," I said. "It is beautiful."

"You earned it," he said. Oh, how my heart soared. I was so proud. "You already use the powers and the eagle energy in your work. You may not know it, but you do." (I did know—but I sure loved hearing this from him!)

We built a fire for the sweat lodge. Joseph generally teaches through experience, but he made an exception in this case. After admiring my ability to build a sweat lodge fire, he turned and looked at me through the smoke billowing between us. "Why does it seem like you've been doing this all of your life?" he asked. When I didn't answer—not that he expected one—he continued. "You know, I used to have all that stuff. I had all kinds of paraphernalia to make medicine with, rattles and feathers and stuff, because people kind of expect it. But what I found out is, all you *really* need to make powerful medicine is your birthday suit. But this feather will come to mean more to you in the future. Maybe in four, maybe eight or twelve years from now."

Joseph taught me later that four was the universal number that represented completion. Four is the number of Sundances one must commit to in order to join the dance. Four is the number of sacred directions in the medicine wheel. Four is also the number of cardinal directions on the compass. It holds immense spiritual and symbolic meaning in other practices, too. For instance, the spiritual yogi goes through four stages of life, divided into 24-year segments—*brahmacharya* (student), householder, forest dweller, *Sannyasin* (renunciant).

I had to wait many years to begin to understand the meaning of the eagle feather. As those years passed, it came to symbolize much more.

What Joseph was saying is that we only really need the pure healing power of intent and belief, unburdened by the paraphernalia of shamanism. We can create a sacred space anywhere, anytime, with focused positive intent. That intent changes perspective. The shift in perspective also shifts consciousness away from fear and obstacles to our healing, which in turn creates the portal for returning to wholeness. Even deeper, Joseph was saying we need to get out of our own way to allow the healing to happen. It's really the power of the Great Mystery acting through us that makes us potent, effective healers. We create an environment and energy in which our clients can find their true self and heal. It's when we become too proud and accomplished that we think *we* are in charge and become ineffective. We are only the channels and the guides.

Collective Shift

Shift also happens collectively. The consciousness of each individual is connected to the collective. Although we heal ourselves as individuals, we are also part of the whole and the planet. If we heal ourselves, we make it possible for all those coming after us to receive that gift. By doing so, we shift the consciousness of the entire planet. When a critical mass is achieved, the planet will heal. Joseph says the war gods will retire, because there will be no need for them. Instantly, people will become more aware. Healing ourselves will heal the planet.

We are being called more and more to this collective healing right now, though it may not seem like it with the social hostility being acted out on a daily basis. Don't be discouraged or distracted by this "dance of Maya (illusion)." In deeper truth, we are well on our journey back to balance and Oneness. The earth is calling for us to heal ourselves and to aid in her healing. We've seen an example of how quickly she can heal, through the many restorative things that have happened during the coronavirus pandemic. Deep down, climate change is a plaintive cry by Earth Mother to restore our balance with nature, with all living creatures, with ourselves. This just happens to be a "darkest before the dawn" moment through which we're passing.

How can we project beneficial outcomes into our future using collective consciousness? One method is to simply "pay it forward." Many may not think of this as pure intent, but it is probably one of the most powerful personal actions we can take. First we "clean our own house," our personal temple, our body. Once we clean our own house and clear the baggage obstructing our accurate sight, our awareness increases. We see outside our issues and ourselves. Our consciousness rises to a higher level. We begin to view ourselves as part of a community, humanity or whole. What will make this easier is to realize we will not all agree and that is ok. What we need is to respect each other's diversity and know we are all in this together. We are all human no matter our color, creed, gender, age or ethnicity.

Taking care of our personal health is more than a societal trend. Health consciousness is now a permanent part of our culture, even if not everyone currently embraces it. This shift in basic human priorities has become a solid societal value capable of changing and transforming community. We are now rapidly awakening to the application of these same balancing holistic methods for healing our community, environment, and most importantly, our planet. Our Mother Earth!

Many have called the 21st century the "New Age." With this comes expectation for change and transition. Certainly, we have seen our share of upheaval and transition in the first 20 years of the century—9/11, the wars in Afghanistan and Iraq, countless school shootings and terrorist attacks, social division in the United States and Europe, the onset of catastrophic climate change, and the coronavirus pandemic, which virtually paralyzed the planet. We may not be done with pandemics, either; the coronavirus pandemic was the third in this century alone. Imagine being a graduating high school senior in 2020; you came into the world just before or after 9/11, and you began your journey into adult life (and, for many, your graduation ceremony) under the social distance mandates.

It's been a tough start to the 21st century. You might think it impossible to expect a large number of individuals to suddenly wake up, change their lifestyles and act responsibly toward the greater continuum of life. We have seemingly insurmountable problems facing us—COVID-19, AIDS, starvation, wars over resources like water, profound ecological imbalances and toxicities, all caused by humans. However, I submit that this New Age is not only a time of tremendous challenge, but also of equal opportunity to bring a greater balance to our earth than we have known. That is what you see when shift happens.

Anytime the scales of the planet or universe are tipped in a direction, *universal law* attempts to restore balance. Awakening is exactly what is occurring all around us. Vast numbers of humans all over the world *are* coming together to meet these challenges through organizations and groups like the World Wildlife Foundation, Bioneers, 4ocean, 350.org, Environmental Working Group (EWG), Amazon Conservation Team, 8 Billion Trees, Leonardo DiCaprio Foundation, Rainforest Action Network, Aid for Africa, Greenpeace, The Great Green Wall and many others. Many dozens of the world's top corporations belong to Sustainable Brands, a group that promotes and shares sustainable business practices, renewing resources and protecting the planet. Back home, many keep the earth's needs sacred by recycling, installing energy-saving devices in their homes, living lives of low carbon footprints, choosing animal-free or regenerative diets, and honoring the earth in prayer and ceremony.

As each person awakens to a greater personal responsibility, they become another voice for peace and balance on the planet. When they become personally healthy, they become conscious of the community and global issues around them. This occurs even if those voices never speak out publicly.

This is the notion of collective consciousness. Just like the spoken and unspoken voices of the mothers and supporters of this country who brought home their sons from Vietnam, we hold the power to restore wholeness and balance on earth. Our planet is a living, breathing being and has always been here to support and nourish us. She is our Mother Earth. Now it is time to return to her some of the energy she has given us through concrete initiatives, beneficial intent, prayer and ceremony. "When we join groups to save the whales, the ocean or the planet—it is because those things are really sacred emanations of us," Joseph Rael told me. "When the earth and the plants and animals and things suffer—we manifest that suffering in our bodies."

Making the Shift

I have seen and experienced many instances of this unity between all things in my years as a physician-healer.

Harold's experience speaks to both unity and the lasting value of creating a sacred space. When he walked into my clinic to see me for kidney pain, a thorough Western medical evaluation (blood count, blood analysis of kidney function, urinalysis) didn't determine the cause. It worsened to the point that he could not sleep, and he worried that something was seriously wrong. "What's going on with work, Harold?" I asked.

"You know, the usual stuff for a guy my age. I'm nearly sixty-four and in the process of retiring. Tomorrow, I'm supposed to finish cleaning out my office and sell my law practice."

"Wow, that's big."

"Not really, I've been working toward this for a while."

"What is happening on the home front?" I asked.

His tone softened. "Well, my wife's mother is dying."

"Yes. I'm sorry."

"I've been trying to support her through this and it's really been hard," Harold said, his voice shaking.

We agreed to administer a CAT scan of Harold's kidneys and abdomen, along with some blood and urine tests to assure that nothing dangerous was developing. If the tests came back clear, he requested the next step was to return for a ceremonial healing.

Harold's tests were negative. Soon, we set the sacred space in my Malibu office and its 180-degree view of the ocean, which it overlooked. We met for the ceremony just before sunset. Sunset and sunrise are powerful times for ceremony, since they are periods of great energy transition and transformation. The veils of ordinary reality are thinner at these transition times.

First, we cleansed the room with sage, which purifies the air—and the energy. I placed Harold on a massage table in the center of the room, with his head pointed to the west for physical healing. I ignited white candles for each cardinal direction as I gave thanks, and called in the energies of the medicine wheel for his healing. We spoke prayers of gratitude to the Creator and to all the sacred directions, and called in the energies. Our prayers started in the east and moved clockwise. We gave thanks and evoked the energies from each direction. Kristie, my assistant, and I chanted healing songs and created a sacred space of loving support, within which Harold's healing could occur.

The energy began to build in the room as the sun set. The candles flickered and crackled in the clockwise (masculine) direction of spinning energy. After many minutes, Harold moved his arms and his legs in a swimming motion. I thought I saw the candles reflecting in water all around him. Harold began to breathe hard and struggle against some unseen force. I glanced up at Kristie; her eyes grew large and round. I indicated for her to stand at his feet (in the east) as I held position in the west (at his head) to maintain the sacred space. We held the energy of the circle as he pushed against some heavy force, his brow furled, sweat rolling down his temples. I felt the concern in Kristie and raised my hand in assurance.

Harold needed to complete his task. He groaned and pressed against the table with great force for what seemed a very long time. I had to stop myself from touching him as I returned to holding the space in support of his struggle.

Suddenly, he relaxed. "Ahhh," he sighed out loud.

A copper-colored new moon hung high in the sky over the Pacific Ocean. Kristie and I sang several verses of a sweet Tiwa moon song Joseph Rael had given me. The moon chant honors the feminine, reflective aspects of the Grandmother Moon. As if dipped in honey, the moon changed the whole energy around us, creating a yellow-orange glow. I moved through the experience as much as Harold did.

The energy turned sweet and reversed into a counterclockwise (feminine) spiral. Harold fell into a deep, tranquil sleep. We didn't wake him until the moon had disappeared into the horizon of the Pacific Ocean.

At first, Harold was a little disoriented and groggy. "Wow!" he said, attempting to smooth his hair unsuccessfully.

"Here," I whispered, "just drink some water first."

He sat up with a big grin, looking out over the ocean for a long time. Then he turned to me. "May I share my vision with you? It was a good one."

"Of course."

"At first I was floating in the water all alone. I saw beautiful rainbow-colored fish and sea animals—so rich and full of life," Harold began, capturing the detail of his vision. "Then I saw things in the ocean that did not belong there—plastics, pollutants and debris I knew were poisoning my children. They choked and upset me. I realized I was a huge old green turtle swimming in the sea and that *I* was responsible for carrying the Mother Earth on my back. I was swimming toward the land, and every time I began to gain my footing on shore, I kept slipping in the sand. I pushed and clawed at the land and pushed and fought until I feared I would succumb to exhaustion.

"Eventually, bit-by-bit, I pushed partway on to the beach, completely spent. As I lay on the beach under the moon, the earth dissolved from my back, giving me more and more land to stand on. Once on land, unburdened by carrying the entire world on my back, my back pain disappeared!" Harold looked happy. "What do think of that, Doc?"

"Wow! How do you feel now, Harold?" I asked.

"Fabulous," he said. "No pain at all! Never better."

"What does it mean to you?"

"I think this retirement thing is bigger than I was willing to admit. I was trying to be such a macho man. I get it. I can't carry the entire world. I know that now. Also I know that I need to clean up my act and get my body clean. I've not been as good about my diet and exercise as I need to be. There is something else interesting about this. What is the meaning of the turtle?"

"The turtle is symbolic for the Mother Earth," I explained. "Some American Indian creation stories tell of Grandmother Turtle bringing in the earth on her back, like your vision, Harold. Very powerful stuff! You are being asked to re-create yourself in just the way you said. Honor the temple of your soul by getting back on your organic diet, exercise program and spiritual practice.

"You are also a reflection of what we all need to do right now as a collective—heal our Mother Earth first by cleaning up our act, and then cleaning up our planet. To clean up our planet and your energy has created the opening we need right now to save our earth!"

"Is there something more the turtle or Mother Earth is trying to tell me?" he asked.

"Turtle speaks of caution in new situations and of being patient in reaching our goals," I explained. "She also tells us to take things slow, to give us time to figure out if we need to protect ourselves or move ahead. Sometimes, the turtle comes to us when we need to go within (into our shell) and wait for our ideas to incubate. She could also be telling you to pay attention to your dreams, or your vision, in this case. The turtle is a potent dreamer. I agree there is more, but a vision like this comes once in a lifetime and continues to reveal itself for years. Do as you have been guided and clean up your diet, exercise and admit where you need support, so we can help you. The other messages will reveal themselves to you when you are ready. You have changed the path for all of us. This is powerful."

Approximately a year later, Harold and his wife, Francine, became the cornerstones for the Chumash Day Intertribal Native American Ceremony in Malibu, which they founded. I was among those helping the initiative. It has since grown into a huge annual event, drawing tribes from throughout the nation. Harold has learned to play the American Indian wooden flute and has become a sought-after local celebrity because of the beauty and natural authenticity of his songs. In addition, he is active in many initiatives to make this world a better place, through teaching and personal contributions to his community. Another benefit of our healing work? We served together on NACCR (the Native American Committee for Cultural Resources).

After almost 40 years of healing others, I've seen plenty of shifts. As noted throughout this chapter, there are several factors in common among people who experience a sudden, unusual or even miraculous healing:

- A 180-degree change in perspective
- Willingness to make all effort needed to reclaim and restore their health
- Change their diet and lifestyle, often including the use of supplements
- Opening to something greater than themselves
- Trust and belief that a Higher Power can help them through
- The loving presence of a supportive family and community of friends
- An increasingly strong spiritual connection

We all can shift! We all can heal. We are all One.

CHAPTER 9
Finding Purpose, Practicing Presence

"There are only two days that nothing can be done. One is called yesterday. The other is called tomorrow. Today is the right day to love, believe, do, and most of all, live."

—The Dalai Lama[21]

We live in a world that keeps us distracted, constantly acting and reacting, often outside the wisdom of our deeper, most authentic selves. Think of how a typical day goes—rushing to get ready for work, hoping traffic doesn't make you late, getting angry at slow-moving vehicles, rushing to get things done, never finding enough hours, then feeding the family and dealing with everything at home. Instead of using breaks in time to breathe deeply, meditate, exercise, or sit and relax quietly, we jump on our email or devices, fall into social media, get trapped by the latest clickbait, or shop online. We never give our minds and spirits a moment's rest. This doesn't take into account the hundreds of advertisements, interruptions, negative news pieces, environmental toxins or other distractors slung our way every moment of the day.

After days like this, suppose you came to my clinic and I asked you, "How many times did you breathe *deeply* today? How long did you sit quietly and meditate, contemplate or pray—or just *sit*? How often did you circle back to your purpose? What motivates you? How long can you sit in the *present* moment and allow that sense of purpose to build? Did you feed stress with an unhealthy food? Or de-stress with some form of exercise?"

What would your answers be? Sadly, for millions, it would fall along the lines of, "perilously close to none."

Equally as sadly, many suffer from anxiety, depression, pre-diabetes or diabetes, cardiovascular disease, obesity, various autoimmune disorders, ADHD and other attention-deficit issues, stress-induced cancers, fibromyalgia, and more. These are the very diseases and conditions that have

119

broken out of a corral like a stampede of wildebeests to become the center of our population's health-care problem. Statistics from the Centers for Disease Control and Prevention are frightening: in 1970, the adult obesity rate in the US was 15 percent. By 2018, it had increased to an official total of 42.5 percent (and an overweight percentage of 73.6 percent)[22], mostly a result of fast foods, processed and industrial factory-farmed meats, and high-fructose corn syrup.

Also of note: in 1970, less than 1 percent of children were diagnosed with ADD or other attention-deficit issues; today, that figure is over 20 percent.

Another number that should alarm us to the core: the child obesity rate worldwide has increased *1,000 percent* since 1975. The child obesity rate in the US alone is 19.3 percent, up from 4.6 percent in 1970. Along with that comes child-onset type 2 diabetes, autoimmune deficiencies, weak immune systems, troubles focusing and paying attention, and a sharp increase in childhood cancer. Our kids should be playing, learning and exploring life. Baby Boomers, Gen Xers and older millennials will remember the President's Council on Physical Fitness tests in grade and middle school, part of our daily physical education classes on the playground. Those are either entirely gone or limited today.

Let's dive beyond these horrifying numbers and some of their physical, environmental causes (poor diet, lack of exercise, too much stress/expectations, toxins in food and drinking supplies, absence of recess and PE, etc.). There's an underlying reason why we can't seem to anchor ourselves, why so many adults and kids walk around aimlessly, over-stressed and in poor health, losing hope that life will ever get easier or better.

Simply put, we've lost our purpose. We have stopped living fully conscious in the moment, in a state of presence. We react to everything around us, and either cave or move forward, always worried about our future, always concerned about the past. Or, just as badly, we choose to push aside present challenges to live in a romanticized past that gave us the greatest joy—because *we were living very much in the present in those moments!* All you have to do is go to your next high school reunion, whether it has been 10, 25 or 40 years, to see former classmates emotionally locked in "the best years of my life." Meaning, the high school years. For those who live in the moment *now*, such a welcome gathering of old friends with whom we shared a campus for 4 years (or 12, if schoolmates since kindergarten) can become a sad observation of raw potential stuck in idle.

This is not how we most of us would envision living to our fullest potential. We need to reach out to be in touch with our minds, hearts and souls, our health and well-being, and our purpose for being on this earth at this time. We need to focus our daily energies on *right now, this moment*, and live in a continual state of presence. We will find that all-powerful, fluid and often effortless place by connecting with a purpose within, leading us beyond ourselves and feeding our very soul.

Practicing Presence

Sue Ann was a 50-year-old single mom with six children. She worked as a nurse for a private practice. Her two youngest children were still in daycare; her nine-year-old was a gem. The oldest boy, however, was 16 and a problem since grade school, diagnosed with Oppositional Defiant Disorder compounded by antisocial, narcissistic tendencies. He routinely sent the whole family into a tailspin whenever he came home from detention. Once, he was expelled from school for attacking a staff member.

Despite being on juvenile parole, the boy challenged his mother in every way. Not only did he steal her money and bank cards, running her accounts to nothing in spite of her best efforts, but at school, he'd started more altercations with both students and staff. Consequently, Sue Ann spent much of her weekends in the bedroom, feeling angry and defeated. To quell her stress, she ate poorly. If that wasn't enough, her son would disappear for days at a time, only to return high on vape oil, with no regard for his family or the terms of his parole.

What happened next? *He reported her to Child Protective Services!* He told CPS she locked him out, forced him to sleep outside and didn't feed him.

Even if a parent is innocent, the CPS can be brutal. They question every parental practice and side with the child. This case was no different, and explained the dark cloud that seemed to hover over Sue Ann.

"I need meds. All I can do is cry," she said.

My heart went out to her. She was an excellent mom with happy, well-adjusted children. Except for the 16-year-old. "I just don't know where I went wrong with him, or what to do about it," she told me. "I've gained twenty pounds, and now I have pre-diabetes."

I put my hand on her shoulder. "That is the least of your problems, Sue Ann," I said calmly. "We can change your diet, get rid of the refined carbs and energy drinks, and get you to exercise. It will give you more energy and, with a few herbs, we can begin to reverse your condition." I paused for a moment to let that sink in. "But, most importantly, you need to do some work to combat this stress."

"How?" she asked, tears in her eyes. "It is relentless."

"Let me share something with you," I said. "You did your best and continue to do your best. You need to forgive your son and yourself, and not take it so personally. It is all his own choice, unfortunately. All you can do is your best. You can't do any better than that. You have five other children and yourself to take care of."

"He loves to get me upset. The more I get upset, the more he loves it."

"Then we need to teach you how to not react. Do not feed his negativity by giving him your power."

Sue Ann's eyes widened. "I never thought of that, Dr. Randall."

I opened up another issue. "Let me ask you: is your job satisfying you?"

"No, but I have to pay the bills."

The time was right to home in on her personal sense of purpose. Not her kids, not the purpose that comes with being a parent, but her own deeper purpose. "What do you really want for *you*?" I asked.

Without hesitating, she said, "I want to have my own business and learn integrative medicine and consult for practices like yours."

"OK . . . then do it! You can do that. Don't wait until everything is perfect to follow your dreams. Everything *is* perfect. Start new; there's no time like the present. Sometimes, we convince ourselves we'll do things when we get more money, or when we get a handle on this or that problem that may or may not be of our own doing. If your heart moves you, listen. Act now. It is the only place we can act. There is nothing like the present."

With that, Sue Ann's eyes began to alight, her hope renewed.

The point of power is in the present. Everything we're capable of achieving, whether great health, works, wealth, contribution or love, grows with the energy we put into it *right now*. We take our first step into the future, as well as our first step out of the past.

When it comes to medicine, practitioners and therapists of all types benefit their clients and themselves most when they are truly present. When I sit with patients, students, staff or colleagues, and before we discuss a case or subject, I already know what will ensure the richest, most beneficial outcome: giving them my fullest attention *right now*. Why? Because I am present for them in body, mind and soul. I bring everything I am, what I know and what I can offer into that moment: my expertise as a healer in more than 20 modalities, the spiritual and emotional depth and experience from decades of prayer, meditation, learning from my teachers and working with thousands of patients. When we live in the present moment, we *are* that powerful, in all the right ways.

Here's the catch: it's the *only way* to fully embrace and express all that we are. "The only place you can truly be and live is right here, right now," Joseph Rael says. "If you try to be in the future or the past, you shrink your own power. Be present and powerful."

When we are in a state of presence, fully in the moment, our aura and inner power grows and expands in waves of inspiration and motivation. We bring the other person into the same stream of light that we occupy. This releases us of distractions from our outside lives, and from being preoccupied with a past that is *over* and a future that has yet to occur. Listening and acting from this space, in our everyday lives, is like dressing unconditional love in plain clothes.

As for Sue Ann? During the following year, she enrolled in integrative medicine courses, joined a gym, changed her diet and lost 25 pounds. She applied to consult for a well-known integrative physician, and then began working with his practice. She loved it and felt great about herself.

When she visited me for her follow-up, she looked fabulous. "Dr. Randall, you were so right!" she exclaimed. "My pre-diabetes is resolved, thanks to seeing you."

"It's really thanks to you, Sue Ann. You have done the work, exercised, followed your diet and taken care of your soul with meditation."

She smiled. "I have, haven't I? I am so happy in my new positive lifestyle. I have more money, but more importantly, I'm following my heart."

"What about your son?"

"I still have problems with him, but I have that under better control. Also," she added, the promise of more freedom echoing in her words, "he will be eighteen later this year."

She shared an exchange she had with her son. "I told him, 'This is your year.'

"'What do you mean?' he asked me.

"'Well, after you turn eighteen, you are responsible for everything you do. It's all on you after that.'"

She looked at me with a knowing grin. "That really affected him. He had an awakening. He's been a lot better since then."

When Sue Ann first came to me, she faced an apparently unchangeable situation with her son. However, she *could* change how she responded to it and take control of her own life by following her purpose and being present in herself. She stopped worrying about the future and lived fully in her present.

"This Is Your Sweet Spot"

One warm New Mexico evening, Joseph Rael and I performed a healing on a man with a neurological problem. While sitting in Joseph's kiva, I used my presence and voice to soothe the man. This anchored him in the moment, the place he needed to be for the healing to be successful.

Joseph leaned over as I worked. "This is your sweet spot," he said. He is right: it is where I am my most powerful, purposeful and serviceful. I have practiced presence and mindfulness since I was a medical student. I found it a natural thing to do, and I've always remained open to learning higher expressions and reverence of being present, which has happened thanks to my teachers.

It is easy to tell the difference between someone living in a state of presence, and someone who defaults to the already-lived past or not-yet-happened future. One is highly focused, resolute, doing high-quality work, healthy in mind and (hopefully) body, and sure of the path they're walking. The other is distracted, scattered, indecisive, often highly stressed, and more susceptible to health issues—and to being manipulated and exploited by others.

Another challenge? We're bombarded by messaging in society, work, home and media, things like "you'll never truly escape your past" or "you'll never have the future you want." Either can turn us into stressed-out, aimless messes, which then opens the Pandora's box of disease. Worse, many of us never take the time to step back, assess how we feel and think, and just *do nothing*. We don't allow the time to recharge, to be in the quietest moments, as Supertramp's Roger Hodgson (a longtime meditator) famously sang when I was a young woman.

It's even worse for our kids. In a revealing 2013 interview with famed TV news anchor Dan Rather on AXS-TV, Rock & Roll Hall of Famer Roger Daltrey of The Who addressed this point to then 16-year-old pop superstar Cody Simpson, who was also being interviewed. "It worries the shit out of me that we're telling these kids to always stay busy, and they spend their lives on their devices, never taking a moment for anything," Daltrey said. "As anyone who has created something or felt something spiritual knows, the inspiration almost always happens when we're doing nothing, just *being present*, not worrying about the past or future."[23]

Prior to that, Daltrey made another strong point: "You may only get one chance, one moment when everything comes together if you take the chance. You've got to take it with everything you've got." Or, as put by famed anthropologist and author Carlos Castaneda (who introduced a generation to Don Juan and the Yaqui way of healing in the late 1960s), "a cubic centimeter of chance." How are we going to recognize that moment, see the opportunity or take that chance if we can't live in the present moment?

One of the healthiest self-caring things we can do is to get beyond all this noise and distraction, connect with ourselves and focus on *right here, right now*. Meditation, prayer and visualization are three great places to start.

Living Purposefully

We are intended to express everything we do in a sacred way. The ancient Chinese regularly lived to the ripe age of 100 years or more, largely because they knew this simple way. This sense of meaning and purpose in life is one of the three primary factors crucial for longevity, according to epidemiological studies (the others are fitness and nutrition). Similarly, my Lakota grandparents told me three things, passed down from their grandparents, that a human being needs to practice daily for a long and happy life: "Sing your song and give thanks every day (prayer and affirmation or spirituality); share bounty with your neighbor (good nutrition and community relationship); and dance (fitness and honoring the earth)."

These are the cornerstones of *purpose*, a most critical element to living a healthy, meaningful life with a true sense of well-being. Purpose is our inner and outer navigator, our compass, the reason we move forward (or try to move forward) every day. It is the oxygen that feeds our actions and our deeds, our works and our accomplishments. Your purpose might be to raise your kids to know how to achieve their fullest potential, to teach illiterate adults so they can read their kids bedtime stories, to create a technology that mitigates the massive carbon buildup on our planet, or to remove plastics from our oceans. Mine is to heal and strengthen the well-being of everyone I touch. That will ignite a greater knowing in those people, who will spread it to others. Ultimately, this increases our awareness of presence and purpose in all people. And that will result in a greater awareness of what we need to do to rescue our planet. Purpose defines who we are in the world, and reflects the inner guidance of our soul, our larger reason for being here at this particular moment in time. In turn, this increases the consciousness of regenerative practices and the higher cosmic consciousness where we can unite to heal the planet.

The notion of deeper meaning and purpose is just now being recognized in medical institutions, even though it's been practiced and emphasized in indigenous cultures and holistic healing circles for thousands of

years. We're also starting to hear more in the media about "sense of purpose" being a vital component of aging, of remaining relevant and making
the world a better place for others. Just a generation ago, the talk in our
society focused on turning 65 and heading off to the retirement pasture
or the Golden Age Retirement Home, our purpose complete, our societal
contributions done. It's the opposite in indigenous societies; they make
sure their elders can fulfill their purpose. They honor them and seek out
their wisdom, expertise and knowledge.

You might ask, "How am I connected with my purpose, and what gives
me meaning?"

For me, waking up with a known purpose is just as important as waking up with a heart and lungs. To feel meaningful and in full emotional and
mental health, we need to have a purpose. As long as your purpose is beneficial to self and others, creates something forward moving, instills your life
with meaning, and benefits others, then it is good. Your purpose can certainly change once, twice or many times in your lifetime, especially in these
days when people change careers often. They can (and should) also evolve.

For instance, when you graduated college, your purpose might have
been to get into your career and make a lot of money. Then, perhaps it
shifted to starting a family. Later, when the kids set forth on their own,
you looked at a more universal purpose, such as working for a cause in
which you believe deeply. A big life event, whether positive or negative, can
change your purpose and focus. Inner reflection is a good way to tune into
your path, your purpose. You might also be one of those souls who knew
your central purpose early on, and evolved as a soul while your core purpose
remained the same.

I'm one of those people. Since my earliest days, I have held a passion
for healing and caring for others, the two-leggeds, four-leggeds, and the
planet. I was given this at birth. Even though my path has changed course
many times, my core purpose governed nearly all of it, beating beneath my
works and steps like a strong, resolute heart.

Recently, I attended "People, Planet, Purpose," a conference at Scripps
Institute Academy of Integrative and Holistic Medicine where I was board
certified. How refreshing to finally see a conference putting these three
elements together (as if they ever belonged apart!). For more than 35 years,
I've pushed hard to bring such initiatives to the forefront. It was especially
sweet to see people, planet and purpose in the same room.

At the conference, my longtime role model, holistic medicine pioneer
Dr. Dean Ornish, spoke about love, trust and healing, while also disputing
the popular notion that fear changes people most. What it does instead is

weaken our individual purpose until we find ourselves flailing, reaching out for a way forward like a drowning person reaches for a distant tree branch.

My lifelong purpose is to heal others with every fiber of my mind, being and soul. Still, I have taken the time to continue my education. I cannot resist the opportunity to learn more. This continuity of purpose makes me a superior physician and healer, not because my ego needs to feel superior, but because I will always go to any extent to help my client or patient—while continuing to learn as much in my field and about people as I can. I love every bit of my work, I love the people who walk into my office and I especially love watching their eyes fill with renewed purpose as we work together.

Why Purpose Is So Important to Soul

My brother Casey died when he was in his late 30s. It was an untimely death. Before we lost him, he was the cofounder and director of Radio Talking Book, a program to help the blind function in a sighted community. Casey did this work despite dealing with an untreatable form of leukemia.

After Casey's passing, the company's new building was dedicated in his name. His gravestone reads, "He made a difference." He lit up every room or situation he walked into. He made anyone he touched or spoke to feel special, because he was so full of purpose. Which filled him with happiness. A sense of purpose in life is a key ingredient to living in happiness.

Our soul is the innermost essence of our Self that exists beyond the space-time continuum. Soul is the bridge between body and spirit, our connection with the universal source. When we develop our spiritual body, we feel a greater sense of meaning, purpose and belonging to life—a factor that contributes most to longevity and happiness. As Ralph Waldo Emerson said, "The purposed life is not to be happy. It is to be useful, to be honorable, to be compassionate, to have it make some difference that you lived and lived well." Emerson wasn't saying that purposeful people cannot be happy; rather, in pouring ourselves into our purpose, and bringing joy, benefit and happiness to others, we give of our own deeper happiness—and the cup keeps running over.

How powerful is finding your purpose—or renewing it? Constantly, we hear stories of mentally and physically ill people healing after they find their purpose. I've seen it happen countless times in my own practice. Their lives change, instantly at times, whether it's the work they now pour their hearts and souls into, or taking their love for a cause and touching hundreds or thousands with it.

The Presence of Renewed Purpose

An initiative in Southern California speaks of this beautifully. It began with Madison, whose central purpose was to empower children with a love of nature and improve their education, health and well-being. Madison was a woefully underweight baby who spent her first years dealing with related health issues. She missed a lot of school and, as a result, was often alone in a wooded environment. Later, she earned two master's degrees and an elementary teaching credential, then married and had three children. Her love for children is so vast and limitless that it expanded her sense of purpose. She wrote an environmental education curriculum for grades two through eight that still serves more than 10,000 North San Diego County kids annually. The kids take daylong field trips to an open space environmental center, where instructors teach marine and plant biology, natural history, ecology, California history and environmental awareness through a fun series of hands-on stations and nature hikes. These field trips are not part of a typical school curriculum. In putting this together, Madison extended her motherly energy toward her three kids into the creative energy and purpose to impact 10,000 each year. Imagine how her work is seeding our future with bright, purposeful and aware lights, focused on healing the planet. All thanks to one woman's vision and purpose.

A new or renewed sense of purpose can elevate our lives from a lower to higher place. Other things elevate, too: the immune system, our mental and emotional outlook, attention to diet and fitness, and sense of well-being. Living purposefully also extends our lives in many cases.

Years ago, a patient came to me for metastatic ovarian cancer, accompanied by her daughter. I told them there were things we could do to help. "However," I added, "the most powerful thing you can do is fall in love with life again. Find your purpose—something you've always wanted to do."

I never saw the woman again. However, her daughter later visited my office as a patient. "You helped my mom live an additional sixteen years," she began, instantly setting the mood for the day.

I was stunned. "How did I do that?"

"You told her to find something she always wanted to do. She always wanted to be a jazz singer. After we left your office, that's what she started doing. She made it a career and did so well she lived vibrantly for another sixteen years!"

Love and purpose in life heals patients—and practitioners!

When we live with purpose, and love for all, we live in a state of well-being. We also put ourselves in the best position to heal—and practitioners who operate like this give their patients some of the greatest medicine of all.

In the December 31, 2017, issue of *Psychology Today*, Stephanie Sarkis, PhD, listed out four ways to achieve meaning and purpose in your life:

1. Achieve physical and mental well-being
2. A sense of belonging and recognition
3. Personally treasured activities
4. Spiritual closeness and connectedness[24]

I'd like to review each of these, and close with practical ways we can bring them into our lives.

- Achieve physical and mental well-being: This happens through exercise and stress-reduction techniques such as conscious breathing, prayer and meditation. A good attitude is vital; think of the glass being half full rather than half empty.
- A sense of belonging and recognition: This is about feeling the way others value you, how friends, family, and coworkers or clients validate you, and the positive feedback you receive from a work situation or group.
- Personally treasured activities: What hobbies or personal passions infuse you with a sense of well-being? A few of mine are walking along the seashore, riding my horse, spending time with my family and cooking. I like to say, "Do whatever makes your duck float."
- Spiritual closeness or connectedness: Become enveloped by something greater than yourself. It is known that people who attend church or a spiritual group tend to live longer and have stronger immune systems than those who don't. You can also achieve this with a feeling of Oneness toward the planet and all of her creatures and beings

CHAPTER 10
Overcoming Fear

"Ultimately we know deeply that the other side of every fear is a freedom."
—Marilyn Ferguson, author, *The Aquarian Conspiracy*[25]

Fear is woven deeply into our culture. When we turn on the TV, go online or pick up a newspaper, fear grips the headlines like an ominous shadow. We're told to fear "bad people" in our communities, the unknown, viruses or superbugs. We also fear the lack of material objects or money, trying something new or starting a new business, venturing into wild nature, traveling outside our country—or even outside our gated community. We're taught to fear God, going to hell, the next storm rolling through or taking care of ourselves because we don't know as much as our doctors. From advertisements to social media, from law enforcement to our well-meaning neighbors, we're bombarded by "fear" messages from sunup to sundown, day after day.

As I see it, FEAR stands for False Evidence Appearing Real.

We live in a fear-based culture. When fear begets fear, events manifest in our lives and create a world on edge due to climate change (fear of releasing our addiction to fossil fuels), hostility between nations (fear *is* power, so dictators and their enablers believe), and fear of stepping forward to stop it (what will happen to our jobs/families/lifestyles?). We often fear for our lives.

Those of us who came of age during the 1960s and 1970s could never have imagined that we'd spend our golden years surrounded by such deep fear. We'd broken open the veil of unconsciousness like The Doors' Jim Morrison famously implied in his song. He swung wide the doors to personal freedom, elevated consciousness, found meditation, yoga, and the ancient arts of healing, medicine and living. We went back to the land, striving for communion with Mother Earth. We carried the peace sign as the Love Generation, the Beautiful People, the Flower Children! Many of us envisioned our adult selves evolving into a society of superbeings, our collective greatest potential creating a harmonious planet, or at least a harmonious country. Fear? What was that?

Instead, in a last grasp for absolute power (darkness before the dawn), those who fear inner freedom and the self-determining power of individuals are trying to clamp us down and stomp out our greater potential. They live in fear, they rule with fear, and create fear-based institutions, limitations and religious interpretations. Consequently, here we are, in a society where school and public space shootings, toxic food and water supplies, and fear of speaking out are the norm. Not quite the society of superhumans we could have seen by now.

Such global fear affects us directly and deeply. It especially impacts our bodies and our health. When I visit with patients suffering from autoimmune, fatigue-based or chronic illnesses, I am pretty certain that after asking a few questions, I will learn that they are in fear of something—which I can then connect to the specific area and deeper cause of their disease.

Fear attacks our bodies with vengeance; think of it as inhaling a plume of toxic smoke, over and over again. It enters our body and seeps through our pores and sinuses into our mind, muscles, bones, bloodstream and cells. The more we feel fear, and the more we tense up, stress out or worry over it, the more our body suffers. When you look at the rapid increase of obesity, diabetes, cardiovascular disease, mental illness and behavioral disorders since 1970, four factors stand out: a fructose-based (corn syrup) food supply; increased conventional and processed meat consumption; the growing toxicity of our food, water and air; decrease in daily exercise; and dysfunctional family units and society driven by fear.

Fear is supposed to be an instinctive response, a survival skill. Something happens, we feel fear, we stand on high alert, we act to rise above the situation, and we elude or overcome it. That's how our bodies are wired. Instead, many of us now live in fear 24/7. Which is entirely unnatural. And a major reason why doctors, pharmacists and therapists are among the busiest people in the world today.

The fear I see in the eyes of my patients, day in and day out, is part of the force that moved me to write this book about an expanded view of medicine and health. They come to me many times as their last shred of hope, their eyes glassing with fear when they say things like:

"I have seen so many doctors. I'm depressed and can't sleep."

"My mother has ovarian cancer with metastases to the lungs. She means everything to me."

"I've been sick for fifteen years and no one can tell me what is wrong with me."

"I've tried everything. Nothing works anymore."

They talk quickly at first, their words bouncing over one another like pebbles falling down the side of a cliff. They are desperately trying to get out all of their pain and fear before I cut them off, hand them a prescription and show them the door. Fear is so malignant to all of our bodies—physical, mental, emotional and spiritual.

When that moment does not come, when I don't respond in the way they expect from a doctor, they relax. Just by my simple act of listening, they begin to release fear—which begins their healing process. They are liberated from the fear that they will not be listened to or cared for because the doctor is too concerned about time or economics to focus completely on them. They are astonished that a doctor actually sits and intently listens to everything they have to say.

The freedom that comes to patients when they are given the attention they deserve fosters trust in the patient-doctor relationship. It is a critical part of overcoming fear in the rest of their lives. This trust begins the flow of healing energy between the doctor and the patient. We doctors are critical people in introducing our patients not only to overcoming the fear of their illness or disease, but to showing them ways to greater inner courage through rebuilding their health and inner power, which has the potential to dispel fear the way light dissolves darkness.

Fear of Illness

"Let us not look back in anger or forward in fear, but around in awareness."

—James Thurber

When we become ill, we may feel fear. We may become even more afraid of the unknown than we already are. We become angry for something we may have done—poor diet, no exercise, working in toxic places, overly stressing—to bring the illness upon ourselves. The future becomes filled with looming, monstrous "what-ifs" capable of swallowing us up at any moment. We feel like we're swimming in a sea of chewed bubble gum or moving from fog bank to fog bank. All of this negative energy only serves to externalize our power, which can reflect back upon us in the form of fearsome possibilities.

Human emotions can be generalized as beneficial, rooted in love and a sense of well-being for self and others, or non-beneficial, arising from fear or anger. All named emotions (happy, sad, irritated, angry, etc.), are different octaves that vibrate from either love or fear. Love has the capacity to heal all things. It cannot exist within fear. On the contrary, fear, anger, doubt and anxiety remove the ability of the body and soul to heal. They often cause us to let our fears simmer inside, freezing us in place and limiting our ability to *move forward*. We give our power away when we choose fear. By externalizing our own power in the form of fear, it boomerangs back to us and drains our life force. When we fear the experience of our disease, often it is because our fear-based egos don't want to give up control over the body.

We must remember that we are powerful spiritual beings who have taken on a physical experience for the opportunity of learning and healing whatever ails us deeply, whatever holds us back from achieving our ultimate identity as rays of the divine light. By understanding this, we can become and remain aware within the challenge, learn the message of our illness, and overcome our fears. We can consciously accept the healing offered through the experience of our illness. The illness has no power over us when we open our hearts to receive and give love and compassion, trust in our own process and that of the universe to provide what we need. This returns our power and aligns us with our soul, which creates the opportunity for healing to take place. Even if you are dealing with health or emotional issues, finding your balance within will help you find your way out. You can also be happy "living with" something that is not within your reach to cure. You can still heal. People can happily live with many things from cancer to a missing limb to living in a wheelchair. It doesn't mean that you give up. Never give up; enjoy what you have. Surrender only to God.

Fear of Releasing Illness

Alan Cohen, the author of *Spirit Means Business* and two dozen other inspirational titles, says, "It takes a lot of courage to release the familiar and seemingly secure, to embrace the new. But there is no real security in what is no longer meaningful. There is more security in the adventurous and exciting, for in movement there is life, and in change there is power."[26]

The idea of no longer living with our disease, or anything we've held near and dear to us despite its negative aspects, petrifies many. Overcoming our disease and returning to balance and holism requires tremendous transformation, including drastic steps like changing our lifestyles, diets or attitudes. Performing an unfamiliar activity, being in new surroundings or doing things in a new way may be terrifying. Change is often frightening. Sometimes the prospect of being in foreign territory—a road to health that involves new living habits—will cause us to remain with our disease rather than face the fear of change. It takes courage and commitment to move against the resistance of familiar sameness into the unknown, even if it is making us sick. Especially when cultural and media messaging *promotes* the status quo. After all, we risk failure whenever we change anything.

However, there's another way to look at healthy change: it is really about overcoming fear in order to take responsibility for our illness. We must be careful not to confuse this with blaming ourselves for causing our illness, which hinders our healing process. Simply take responsibility for the illness and the process of healing: "OK, I have adult-onset diabetes, it happened, now it's time to move beyond it . . ." This very movement against resistance propels us into the future and toward holism.

When I was working at the UCLA Cardiac Care Unit, a cardiology professor came to speak with the residents. He said, "If something unexpected happens to one of the patients, call me immediately, but *do something.*"

What did he really mean? Simply, that trying *something* would bring us closer to the right path, even if it were not the exact correct choice. When we find ourselves stuck in a particular pattern causing ill health, the same holds true. If we take a risk and try *something*, we move against the resistance of fear, and break from the inertia holding us in that pattern. Sometimes, doing the "wrong" thing leads us to the right thing. It's all about taking a step forward.

The case of Annie illustrates the art of overcoming fear. Annie was 58 years old when she came to me for severe back pain, which she had suffered for five years after rupturing a disc at work. She was an accountant for a large bank, and her superior ordered her to move heavy file boxes to storage. Lifting heavy boxes wasn't part of her job description. She asked to be relieved of the duty, since she felt it was too much for her. Instead, her superior punished her for asking by canceling her vacation. This superior had a reputation for extreme cruelty, and nearly everyone in Annie's original department quit or transferred out because of her oppressive behavior.

Annie returned to work the next day. Her superior again demanded she move the heavy file boxes into the storage closet—or suffer the consequences. Annie acquiesced and began moving boxes. Later that same day, she experienced a ripping pain in her back. She was diagnosed with a ruptured disc. She took medical leave because of her disability and did not return to work. The pain was too great.

Two years and many physicians later, she sat in my office. Her other doctors had tried everything they knew—pain meds, X-rays, MRI scans and epidurals. She was also seeing a counselor for panic attacks and agora-phobia, which she had developed as a result of her injury. Annie confided that she saw visions of bloody monsters whenever she closed her eyes, and the visions made her terrified to sleep; add sleep deprivation to her situa-tion. "I cannot get that horrible woman out of my mind," she said, referring to the bank supervisor. "When I think of her, I see those monsters with blood dripping from their faces. Sometimes they have *her* face!"

It was clear to me that "monsters" were a result of Annie's anger toward and fear of her cruel boss. I also realized she suffered from PTSD, compounded by night terrors. I found her a PTSD specialist and taught her guided meditation to deal with the fears and monsters. We also did acupuncture for her back pain, along with meditation and Aura-Soma, a dynamic color aromatherapy.

One of the things that helped Annie most was learning to release her anger toward the cruel superior through breathing mediation. The monster visions stopped after two or three months of practicing a clearing medita-tion. While her acupuncture treatments relieved her back pain for up to a week, it always returned. Her right leg had felt painful and numb since her disc rupture.

Once the horrible visions stopped, we moved onto the next phase—getting Annie ready to consider a surgical option. Before that, she was too frightened to consider it. She began a meditative process to quiet the mind, one that also involved prayer. So traumatic and fear-driven was the abuse of her superior that it took six full months of PTSD psychotherapy, meditative practice and prayer for Annie to believe that it was safe to have surgery. She also felt more comfortable when her visions of monsters were replaced by healing dreams of angels, a sure sign she was overcoming fear in her deeper subconscious and psyche, right down to the cellular level. "If you have the power to turn anger and fear into monsters and then let them go, you have the power to make angels and get through this surgery," I told her.

We scheduled Annie for a laparoscopic discectomy. To perform this pain-alleviating procedure, I called her orthopedic specialist, who had been waiting for the "go ahead."

On the day of the surgery, I accompanied her to the operating room and helped her to focus on her meditation. She visualized a beautiful, lush forest meadow with fragrant, brightly colored flowers and birds singing. The sun shone on a soft bed made for her in a clearing. She padded across the lush green grass and lay in her special bed. She knew all was well; her surgery would go perfectly. I left her side and took a seat in the recovery room.

When Annie got out of surgery, she was calm and still, her focus in the lush forest. She was surprised the surgery was over. "Dr. Randall, the forest is so beautiful," she said.

"That's good. How do you feel?"

"Great. I'm ready for the surgery."

I smiled and rubbed her shoulder. "Annie, the surgery is over. It took two hours."

A few hours later, she lifted herself off the bed without assistance and walked out of the recovery room without pain. She never required more than ibuprofen during recovery. A year later, she remained pain-free. Annie learned the power of her own mind to overcome fear and continues to use her meditative skills to handle the stresses in her life.

Another patient, Nan, suffered from kidney cancer. She dealt with her fear in a different way, an excellent example of "living with." She kept a positive attitude through many surgeries, chemotherapies and a lot of discomfort. Finally she told me, "I'm done with all that, Doc."

"OK. No problem, it's your choice."

"I'm good! Still enjoying life and my friends. I go to hula class three times a week and it keeps me going. Great group of gals! You should join us sometime!"

Nan demonstrates how a good attitude, physical activity and community can make all the difference. She squeezes every drop of joy out of life and is an inspiration to all of us!

I also think of Eduardo, a young man in his 30s who came to me a month after a colon resection for colon cancer. He brought his sweet wife, Lucy, with him for the appointment. "We have three girls, Doc, and are a very close family. They and my wife are worried about me," he said. "The oncologist and primary are pushing me to do chemotherapy."

Eduardo and Lucy were scared by the word "cancer" and by what the oncologist told them. They wanted guidance and a plan to move forward. I coached him on how to ask for the statistics regarding chemotherapy.

The next week Edwardo returned. "I did it, Doc! There's an eighty percent cure rate chance with surgery, and ninety percent with chemotherapy. I don't want to have chemotherapy. What do you think, Dr. Randall?"

"It's really up to you and your family, Eduardo. If you are willing to make some very strict lifestyle changes and follow an intense supplement program and do IV vitamin C drips, I think we can do it," I said. "You have to really be into it and believe. If your markers become positive, we can always do the chemotherapy."

We gave him the protocol, and he studied everything he could find about colon cancer. He watched many documentaries, like *Chris Cured Cancer* and *Radical Remission*. He also meditated, worked out five times a week and kept a pristine vegan diet along with his entire family—which he and they still do.

It has been three years since Eduardo's resection. He is still free of cancer, with negative markers and scans. "I have never felt better, Dr. Randall," he told me.

Combining a personal education with a solid plan and strong family support gave Eduardo the positive attitude he needed to overcome all fear and to heal.

Doctors in Fear

One of the biggest challenges facing patients today actually comes from well-meaning doctors. How are physicians, surgeons, therapists and clinicians supposed to help patients overcome fear when they fear "the system" itself?

It is understandable that physicians are fearful when they constantly have to be on the lookout for denial of benefits by insurance companies and HMOs, Medicare and Medicaid billback costs and threats of malpractice litigation. Our health-care system is broken as politicians fight over what it will look like in the future—or if the government will even provide a decent one. One of its greatest tragedies is that many doctors fear the types of treatments they can give patients. Restrictions by health-care insurance providers limit their tools and further weaken our health-care system and our public health.

Economics largely drive this fear. If the third-party payment system does not approve payment for a treatment, then the doctor cannot supply it. And those approval lists are limited, in many cases to the most basic care. Take the things in which I also specialize besides allopathic medicine, like integrative and functional medicine. So-called "alternative health care." Often, allopathic doctors tell their patients that complementary alternative treatments are not "standard of care," and suspect at best. Why? Most have been around much longer than Western medicine. Is it because these doctors never learned about them and are ignorant of their benefits? Or that they promote *healing*, moving beyond symptoms with diet and lifestyle changes . . . and thus reducing the need for office visits, hence billings?

Those of us who practice integrative medicine often hear, "there are not sufficient Western studies to prove the effectiveness of alternative therapies." Many think them worthless and invalid. Never mind that most "alternative therapies" date back thousands of years, their proven efficacy embedded in the age-old literatures of the cultures from which they came. The namesake of the Hippocratic Oath, which all medical doctors take, was writing about them in ancient Greece *2,500 years ago*! Just because someone in the United States didn't research a particular therapy until recently, under the strict peer-reviewed guidelines of the American Medical Association or others, doesn't make it less valid. Not by any means.

Fortunately, in the past few decades, many more solid research studies in integrative medicine have been conducted. I think of the works by Dean and Anne Ornish at the Preventative Medicine Research Institute at the University of California, San Francisco. Their lifestyle program reversing chronic diseases is now paid for by many insurance companies, a huge leap forward for the medical health system. Thank you, Dr. Ornish! Also, a growing body of evidence-based medical data on integrative and functional medicine is finally showing up in reputable journals, including *New England Journal of Medicine*, *Archives of Internal Medicine*, *Journal of the American Medical Association* and others. These include studies on subjects such as herbs, vitamins, patient-doctor relationships, healing touch, acupuncture, energy medicine and more.

The other issue in overcoming this fear is the communication from physicians to patients. Some physicians have responded to their patients' desire to consider alternative therapies with scorn, even scolding them. What does negative communication create, especially by an authority figure like a doctor? *Fear.* Patients either fear pursuing that health care, or dread telling their doctors about seeking it. The result? Patients withhold vital information from their doctors, never a good thing. A healing relationship tainted by fear is not likely to be successful.

Many doctors fear that associating with practices outside the Western medical model may tarnish their careers. They worry their reputations will be damaged by associating with non-traditional "quacks."

It is now time to awaken doctors and other practitioners with separatist mentalities. Or for encourage them to overcome their own fears and awaken themselves. We have learned the gift that "mind and body" medicine has given us, and it is time for holism to be born anew. It will dissolve much of the fear we face in our health and healing choices. The medicine of the future is a combined medicine where all disciplines are respected. That is where the real power to heal resides.

CHAPTER 11
Mental Health Is Like an Iceberg

Mental health has been an increasingly serious issue in the US for decades, but the COVID-19 pandemic has made it worse. Between January 2019 and July 2020, about one in ten people reported anxiety and depression—an alarming enough number. Since then, however, that number has jumped to four in ten, or 40 percent.[27] And that's just reported cases; many others suffer in silence. Economic and housing uncertainty, social isolation, rising inflation and job loss have created new barriers to people with mental health issues and addiction problems seeking help.

When I discuss mental health, I think of an iceberg. What you see on the surface, or the tip of the iceberg, is just a small indication of what is hidden. The body of the iceberg beneath the water represents the subconscious, where we stuff and hide many of our feelings, wounds, traumas and fears. When you recognize, identify and address those hidden issues, you will likely feel greatly relieved, energized, more positive about life in general—and thus much more able to do the work you need to handle and integrate those issues.

The first step to healing, any kind of healing, is always to believe you can and will be better. It all begins with a strong, positive attitude, and trusting your body and your healing process. Your attitude is key, as we discussed early in the book. It can literally make the difference between life and death. How many times have you seen or known someone who has suffered greatly or died from the effects of severe depression, while another finds a way out of that depression, changes their attitude and then thrives?

The tip of the iceberg expresses the results of what's hidden beneath: fears, traumas, anxiety, wounds. And illness is the result. Remember: no amount of anxiety and worrying ever helped anything.

Then there's stress—a silent killer that attacks body, mind and soul equally harshly. Stress is the result of stuffed emotions, resentment and frustration, external pressures, and the pressure we put on ourselves. There are two kinds of pressure: positive pressure, when you push yourself to perform at your best on a job or task, to which tennis great Martina Navratilova says, "Pressure is a privilege." Then there's negative pressure, that we allow others or outside factors to put on us—or heap on ourselves through unmet self-expectation. That form is *the* most damaging force to health and happiness, because it produces high levels of fight-or-flight neurotransmitters, cortisol and alarmins. Those literally tear down your tissues through increased inflammation and DNA damage. They also activate damaging CHIP cells, which cause cell death. Think of them as microscopic assassins.

The unwelcome results of all this self- or socially induced pressure and stress are chronic disease, greater potential for cognitive decline, mental health challenges, and a decreased life and health span. The opposite is what we want to achieve. To promote health and well-being, need to deal with stress-causing issues in the subconscious, relieve and then mitigate or eliminate it, and shift those stress-laden survival mechanisms to fundamental cellular balance.

How do we shift mental health issues into ways to achieve long, happy and purposeful lives? Let's look quickly at the blue zones (see Chapter 16). These micro-societies and communities of superagers achieve mental balance through spirituality, social activity, physical activity, attention to and participation in nature, a plant-based Mediterranean-type diet, and putting family and community before their own needs. They also do something else key to balanced mental health, especially in this hyper-fast, "gotta get it done now," distraction-filled society—they always seek to reduce or eliminate the sense of urgency. Whether at work or play, they pace themselves, and live a slower lifestyle in general. They share their problems with their friends and family, and do not feel a need to bury them.

As we go through life, we realize we need a lot of friends. It is known that people who have an abundance of friends are healthier. If you have a stressful or pressure-filled situation affecting your ability to work or live in balance, share with a family member or friend whom you trust and feel most comfortable. Choose a supportive confidant to talk about what bothers you. Ask them if they feel comfortable with you sharing your issues. This person is probably most supportive and uplifting. Your heart usually knows the answer to this question. If you don't have such a person in your life, I would recommend seeking out a life coach or therapist, depending on how upset you are, and how much it is disrupting your life.

Past Wounds and Traumas

A more chronic and major mental health issue concerns our past wounds and traumas. In this country, we often do not deal with either. That's dangerous to our mental well-being. If you do not deal with old wounds, they become like secrets. You want to hide them, and hide them some more, and knock them down whenever they try to surface—because you don't want *anyone* to see or touch them. The effect is like throwing a heavy coat over a lamp. It eliminates the "light," and lessens the likelihood of bringing the wound into the open. This creates what I call "thought viruses," and we develop whole new defense mechanisms and behaviors to keep them hidden. In *The Mastery of Love*, Don Miguel Ruiz talks about how we hide our wounds.

The best way to heal our wounds and traumas is to take responsibility for their existence, regardless of how they occurred. For example, when a child, if you suffered the source trauma for what became PTSD from your parents, and they are either no longer with us or inaccessible, take responsibility that it exists within you—without assigning any blame. If you're dealing with social anxiety disorder, first of all know you're *not alone*. Then, admit it exists within you, assign zero blame, only be responsible for integrating it. Then you really begin to address it.

From there, we just get rid of the issue, right? Well, It's a little more complicated than that.

Instead of trying to push away the wound, we need to learn to *integrate* that trauma into our own psyche. Open that heavy coat, and let the light of love shine in to heal the wound. While burying wounds and traumas only cause more fear and anxiety, exposing and releasing their hold creates the opposite—more joy and confidence, and much less stress. It might be painful at the outset—you're picking off a scab and exposing a deep-seated wound that may not have felt any "air" of healing or resolution since the event that caused it. We could be talking decades, in some cases. Once that wound is exposed to the oxygen of the soul doctoring you're doing, though, the healing has begun. If you don't take time to work through your most difficult traumas and experiences, they hold power over you and make you sicker.

There's another health issue we don't often associate with mental health, but is tied to it in many ways—various physical aches, pains and challenges. Joint pain, abdominal distress, skin rashes and headaches can really be physical expressions of what is hidden in your subconscious. The way to get out of chronic disease patterns and troubling symptoms is following the functional medicine map to find the root cause and see the connections between your subconscious, your brain, your gut and your body.

What You Do to Your Body, You Do to Your Brain

The treatment of mental illness is not completely addressed by big pharma antidepressants, antipsychotics and antianxiety medications, psychiatry, and psychotherapy, today's standard medical approach. We need to treat the body, and especially the gut, to communicate to the brain. Remember this simple maxim: *what you do to your body, you do to your brain.* Foods that negatively influence stress include sugary drinks and foods, fast foods, conventional meats (full of inflammatory omega-6s, glyphosates and other chemicals and hormones), conventional cereals, and refined carbohydrates. Foods and supplements that positively impact stress can be found in the Mediterranean-type or whole-food plant-based diets, olive oil (anti-inflammatory oleic acid, oleocanthal, polyphenols), organic foods, and lots of fruits and vegetables. Also, look into regeneratively farmed meats and poultry (always organic, grass fed and toxin-free).

Also, look at a couple of key nutritional supplements. Use omega-3s, but try to obtain them from plants or algae oil, as omega-3s derived from fish are too toxic. Also bring turmeric, the great anti-inflammatory herb, into your life. The best type of turmeric is water soluble, which creates the highest levels of free curcuminoids in the bloodstream. Curcuminoids then go to work on systemic ails. Melatonin, a good sleep remedy, also protects the gut by preserving the mucosal integrity and inhibiting the accumulation of neutrophils or inflammation. Be sure to attend to your sleep: sleep deprivation or inconsistency is a significant contributor to gut problems, cardiovascular disease, hypertension, weight gain, depression, anxiety, brain fog and neurological problems.

The best anti-inflammatory of all? That's simple: deal directly with your issues. When you do, you will also reduce stress and gain greater control of your mind, life and energy. If talking with family and friends is not enough, get help from a therapist, life coach, neurolinguistics programming therapist (NLP), or hypnotherapist. Use prayer, meditation and visualization. Return to your simple daily tasks and habits that make you feel safer and more balanced. What activities leave you feeling lighter, happier and more optimistic? Which seem to add to your stress or anxiety level? Sort these out, go with the activities that feed you, and start unlocking your longevity potential (life span and health span). Go for walks in nature, have meals with family or friends, eat regenerative foods from your garden or the farmers market, and give gratitude for what you do have.

Finally, I leave you with something to reset your attitude and perspective daily, a great saying of the Buddha:

> *What you think, you become*
> *What you feel, you attract*
> *What you imagine, you create*

CHAPTER 12
All Work Is Worship

"The best things in life are nearest: Breath in your nostrils, light in your eyes, flowers at your feet, duties at your hand, the path of right just before you. Then do not grasp at the stars, but do life's plain, common work as it comes, certain that daily duties and daily bread are the sweetest things in life."

—Robert Louis Stevenson

Paul was a bright, handsome, hard-working entrepreneur and founder of many tech companies. He worked tirelessly, despite being the heir to a fortune. He originally entered business with enthusiasm, dedication and great passion that he shared with his employees. As time wore on, though, business became business, and economic concerns won out over his desire for a more impassioned community spirit at the workplace. He folded his companies and sold out to a corporate management group.

This made Paul even wealthier, but not happier. He ended a relationship with his longtime girlfriend and began to self-medicate with drugs and alcohol to quiet his soul. He got into trouble with the law and lost many long-term relationships. Then his body began to fail him. Paul developed a severe neuropathy. His limbs, hands and feet were painful and numb, making it impossible for him to write, open packages and envelopes, or do daily chores and self-care.

He came to see me while in this condition, his eyes dulled by drugs and physical and emotional pain. "Please, Dr. Randall, I need you to help me. I am only thirty-six years old and I feel like I'm eighty. I'm ready to give up all the drugs, the fast life and alcohol, but I need help. I can't even feel good about anything. I don't even get high anymore. Help me get sober, please."

"Of course," I said. "When you get on the other side of sober, you'll realize that that was the easy part. It's whatever broke you and sent you to drugs and alcohol for comfort that is the real problem."

He looked at me with a moment of clarity through his pain and drug fog. In his heart, he knew I'd hit on the deeper issue.

We enrolled him in a top-of-the-line detox rehabilitation center for two months. He saw a neurologist, who treated him with pharmaceuticals after his tests showed widespread peripheral neuropathy. On the third month, he was ready to start making amends to all he had injured and cast aside. He contacted as many people as would speak to him and achieved closure.

On the fourth month, he came back to me. "I'm ready for the next step. I realize I can't go back, but I can move forward," he said. "This neuropathy thing is really hard, Doc! It stops me."

"How about we try some outside-the-box therapy?" I asked.

"Sure! Anything. I am ready."

I leaned in close. "You need to be ready to forgive yourself and get to the root cause of all this."

"I am."

"OK. First, start meditating on how you got here. Keep a journal. Be real. Be you. Be personal. No blaming of yourself or others. The best thing you can do is forgive yourself and others. You have done your best."

We built a program of supplements focused on the brain, nerves and nervous system, and enrolled him in physical therapy. He purchased an electromagnetic device to work on his microcirculation and nervous system. We also sent him to a therapist for electromagnetic frequency therapy and cold plunge alternating with a hot pool for microcirculation.

After a month, he came back, astonished at his progress. "I want to revisit the idea of creating a company with soul and community," he told me, "one based on service to others while creating a sustainable environment for all those who work there to serve others. They will also be served." I smiled warmly and he continued, "That is it! That is what I was meant to do! The neuropathy was my body's way of stopping me until I moved into the right direction. Now I am in sync and healed."

Even I was astonished.

Paul opened the company, and today remains healthy and truly successful, fulfilling his purpose and work in a sacred way.

Applying Sacredness to Our Work

It is more vital than ever that we apply sacredness to our work.

Our work environments have become fear-driven, bottom-line cultures that jeopardize the health of millions by treating them like robots or factory automatons. Their bodies are environmentally and emotionally toxic from poor workspace practices, where competition is valued over collaboration, allies turn into rivals and communication is broken. We're left to wonder, what happened to the spirit and purpose we felt at the beginning of our jobs or careers?

Think of public school teachers, who enter the educational system full of purpose to infuse children and teens with a lifelong love of learning and the tools to create enriching lives. All too soon into their careers, though, many feel blunted and muted by restrictions on curriculum, what they can say in class, what they can assign (or not assign) their students, and the pressure laid on them for conducting multiple standardized tests—to which school funding is tied.

When this happens, it often leaves us in a dark pool of physical and emotional distress, the stress so intense that it makes us question the purpose of our work—or if we should even work at all. When that happens, we have lost the deeper meaning and sacredness of work, but also, of our place and purpose on the planet.

Right now, this is a very big problem. How big? Let's go to the data and look at a few numbers that show a working world in desperate need of sacredness, and a workforce that needs to feel more purposeful about their jobs.

According to the University of Massachusetts Lowell, job stress costs the US economy and corporations $300 billion per year in the form of health costs, absenteeism and poor performance. Job stress is also a leading factor in job turnover, can cause depressive illness and causes more health complaints than financial or family problems.[28]

We are seeing this play out in front of our eyes. The quality of life in the US has dropped consistently since 2014—while the rest of the world's continues to rise overall. There are many factors for this. Lack of feeling safe partly from COVID, the ongoing opioid crisis increased stress, anxiety and depression are causes, according to the Centers for Disease Control and Prevention. All speak to the loss of purpose and direction in life, and the loss of meaning and sacredness in work.

"The problem with stress is that it's such a big concept," said Dr. Elizabeth Brondolo, PhD, of the American Psychological Association. "When people think about it, they often get overwhelmed or they're not sure how to measure it or how to think about what the clinical implications are."

Adding Sacredness to Multiple Careers

It's essential we find the sacredness and purpose in our work, because it is also a far different work climate than a generation ago. Multiple career paths are the present and future. Job descriptions are changing as fast as we can blink thanks to automation, the gig economy and digital technology. Today's middle school students are 10 years away from entering a workforce in which up to *50 percent of the jobs and careers they will apply for do not yet exist*, according to CNN technology reporter Lori Schwartz.[29] Also, since these paths are changing and shifting so quickly, teenagers and young adults must plan for eventual work in many fields. Mom and Dad's one-career culture has gone the way of the printed atlas and the VCR.

"The days of going to college, getting a degree, putting in 40 years as a loyal employee and leaving with the pension are basically over—especially for people in school today. It doesn't work that way anymore," said National Geographic Channel correspondent, social justice activist and neuropsychologist Cara Santa Maria, host of the popular *Talk Nerdy* podcast. "We have to be scrappy. Right now, the average millennial is changing careers every six or seven years—but the coming-of-age generation will be changing every four or five years. We have to wear different hats, be more multidisciplined, and have more life and business skills. *And we need to feel a strong sense of purpose in everything we do*" (emphasis mine).[30]

Santa Maria, who is in her late 30s, advocates bringing more girls into STEM (science, technology, engineering and math) courses and eventual STEM career fields—highly purposeful work shaping the world ahead of us. Her work is beautiful and sacred, not to mention empowering millions through her media platforms. She believes the time to start looking at work as worship is the day we get out of school—as she points out to the young people she influences.

"You are alive *today*," she tells them. "This is important. Life does not start *after* the education ends or you've established yourself in your career. Kids get so caught up in 'once I get out of school . . . once I settle in . . .' Don't go there. Start living *now*. You might write a book, help make a movie, experience tragedy, love and joy, get married or even have a kid while still in college. It's a negative psychological block to delay living until we think we're prepared to live. For my PhD, I studied what's called 'dying research,' the life review when dying people look back on their lives. When you're in that dying phase, what will matter most to you about your life?

"Your life doesn't start at forty. It starts when you come out of the womb."

That is very sage advice.

To this point, I tell my students and patients that life is like a spiral. Sometimes things don't work out the way we thought they should. We do not have to go back to square one. We carry forward with the experience and gifts we gained along the way—and do similar work at a higher level. No work is ever wasted. This is what Cara is suggesting as she discusses preparing for multiple career paths—and making the most of whatever life throws at you.

Many Paths, One Central Purpose

You can also bring worship into work by walking many paths within your central purpose, your sacred purpose. In other words, one career path morphs into many trails serving the same objective. This book brings forth the many ways I help and heal patients who walk into my clinic, plus my work with the planet. All of these "many ways" come from my sacred purpose: *heal yourself, heal the planet*. My purpose is to bridge the gap between various Eastern and Western modalities to heal the health-care system, the individual, humanity and by extension, the planet.

This began when I first worked as a nurse's aide at age 15. Shortly after that, I became a horse trainer, one of the early "horse whisperers," because I never believed you train a horse by breaking them. It's about establishing communication, trust and a relationship, which has served my work since. I next worked as a dental assistant, and then a surgery technician. During medical school, I organized an innovative "group practice" of students that did admission histories and physicals on cardiology patients coming in for heart catheterizations. After that, I moonlighted in ERs and worked as an intern during the day, plus my experiences on the Lakota, Tiwa and Yaqui reservations. Then I came on staff at UCLA in internal medicine, followed by taking a gastroenterology fellowship. Then I was asked to come on staff at UCLA in the medical professorship program.

Every bit of this work was sacred and purposeful.

My attending physicians used to ask, "What kind of drugs are you on?" because I was always smiling. I was so happy to be doing what I wanted to do. *My sacred work.* Even though I've done many things and worn many hats since, I found something in each station that I loved, and something I loved within each person I've seen.

We can all have this in our work. We need to find what gives us a sense of purpose and sacredness, whether in the job we hold now, or work we have yet to do. What gives you that sense of purpose? Some organizations have taken steps to address this by giving employees places to retreat within their buildings, small sanctuaries such as publishing company Rodale's American Indian-style kiva room. Others encourage meditation, positive affect training and how to bring a sense of spirit into the workplace. The numbers of hospitals and businesses in America addressing employees' spiritual needs are slowly increasing. But they still have a long way to go.

Dr. Mimi Guarneri is a great example of one who sees her work as sacred and has built a facility to encourages all involved, patients and staff alike, to include spirit in their healing processes. Her passion has been a driving force in the growth of integrative medicine. Mimi began her career at a state-of-the-art allopathic cardiology department at Scripps Institute in San Diego. Later, she founded the Academy of Integrative and Holistic Medicine, establishing her mission to heal others through a combination of solid science and deep compassion. She also worked with philanthropists Penny and Bill George, founders of the Bravewell Collaborative in 2001, to create more sustainable environments for holistic health practitioners and treatment practices. In 2005, the Bravewell Collaborative honored Dr. Guarneri for her work in driving the evolution of integrative and holistic medicine over the past decade.

In order to heal ourselves and participate in the healing of our society, we must turn back the clock and practice as our ancient forbears did: Tying together mind, body and spirit in the workplace. We also need to rise above the limitations thrown upon us by our increasingly oppressive government, and also rise above our own limited definitions of what work constitutes.

Sundance Ceremony: a Living Metaphor

The Sundance Ceremony offers a great metaphor to finding purpose and sacredness in our work. The ceremony begins long before the drumming and dancing. Everyone joins together, watching the chief choose the tree, making prayers to it, and we all work together to take it to be erected in the center of the dance corral. Branches from the tree are tied over the edges of the circle to provide shade for the dancers. Everyone—weak and strong, old and young—does their part, from preparing tobacco and corn meal–filled belt ties for the tree, to handing rope ties to those suspended from the dance corral, to lashing down branches. Everyone is involved, which makes the ceremony itself even more sacred.

Not surprisingly, one of the biggest culprits of sucking sacredness out of work is modern medicine. Ancient healers included the sacredness of all things in their practice. They tended to the body, but also the spirit. Today, after centuries in the other (and wrong) direction, a slowly increasing number of doctors are reconnecting with the sacredness of what we do, as these practices are more accepted and sought.

The time has come for us to understand and accept a core issue of healing and working: the issue of *spirit*, which, by its very existence, mandates the sacred nature of healing. This precept is more ancient than any medical discipline, even though it has been largely ignored since Descartes and Newton changed the medical world when they essentially separated the scientific from the phenomenal, or spiritual.

The Problem with Separating Work from Spirit

More recently, the explosion of technology-driven scientific information created more distance between doctors and patients. Modern medicine also narrowed its focus into specialties, pressuring young doctors to focus on one type or another. Now you walk into a doctor's office, clinic or hospital, and a person behind a computer or tablet meets you. They locate your name, enter your arrival and place a band on your arm to identify you. Everywhere you go, there is more staff armed with tablets, more forms to read and sign, and more data to enter. Often, they do not ask how you're doing, feeling, your symptoms or what brought you in—such basic caring questions. Finally, you see the doctor, who takes your history on a tablet or, worse, by dictation.

This new culture was created on the basis of natural order. New ideas grew from the concepts that science would lead us into a better world, away from ignorance, primitive notions and foolish beliefs. Technology provided the scientific community with compelling answers, but the ensuing tech explosion pushed aside family, community and consideration of spiritual or emotional matters in healing and caring.

For those of you who are raising kids, a quick question: How often and routinely do you sit down to a family dinner? A family conversation? A family activity? When I was a kid, the answer was, *almost every night*. Today? Not so much. Often, it's because we're all too busy with something else, engaged by a device in that busyness.

Going further, technology brought about the sharp decline of the family farm (replaced by agribusiness); the small corner grocery (replaced by supermarkets); hardware, toy, garden and department stores, and entire blocks of downtown "mom-and-pop" shops (replaced by Wal-Marts); and family-run bookstores with lovingly selected titles (replaced by chains and digital books). (Thankfully, independent bookstores are on the rebound; they and libraries always were the soul of the reading experience.)

It was often a simple act of *worship*, a sacred act for many, to walk down Main Street on a Saturday morning, buy a fountain soda, then shop from one store to another for groceries, fresh fruits and vegetables, clothes and other items—and have meaningful interaction with the store owners or salespeople. We have lost much of that *spiritual* connection between the product, the salesperson and the customer.

We can learn from our past. We need to find that sense of spirit again in order to restore our community culture—and ourselves—to health and to the planet.

Looking Again at the Nature of Work

Science is important and well intentioned, but we know now that it does not replace the importance of spirit and sacredness inherent in true healing, the nature of ourselves or nature on the planet. This translates to our sense of worship in work. We get into trouble when we think we are smarter than nature, and that goes for the nature of work as well. As medical intuitive and author Dr. Caroline Myss points out, "Our 'spirits' are longing to be recognized as legitimate, meaning they are every bit as real as our physical selves. Beyond the religious and poetic acceptance of the human spirit, our spiritual natures are breaking through the barriers of our psychological and emotional language, demanding to be identified as the underlying force of life from which all else flows."[31]

The *Somon*, a classic Chinese medical book written over 2,000 years ago, speaks of people that lived to be healthy centenarians (over 100 years old). They attributed such healthy life journeys to balanced living, tending to the body, mind, spirit (or religion), emotions, community and planet. An old Chinese proverb best describes this balance:

> *If there is light in the soul,*
> *There will be beauty in the person.*
> *If there is beauty in the person,*
> *There will be harmony in the home.*
> *If there is harmony in the home,*
> *There will be order in the nation.*
> *If there is harmony in the nation,*
> *There will be peace in the world.*

Similarly, in Ayurvedic thought, balance of body and spirit provides the key to healing. The body is a mini-universe governed by the same forces that govern the external world. As life enters our material body, three vital catalysts, or doshas, work in harmony to maintain health. They are vata (air and ether), pitta (fire) and kapha (water and earth). Disharmony among the doshas creates disease. A good diet, exercise, proper deeds and spiritual practice will help to keep the body balanced, enhancing our ability to live and work in a harmonious, sacred way.

According to Ayurvedic philosophy, our life is the sum of a series of relationships: with significant others; with work; with our body, mind and consciousness; with spirit; and with community and planet. Clarity in these relationships brings compassion, another form of love. Without clarity, there cannot be true insight. Ayurveda feeds the insight that brings harmony, happiness, joy and bliss in our daily lives and relationships.

The view of Native peoples is much the same. Revered medicine man Frank Fools Crow (1890–1989), ceremonial chief of the Oglala Lakota, spoke of the nature of the healing power:

> Even our physical bodies cannot contain us, because our spirits can step out of our bodies and spirit-travel. We dream and vision and have fantastic thoughts. This begins while we are still children. Because of it, we are always ready for *Wakan Tanka* (God) and the *Helpers* to take us places and show us things that others, because of their closed minds, may never see. The *Power* that we receive is for curing, healing, prophesying, solving problems and finding lost people or objects. It is also for spreading love, transforming and assuring peace and fertility (all aspects of sacred work). It is not to give us power over others, because the source of power is not ourselves . . . The power and ways are given to us to be passed on to others. To think or do anything else is pure selfishness. We only keep them and get more by giving them away, and if we do not give them away, we lose them.[32]

My teacher, Joseph Rael, taught me, "Work is worship." All work is worship. If it's not, we may need to change our workplace type of job, or method of worship. In our hyper-accelerated, 21st-century lives, we have to remember that all of life is sacred. Its very existence in our minds and on the tips of our tongues can bring about a sense of inner peace and healing, and provide deeper meaning to our work.

Take the farmers of Nepal's central highlands. The men and women work the millet, lentil and buckwheat terraces from dawn to dusk while chanting and chattering. Their work is vitally important: if they don't produce food, their communities don't eat. It is also part of a daily worship that integrates their Tibeto-Burman mixture of Hinduism and Buddhism, the land, each other, and their community. Life and work are equally sacred; there is no separation.

This is what we are intended to do, and to be.

As I mentioned before, my Native grandparents told me three things a human being needs to practice every day for a long and happy life, which was passed down from *their* grandparents: "Sing your song and give thanks every day (prayer, gratitude and spirituality); share bounty with your neighbor (good nutrition and community relationship); and dance (fitness and honoring the earth)."

At the time they told me these things, I asked, "Why isn't work on the list?"

They laughed. "Work is a prayer form, too. You have to work to grow and prepare the food to share with your neighbor. Before you dance, you need to clean your house and prepare the grounds for the people to come. Every day, we work and put prayers and thought into the work we are doing (mindfulness). We make offerings to our Mother Earth. When we have work like this that we enjoy, we are happy to be alive."

We all possess the gift of being alive and part of a greater circle of human beings, or "the collective," as psychic Edgar Cayce and psychologist Carl Jung put it. Some realize the gift of being alive from the beginning and lead very purposeful, sacred lives, while others come upon it later. In their work on this matter, Cayce and Jung spoke of the storehouse of universal symbols, knowledge and wisdom, closed to ordinary consciousness but accessible through the individual unconscious mind or spirit.

Let us take back our aliveness and mend the sacred hoop of living in harmony and balance with each other, the cosmic consciousness, and the planet. Let us open our eyes and see that life *is* sacred.

Worshipping Work in the Clinic: the Prayerful Practitioner

The power of prayer has been well documented. Author and esteemed medical expert Dr. Larry Dossey has compiled numerous studies demonstrating the beneficial power of prayer on subjects varying from bacteria in petri dishes to patients in cardiac care units. I wholeheartedly buy into this, right down to how I practice medicine. Praying for my patients has been part of my daily spiritual practice since I was at UCLA, and before that as a medical student.

I continue this tradition today. I pray for the clarity to serve in the highest way. I begin every day of work with a prayer and song. I pray mostly for humanity, the community and my patients to receive everything they need for wholeness and balance, and that we come with permission and a willingness to heal. These are necessary elements for healing. I pray that we learn to look to the earth as our forebears did, and to learn the recipes of nature, which hold the secrets of healing, with balance and sustainable medicine to keep ourselves and our planet healthy.

I think this approach needs to be adopted across the medical spectrum. The practitioner must be sensitive to each individual's belief systems when prayer is discussed or suggested. Prayer can be woven into whatever belief system is involved, even for those who do not believe in a higher power. Most people would agree that thought is a form of energy. Matter follows energy. A tree sends up branches to the sky and takes in light. The tree sends roots into the earth and draws energy from the soil. This process produces matter in the form of leaves, branches, trunks, stems and roots. All are forms of manifested energy.

The same interactions are possible for us. Energy can be directed to the body by thought or prayer, and matter can be changed, transmuted. The matter that makes up our body can be shaped by our conscious intent. Healing energy can be delivered to our bodies through the focused energy of prayer. We can also send this energy outward to affect others. Dr. Dossey meticulously described this phenomenon in his book *Healing Words*. He looked at prayers that faith-based individuals directed at unwell subjects, and at the prayers of individuals of no particular faith who also prayed for others. The result? All prayers were equally effective in creating beneficial outcomes.

Often, I send prayers for my patients, family or friends when I know they may be in special need. I focus my intent more if a person is having a hard time or going through something difficult like surgery, chemotherapy, loss of a loved one or divorce. I pray daily for all who come to me for guidance. Also, I pray to have the clarity and strength to see how to walk now with God, and to go where spirit is leading me. Through studies and compilations like *Healing Words*, and the work of people like William Braud, we know that prayer, remote healing and energy medicine have measurable physical effects. MRI studies show that activity increases in certain parts of our brains when distant deep, focused prayer is involved.

This power is demonstrated by Suzanne, a 46-year-old married woman with two children. Suzanne came to my office after being diagnosed with breast cancer for the second time in five years. Two weeks prior, she had reported to her doctor for her checkup. A five-year survival rate with breast cancer is typically a major milestone toward becoming fully cured. During this checkup, however, her doctor found a tumor in the remaining breast. Further, her doctor said there was a good chance the cancer had become metastatic and spread outside of her breast. A blood test revealed that the tumor markers specific for breast cancer, CA 15-3 and CEA, were elevated. Another showed abnormally elevated liver enzymes, suggesting a possible spread of her cancer to the liver. Worse, the pathology of her tumor biopsy showed a very aggressive type of breast cancer.

Suzanne was devastated when she visited my clinic. "Dr. Randall, what else can I do beside conventional therapy?" she asked. "I want to do everything this time."

I began to share options outside of the traditional surgery-chemo-radiation treatment triad. "The therapies I suggest will not interfere with your conventional therapy," I said, making sure I eased her mind. "Some small studies have even shown conventional therapy is more successful with the use of some alternative medicines. However, there are no guarantees."

I suggested tonic mushrooms (reishi, maitake and shitake) and astragalus to increase her immune response to cancer. I added antioxidants, herbal adaptogenic teas for stress (cordyceps and ashwaganda) and nutrient-based supplements to use in conjunction with her Western medical regime. Nutrients such as curcumin and boswellia serve to reduce the inflammation that comes with all forms of cancer.

Suzanne was scheduled for a right breast mastectomy the following week. "Are you spiritual?" I asked.

"Yes, I attend church."

"Contact your family, good friends, loved ones and the church where you belong, and ask for them to pray for you."

"Yes, they will put me into the prayer circle."

A week later, she underwent surgery. She healed well and began the natural regimen we designed. Two weeks after surgery, she visited her oncologist for a consultation about chemotherapy. When she walked into the office, a startling surprise waited: the pathology report showed her lymph nodes to be free of cancer. No signs of spread were found.

When she called me, she was so excited she could hardly get the words out. "Dr. Randall, Dr. Ra-Ra-andall! It's a miracle!"

"Whoa . . . slow down, Suzanne! What's happened?"

"My blood test showed my liver was normal, and the tumor marker has dropped into normal range." She and her family chose to wait and only do chemotherapy if signs of spread arose. Luckily, they have not to this day.

I smiled from ear to ear. "That *is* a miraculous turnaround."

Needless to say, Suzanne and her family were thrilled. They attribute this little miracle to the allopathic and natural medicine we practiced on her, *and* the power of prayer. She also worked on her own healing, energized by the greatest of purposes—to keep on living. And I had the honor of facilitating this. Work doesn't get much more sacred and worshipful.

I do not pretend to know all the ways we can pray and heal. My experience is all I can draw upon. We do need to be far more tolerant and respectful of the practices and religions of others because, let's face it: while we might call it different things or focus on different aspects, *all truly spiritual prayer is directed toward the same all-encompassing source that breathes life into all living things.*

The practice of prayer involves a communication with a greater energy force, both within and outside us… a higher consciousness. To some, this all-encompassing energy force is God; to others, it is Universal Intelligence. Some know it as the Great Mystery; those in India or sometimes in Catholic practices call it the Divine Mother. To others, it is something else. These names are simply different reflections of the greater force of the universe, which is available to all of us. We can pray alone or with others, which increases the power. Prayers may be practiced out loud, or in silence. No specific tools or paraphernalia are needed; the words or intent are left up to the individual or group doing the praying.

Giving thanks is a crucial part of prayer. Gratitude sheds a positive outlook and golden light on everything for which we give thanks. Appreciation for our gifts and lives places us in a state of mindfulness and changes our biochemistry, resulting in a higher vibration. According to the American Psychological Association, if you express pure gratitude or joy for 90 seconds, your immune system is strengthened for *up to 24 hours.* However, if you express pure anger for 90 seconds, it is weakened for *up to 8 hours.*[33]

Joseph Rael taught me that all of life is a prayer form. Gardening is a prayer form. So is cleaning the house, sweeping the floor or washing dishes. Your job and your work are a prayer form. How we keep our kitchens and prepare our food is a prayer form of the highest degree. Yogis give it a sacred name, *karma yoga.* When we do this with complete attention and honor for all living beings that gave of themselves so that we can live, we honor the plants, animals and the planet. This is the sacredness of work in action, the practice of work-as-worship in our deeds.

Some spiritual practices that help us to tune into our bodies included one-pointed silent meditation, walking in nature, reciting affirmations, visualizing the highest outcomes of any endeavor for ourselves and other active forms of mindfulness such as martial arts. You will know the spiritual practice that suits you by the deep sense of passion and vivacity you will feel during regular practice, and the deep peace that follows. A saying describes this: "calmly active and actively calm." If you have not meditated or practiced a prayer form, it may be awkward at first, just as with any new activity. With practice, it will become easier to drop into a relaxed calm state and clear the chatter from your mind.

Sometimes, when we become well-practiced, we enter a state of rapture like Bernini's famed the *Ecstasy of St. Teresa* sculpture, depicting St. Teresa's famous vision. An angel pierces her heart with a golden shaft, causing immense joy and pain. She is overcome with divine rapture.

Practicing Worshipful Prayer

How do we open our hearts and fan the passion of sacredness in our lives and our work? Begin by finding a calm, quiet place in your home where you will not be disturbed for 20 or 30 minutes. Sit in a comfortable chair or on the floor. Close your eyes and focus on your breath. If you feel any tightness in your body, use your breath to gently release it. Breathe in slowly through your nose to the count of five, then exhale slowly to the count of six. Whenever random thoughts enter your mind, allow and observe them, then use your breath to clear them away. If you're having trouble keeping your mind clear, don't worry; a busy mind is completely normal at first. The counting helps keep other thoughts out.

Some people find that meditating after exercise makes it easier to achieve the quiet mind, since the body is relaxed and emotional and physical toxins of stress are released. Release all obstructions to spirit. Allow yourself to be in the child-like space of giving and receiving. Once you are practiced, use visualization to clear your mind. I like to visualize a clear blue pool of water. Thoughts are ripples on the water and smooth out with the breath.

Other suggestions include drumming, dancing, mood music, concentrating on the flame of a candle or fireplace, sitting in nature, or watching the ocean or a river. There are also many classes and meditation apps or videos. I find that meeting with Mother Earth, whether inside or outside, helps me quiet my mind, ground myself and get into a higher consciousness—from where I do my best work.

CHAPTER 13

Mediterranean Diet: What's Good for the Planet Is Good for Us

What if someone approached you and made you an offer: *if you change the way you eat, you can save the planet.* Would you do it? Would you even believe it?

First of all, this statement is very real. If you switch to a primarily plant-based diet right now, and vote with your dollar on food-related issues, you can begin to change the planet *right this second.* If we had a switch *en masse,* we would significantly improve the planet. By looking at our earth and oceans in a sensitive way, we can see and sense messages the earth is sending us about the damage we are doing to our world and our health, and the way we should be eating.

Let's start with who we are in our deepest, most primordial selves. We used to be the same on the *inside* as our environment was *outside.* Our deep ancestors were one with the earth and environment. They nourished us and strengthened our bodies and immune systems by simply eating off the trees, bushes and the land, even ingesting a bit of soil. There are more microbes in one handful of healthy soil than there are people on the planet. This way of drawing sustenance and balance from the earth created and maintained harmony between humans and the environment. Our ancestors knew how to find this dietary balance. It reminds me of a refrigerator magnet I once saw: "Eat organic food, or as your great-grandparents called it, 'food.'"

Let's explore what eating wholesome food really looks like, inspired by the Mediterranean diet, which has been the mostly plant-based rage in recent years. I am also going to share the deeper story of why this is such an important way to eat today, for our health—and our planet's.

An Italian *Festa*

I have enjoyed the good fortune of traveling to Italy several times. I love the country, the food, the people and the history. One time, my good friend Mike asked his friend Ron to make all the arrangements. We traveled to Venice and they introduced me to Roberto and Roberta; we all immediately became close friends. Roberto and Roberta invited us into their lives and showed us the rich inner magic of Italian life—their love of food, music, family and friends. It was a most beautiful experience. They prepared meals for us, took us to community gatherings, introduced us to their two wonderful sons and much more.

One of the most stunning events was our midnight gondola rides. Night after night, we were the only boat on this section of the canals. So romantic! The flickering lights of the centuries-old *palazzi*, waterside cafés, boathouses and upscale *pensioni* (hotels) reflected off the perfectly smooth Grand Canal. Roberto's songs floated over us like a male loon, his voice backdropped by the muffled happy sounds of people enjoying themselves and laughing from the buildings. When he pulled up to docks at the backs of hotels, dashing Italian men ran out and passed us champagne and luscious snacks over the side of the gondola.

It was truly magical.

When we ate at their family home, it was so wonderful to witness and taste firsthand the most classic example of the Mediterranean diet. Roberta prepared a five-star meal and presentation in a three-foot by five-foot kitchen with one stove. She was a wizard. The meal was fancy and involved several courses. Let me tell you, it was nothing like the food that visitors and locals eat in the Italian *ristoranti* for the tourists that passes for authentic Italian. Not to mention the American versions. Eating is an event in Italy. It is designed to take several hours, involve several courses, lots of socializing and as many people as possible that fit around the table. Several members of their community and family joined us. We were treated as part of them, and there was much laughter and smiles all around. A perfect Italian red table wine accompanied our delectable meal, and an optional liqueur after the meal.

If you ever are so lucky to be invited to a native Italian's house, then remember to pace yourself—for the five or six courses that will be coming your way. Roberta started us out with finely spiced lentil carrot soup garnished with basil and breadstick crisps. Next was a huge platter of thinly sliced pieces of freshly roasted beef and poultry, garnished with thinly sliced onions and fermented vegetables. Then came my favorite, shrimp as big as lobsters and smothered with olive oil, garlic and fresh Italian spices. *Oh my goodness.* We feasted next on classic Italian semolina pasta, which comes from the original seed with a natural anti-gluten or gliadin ingredient. (Sadly, in America, our hybridization of wheat has removed that nutritional advantage and some of the taste.) The sauce was simple and very tasty, made from fresh tomatoes, onions, garlic and fresh herbs— but not too much. The bread was also fresh baked from semolina, crusty on the outside and soft on the inside. We dipped our delectable slices in locally sourced olive oil and thick aged balsamic vinegar, from the northern province of Modena. Following that was a gigantic plate of mackerel oven roasted in olive oil, stuffed with mushrooms and fresh herbs and garnished with basil. This dish was full of beneficial polyphenols and omega-3s, typical of the Mediterranean diet.

Finally, our last course came—a beautiful crisp dark green and purple lettuce salad freshly tossed with olive oil, balsamic and a touch of Mediterranean salt. Even though this seems odd to us Americans, having greens at this point was amazingly delicious and satisfying, cleared our palates and calmed our stomachs before dessert.

Dessert is not an everyday pleasure for most Italians, but we certainly were treated with a pomegranate pudding sprinkled with whole seeds and dark chocolate pieces on a flaky crust, warmed before the pudding was placed on big chunks of chocolate. Both pomegranates and chocolate are full of healing anti-inflammatory polyphenols.

I will always remember this taste treat. This meal typifies the health benefits of the Mediterranean diet, which also features community, family, good humor and love. Nutritionally, everything was locally sourced, full of polyphenols and omega-3s. It could not have been more delicious.

What Is a Mediterranean Diet?

A Mediterranean diet refers to the native foods of countries surrounding the Mediterranean Sea, such as Italy, Greece, Croatia, Egypt, Spain, Israel, Lebanon, Morocco and others. Many studies have shown that the diet is associated with significant health benefits against cardiovascular disease, stroke, diabetes, cognitive decline, obesity, osteoarthritis, cancer, hypertension and gastroesophageal reflux disease. In other words, it helps us to sharply mitigate or completely eliminate all the inflammation-based chronic diseases that result from the standard American diet (SAD). That diet is full of saturated fat, refined sugar (specifically high-fructose corn syrup) and refined carbohydrates—usually nonorganic and full of glyphosates, hormones and other poisons used in industrialized farming.

The principal aspects of the Mediterranean diet include a proportionally high consumption of olive oil, legumes, unrefined whole grain cereals, seeds and nuts, vegetables, green leafy vegetables and fruits. Some consume a high amount of fish, along with a moderately low amount of dairy, mostly in the form of yogurt and cheeses. Consumption of refined carbohydrates, sugary foods and red meat is also low. The cereals, fruits, vegetables and legumes not only have antioxidants, but fiber well known to benefit health by promoting a healthy microbiome and reducing gut and health problems. One more thing: those on Mediterranean diets sometimes consume a moderate amount of red wine, which contains health-promoting resveratrol.

Why is the Mediterranean diet so healthy? First, consider where it originates. As a whole, the Mediterranean region is sunny and mild to hot, and only humid for a few months per year. For much of the area, its climate is similar to Central and Northern California. Now think of eating food infused by all of this sun, added warmth and *light*, which *is* ingrained in the plant cells. When you eat a Mediterranean-type diet, you are absorbing the healing and restorative energy of the sun in ways people on the SAD or other less healthy diets do not.

When you further break down the Mediterranean diet, a great place to start is with the substance everyone in those countries puts first in the pan—olive oil. Olive oil is loaded with polyphenols, important and beneficial molecules for our bodies and brains. If grown organically in microbe-rich soil, they are abundant in nutrients, too. If the soil has been treated with chemicals, such as the glyphosates found in both agricultural and home gardening products, there are no microbes—and therefore no nutrients or polyphenols. The other huge health point to mention about polyphenols is that our guts need to have a balanced microbiome to digest these large molecules into smaller, potent antioxidant metabolites so they can be absorbed and utilized. They are active in preventing cognitive decline, heart disease and other inflammatory diseases.

By comparison, saturated fat from animals is associated with cardiovascular disease, diabetes, cancer and cognitive decline. Monounsaturated fat from olive oil does the opposite. It cannot be turned into an inflammatory molecule. Many studies have shown conclusively that a Mediterranean diet can reduce and even arrest progress of cognitive decline in people who already have it.

Another key Mediterranean diet ingredient is whole unrefined grains, whether cereals, pastas or cooked grains. Farmers have grown and fed grains to their livestock and families in the larger region for more than 5,000 years; archaeological digs show the earliest farmers were cultivating the land in parts of what is now Turkey, Syria and Lebanon up to 8,000 years ago, based on carbon dating of seeds found in ancient urns and containers.[34] Some of these are the "ancient grains" you see on food labels more and more—spelt, sorghum, amaranth, quinoa, millet, and kamut. Rice, wheat and barley also originated in the region; barley was the breakfast of choice for the famed Spartans of ancient Greece. However, unless you buy wild, colored or long-grain rice and original seed wheat, or buy any of these grains organically, then you won't receive the full benefit.

Then there is fish, one of the principal protein sources of the classic Mediterranean diet, full of omega-3 fatty acids. Things have changed—as in environmental and climate change. The ocean is struggling from toxicity, global warming, reef bleaching, overfishing and the dangerous prevalence of nanoplastics in every living sea creature—most especially fish, who are always on the move, and bottom-dwelling scavengers like shrimp and lobster, which also ingest heavy metals and toxins that reach the sea floor. For these reasons, it is important to know you don't have to eat fish for omega-3s.

I found a company that grows algae organically in man-made salt seas in the desert. Algae oil is better than fish oil because it is clean, organic and contains all the same beneficial omega-3s, DHA and EPA. IWI is an innovative company that creates and sells healthy nontoxic algae oil. Many of us also have metabolisms that can convert flaxseed oil to omega-3s, although it also comes with a complement of omega-6s. Another source of omega-3s is in grasses, such as wheat grass, but our bodies and cells do not absorb the omega-3s from flax seed and wheat grass as well as they do algae oil.

The Argument for Avoiding Fish

The ocean is one of the most toxic areas on the planet. The extreme toxicity of fish and the oceans comes from the heavy metals, toxins, glyphosates and other poisons dumped into the oceans from industries. Worse, these toxic substances bind tightly to the nanoplastics. Nanoplastics are about the size of a molecule, so they cannot be filtered out by any current filtration systems or methods. Which means that *all fish* are contaminated. It doesn't matter whether the fish was wild caught or farmed, large or small, deep ocean or shallow, warm Mediterranean waters or frigid North Atlantic seas. There is no escaping it.

The other huge problem in the Mediterranean Sea, as in all large seas and oceans, is the egregious open-water commercial fishing practice that is stripping our seas of fish, sharks, turtles, dolphins, whales and many other creatures, and making endangered species of them. Nets up to seven miles long drag along the bottom of the ocean, scraping out the coral reefs and sand-dwelling creatures. Oceans are already suffering a vast loss of life-producing coral from the increase in water temperature. Nets, when dropped to shallower depths, catch anything that swims past in the open sea, which accounts for much of what is called the bykill. Today, the bykill is three to one; in other words, for every intended fish they catch in the nets, three other creatures are captured and die as well. The nets kill them before they can be untangled and released. The tragedy here is this: crucial and endangered species that balance the ecosystem and ocean food chain are dying because of the vicious nets, including whales, dolphins, green turtles and others. The nets dropped into the ocean keep killing sea creatures long after the commercial fishing boats return to port, and are the largest contributors to ocean plastics and nanoplastic toxins. If stretched out, the nets would encircle the earth *500 times!* This practice should be outlawed, and a global ban enforced.

Ocean specialists say that, if commercial fishing continues unabated, we may not have any fish at all by the year 2040. Which presents more ramifications than I can count, including one you might not have heard about. The constant swimming motion of the fish, and the up-and-down flapping of their tails, actually keeps carbon dioxide embedded in the bottom of the sea floor. Without them, that carbon will join our already over-the-limit carbon debt.

What can we do? Well, ideally, the ocean needs for us to take a pause from our seafood-eating habits to regenerate. If the market for fish dries up, there will be no human need for gillnets anymore. In this case, vote with your dollar by not buying fish.

It is apparent to me that the health benefits of a Mediterranean diet are undeniable. I believe the secret "fountain of youth" formula within this style of eating is the high proportion of foods containing polyphenols and omega-3s, which protect us against the effects of stress and chronic inflammatory diseases. Another part of this diet is red wine, which contains resveratrol, another polyphenol known to lengthen telomeres on the ends of chromosomes, associated with longer lives. People who don't want to drink can eat the grapes. In addition to olive oil, this diet contains other polyphenol-rich foods, including pomegranates, chia seeds and cacao.

CHAPTER 14
Let's Talk Sensibly about Food

We need regenerative lifestyle practices to heal ourselves and the planet. What we mean by regeneration is the act of healing ourselves, others, community, humanity and the planet in every choice we make. This starts with us. How do we align our mindsets, eating and food buying practices, health and wellness choices, activities, relationships, and work to continually regenerate them, and in doing so, assist the regeneration of others/community/humanity/the planet? And what can we change in our current lifestyles to make that happen?

So let's focus on food: how do we nourish ourselves in a regenerative way and protect ourselves from the overall tainted food supply that we deal with every day?

We have moved so far away from the diet our predecessors ate and that packed our ancient genes with the instinctive memory of eating to live, rather than eating for creature comfort. Our bodies evolved to metabolize this moderate-protein, moderate-carb, high-fiber, plant-based and free-range diet over thousands of years. "What should we eat?" has become a complex question clouded by food fads, fast foods, industrially raised and processed foods, protein and fat controversies, and the latest diet-of-the-month offering miracle weight loss and health.

Let's talk about food sensibly. *Sensible* is the operative word here. However, most of us don't care about sensible; we want quick results and ease of preparation. A quick look at the diet section in any grocery store sheds a lot of light on the situation. Now, even low-carb stores capture the consumer dollar by demonizing a particular food group. It's not a new strategy. But we keep falling for it. Remember when all fat was considered bad? Now we know that some fat is good and essential for metabolic needs, though recent studies have shown any fat in excess raises insulin resistance, especially saturated fat. Remember the saying, "All things in moderation, including moderation?" How can *all* carbs or fats be bad? Or *all* protein be good? By simply mimicking our hunter-gatherer ancestors, known as biomimicry, we would eat primarily whole, plant-based foods that look like what they are: roots, vegetables, fruits, berries, maybe a few bugs. All coated with natural probiotics. It's really pretty simple.

The Problem with Industrialized Farming and Our Food Supply

Today, though, most of our nation's food supply is the opposite of organic. Or simple. Factory industrial farming is very damaging to the planet, and us. Most industrialized farming is dependent on chemicals, such as glyphosates, which eventually strip the land of microorganisms. Those microbes are key for fertilizing plants and keeping carbon trapped in the soil and plant roots. In addition, glyphosates and other chemicals are proven to cause cancer and other chronic diseases.

Industrialized farming should be legally prohibited. Our meat, feed crops and basic grains (wheat, corn, soybeans, white rice) are processed in ways that renders them almost devoid of nutritive value and toxic. Not to mention sterilized of healthy microbes, irradiated, plastic-wrapped, pasteurized, microwaved and made extremely harmful to the environment. According to a 2017 video on *The Atlantic* website, if we in the United States merely replaced meat with beans, we'd mitigate much of the *world's* greenhouse gas and global warming problem.[35]

Factory farming magnifies climate change by releasing huge volumes of greenhouse gases, in particular CO_2 and methane. Standard livestock production accounts for *14.5 percent* of all human-caused emission.[36] In addition to factory farming impacting climate change so negatively, we also end up with nutrient-poor food with little of its natural taste. (For a quick taste test, compare a store-bought tomato or cucumber to one that is garden raised or organically grown.) Or, our foods are overwrought with additives, preservatives and artificial sweeteners. The central additive, high-fructose corn syrup, approved by the FDA in 1972, is a perfect example. It is a major contributor to obesity, cardiovascular disease and type 2 diabetes, among others.

So, I ask once again: why are we putting our food supply through these unnatural processes? For the past century, chemicals and pollutants used to increase food volume and income for agribusiness, primarily through the creation of pesticides and fertilizers, have contaminated our environment. They are literally killing people by acting as carcinogens and potent neuroendocrine disruptors! Isn't food supposed to *sustain us*? The chemicals we place on the land also attack microbes, which results in produce with beautiful polish and shape, but totally lacking in nutrients.

Which leads to the big question: what is the right diet for you and your family? Is it a standard American diet of bread, pasta, meats, potatoes, fast foods, and white and processed foods? Along with sugary desserts or sodas? And are those regular or diet sodas? Regular soda increases inflammation, insulin and glucose levels, and increases diabetes risk. Diet soda contains aspartame, which converts to formaldehyde in the body—and spikes glucose and insulin, also leading to pre-diabetic conditions. Most of us know this is not the best way. Gluten can also be inflammatory, especially if derived from industrially raised wheat (which contains glyphosates). Nonorganic, hormone-laden meats are carcinogenic and inflammatory because of the animal fat, which contains herbicides, fungicides, pesticides and hormones.

The best food style choice is a mostly plant-based diet, with meat if you feel the need. If so, go with organic grass-fed pasture-raised meats (regeneratively farmed), fruits and vegetables, and some healthy grains. "Grass-fed" or "free-range" meat or poultry is not the same as certified organic, nor the same as regeneratively raised, which is best for you, your family and the planet. Be sure they are both.

My personal favorite diet is a whole-food plant-based diet with organic fruits and vegetables, along with organic non-GMO soy and pea or other legume proteins. There are many good sources of amino acids (proteins) for vegans; the best are peas and soy. We've all been brainwashed to think our bodies need protein in the form of animal products. Not true. It is really about getting enough amino acids, the building blocks of protein, in the right complement. Our bodies were designed to make protein out of plants. How do you think the cow does it? That said, I do feel if people feel they need meat, it should be regeneratively raised.

Many people worry about lectins in legumes, an amazing source of amino acids. Legumes and lectins have been vilified. In fact, one form of lectin is toxic and can contribute to leaky gut (see Chapter 17), the phytohemagglutinin found in raw kidney beans. However, you would have to consume massive amounts, and the toxic elements are removed easily by soaking overnight and cooking slowly. If you are concerned use red beans instead. Legumes are excellent plant-based foods. You can also use a pressure cooker—main thing is to cook them at the correct temperature for long enough. Boil unsoaked beans for at least 30 minutes or presoaked beans for 15 minutes, cook for 2 hours at 176 degrees, or cook in a pressure cooker for 45 minutes at 15 psi. (Note that slow cookers do not get hot enough to kill the toxin.)

Don't We Need Animal-Based Proteins?

Some vegans consistently seek protein through animal substitutes, like new plant-based meat replacement patties available in fast-food restaurants and stores. These are often unhealthy as well. Beyond Meat is a good choice for amino acids for legumes and spinach, but it is not organic—and each patty contains 280 milligrams of sodium. It is non-GMO, true, but nonorganic is a deal breaker for me. I do not recommend any food containing toxic chemicals. Dr. Praeger's burgers are organic, but they contain a substantial amount of gluten. The Impossible Burger, made of GMO soy (watch out for GMO!), has more cancer-causing glyphosates than Beyond Burgers. Like they say on *Shark Tank*, "I'm out!"

I am still looking for a good, clean organic patty to recommend to patients.

I like to pose a question to those who are convinced we just *have to have animal protein:* if it were true that we need animal protein to survive and be strong, then why do silverback gorillas have so much muscle? Every day, the silverback eats about 60 pounds of food, drawn from up to *142* different sources, primarily bamboo shoots and berries, leaves, and other plant matter. They never touch meat. Other vegetarian animals that far out-size and out-muscle humans include whales, hippos, horses and dolphins.

I always teach my patients to eat non-processed food. Processed meats have been shown to be highly associated with diabetes, heart disease and cancer. This is primarily due to toxic, inflammatory chemicals they ingest in the nonorganic grains they eat in feedlots or on farms. These meats fill with cytokines, which initiate the inflammatory response in humans. And remember: inflammation is the biggest killer of all, or at the least a major contributing factor, regardless of the disease or illness.

Let's look for a second at regenerative ranching of animals, which is finally starting to catch fire. Regeneratively raised cattle eat grasses high in phytonutrients and completely empty of chemicals. This is healthy beef. If your choice is to include meat, make it regeneratively farmed, or at the very least, *organic* grass-fed and pasture (free-range) raised meat, poultry and dairy. However, often these are tough to sort out and our labeling does not help. Grass fed could still be penned up and abused animals, or just grass finished.

We would greatly reduce greenhouse gases if we substituted beans for meat as a population. We could reduce the allocation of 70 percent of health-care dollars to chronic diseases by leaning toward a plant-based diet. Also, it has been conjectured that if we invested as much money and acreage into plant crops for *our* food purposes, as we do for growing livestock, we could feed the world.

Studies have shown that a whole-food plant-based diet can reduce and "click off" your genes for breast cancer, prostate cancer and heart disease in only three months.

Whole means *complete*, and not *broken down*. Try to avoid foods ground down into a powder and pressed out into flakes, loaves, bars, crusts, cookies, chips or crackers. They are processed, which converts to sugar in your body more quickly and makes those foods too glycemic. Gluten-free organic whole grains like colored rice, quinoa, buckwheat, sorghum and flax are excellent sources of nutrition.

Be mindful and wary of new diet crazes. Make sure your choice is wholesome and works for you. I knew about the keto diet before it came out, but then watched it become a fast-spreading national sensation. Personally, though, I believe it more a fad than a way of life. It may be good for temporarily losing weight and perhaps cleansing. However, anything that makes you *ketotic* also makes you *acidotic*. (We should try to avoid acidic diets, because they promote inflammation and dissolution of healthy bones. Significant inflammation is a common denominator of *all* fatal diseases.)

The only reason a ketotic diet works is because your body has learned a way to survive and feed the brain during times of emergency. However, we do not want to keep our bodies in that alarming state. Many doctors have seen patients on keto diets have developed elevated cholesterol levels, increased CRP (C-reactive protein levels) indicating inflammation, and decreased bone density on DEXA scans. None of these are desirable. Newer studies have shown any fats in excess cause insulin resistance, including healthy fats. In conclusion, the best foods are primarily organic plant based, low refined carb, moderate fat (for good fats see below), and occasional regeneratively farmed meats, poultry and eggs.

The Benefits of Fasting

Intermittent fasting is a fantastic way to detoxify and purify your body, while giving your digestive system an occasional rest from its endless work of breaking down our food. Plus, it saves on food bills!

Which leads to the first bit of good news: *you don't have to fast for two or three days to achieve effective results!* I usually choose to fast 12 to 14 hours per day, including my sleep time, and try not to eat from dinner until the following mid-morning or lunch. Whatever timed eating pattern works for you is best. We are all different. There are even genetic tests that show what is the best way and best food for each person. The key point is fasting reduces insulin resistance and increases sensitivity to CCK and insulin—reducing HbA1C, blood sugar and weight.

Healthline listed these most popular methods of intermittent fasting:

- The 16/8 method: Also called the Leangains Protocol, this involves skipping breakfast and restricting your daily eating period to eight hours (say, 11 a.m. to 7 p.m.). Then fast for the 16 hours in between.
- Eat-Stop-Eat: This involves fasting for 24 hours, once or twice a week. One suggested interval is to not eat from dinner one day until dinner the next.
- The 5:2 diet: Consume only 500 to 600 calories on two non-consecutive days of the week, but then eat normally the other five days.

These types of timed eating are effective for weight loss, weight control, lowering blood sugar, increasing insulin sensitivity and increasing your metabolic function. They have also been credited for remediating cognitive decline. Make appointments with yourself for mealtimes, keep the appointments and eat mindfully. Eat slowly and appreciate every bite. Don't skip meals, and do not eat outside of your scheduled times. Anything you eat after dinner, you wear.

Overcoming Emotional Eating

Recognize and gain control over emotional eating. If you are feeling stressed out, pressured, depressed, anxious or bored, then ask yourself, "Am I using food to soothe or stuff my feelings?" Instead of reaching for that bag of potato chips, cookie or candy bar, ask yourself, "What's eating me?"

Now, change the channel when it comes to your emotional eating. Go for a walk or run, put on some music, call a friend, do some yoga postures or stretching, take a 10-minute prayer or meditation break, or play with your dog. Then, get into the habit of drinking half your body weight in water daily, as measured in ounces; if you weigh 140 pounds, drink 70 ounces (just over one-half gallon). This is a lot for me, but I too shoot for it. I weigh about 145 pounds, and drink three 20-ounce cups of pure filtered water per day, plus tea. That adds up to about 68 ounces, a little short of the 72-ounce "halfway" mark. My point is, get into that range with your daily water consumption.

Another good step is to count to your age before you "*ch*-eat." You always have a choice. If you do choose to ch-eat, enjoy it thoroughly. Here, I turn to Randall's Rule: It's not what you do 10 to 20 percent of the time, but what you do the other 80 to 90 percent that creates your health. If you are truly on goal 80 to 90 percent of the time, then you can indulge in those treats once in a while. But I also caution you, do not feel defeated if you fall off the wagon. Everyone falls now and then. If you beat yourself down, you are more likely to continue a downward cycle. Learn from your mistakes and cravings, whether chemical, emotional or both. Be gentle to yourself and know you can improve with help and good intention.

Do whatever it takes to distract yourself from craving and eating unhealthy food.

Are Carbs Truly Demons?

Refined carbohydrates are not healthy when eaten in excess. This is nothing new. Still, it's a huge problem in wealthier countries, including ours, and it results in the high obesity rates we experience today. It begins with the way we refine grains like corn, soybeans, wheat and other crop plants. Man has altered these seeds and grains to extract the sugary portion, leaving the much more nutritious roughage and protein behind. Grains are also ground down into a paste, which partially "digests" the food for us, allowing our bodies to convert it to sugar all too easily. Take the high-fructose corn syrup found in much of our food supply. By the time the amylase enzyme in our saliva starts breaking down the corn syrup and it arrives in our intestine, it has already been converted to pure sugar.

Health practitioners have long counseled weight-loss clients to avoid refined sugars (desserts, cakes, pastries, candies), wheat products (refined breads, pasta, crackers), white rice, and bottled juices. These are high glycemic foods. *Glyc* is the root for sugar and *emic* means "in the blood"; literally, *glycemic* means "sugar in the blood." This acidifies our body (adding to inflammation), leaches calcium out of our bones (promoting osteoporosis), causes insulin levels to spike (leading to syndrome X—obesity, hyperinsulinemia, insulin resistance), and contributes to hypoglycemia (low blood glucose from insulin overshoot), obesity and dysbiosis.

Dysbiosis is an imbalance of the bacteria and flora in the gastrointestinal tract. The sugar promotes growth of unfriendly bacteria, candida or yeast and other organisms, which crowds out and decreases the healthy normal organisms, or flora. It disrupts the brain-gut axis and affects our immunity. Over time, this can lead to illness, arthritis, irritable bowel syndrome, inflammatory bowel disease, and other chronic inflammatory diseases and autoimmune diseases. *Avoid refined carbohydrates.*

What about unrefined carbs? They are highly desirable in the form of fruits and they help to prevent cancer, aging and chronic diseases, loaded as they are with antioxidants and fiber. Epidemiologic studies have shown significantly lower rates of colon and breast cancer, type 2 diabetes and cholesterol levels in people who consume five or more servings of fruits and vegetables a day.

Many beneficial nutrients exist in fruits and vegetables to keep us in a state of balanced health. Violet-, blue- and red-colored foods contain anthocyanidins, potent antioxidants. Eggplants, grapes, raspberries, strawberries, turmeric and green tea contain phenols, which protect our DNA from damage by cancer-causing chemicals. Foods containing thiols from the *Allium* family are antiviral, antibacterial, antifungal, anti-inflammatory, anticancer, antimutagenic, and cause tumor inhibition and improve immune responsiveness and circulation. These foods include garlic, chives, leeks, onions, shallots, and cruciferous vegetables (broccoli, cabbage, cauliflower, turnips, bok choy, collards, kale, chard, kohlrabi, mustard greens, rutabaga and watercress). People in Mediterranean countries consume large amounts of these types of foods, with olive oil, which includes polyphenols that are processed by gut bacteria, making them bioavailable. They also develop less coronary heart disease.

Cruciferous vegetables contain glucosinates and sulforaphane, substances that block tumor-promoting enzymes and are antioxidants. Grains, green vegetables and soy contain terpenes, which protect against free radicals that contribute to aging, chronic diseases and cancer. Soy-based foods such as tofu, tempeh, soy milk, soybeans, and soy nuts have also been shown in vitro studies to switch off the growth of cancer cells, while providing phytoestrogens (plant-based estrogen-like products), which can ease the symptoms of menopausal transition.

Fruits also contain abundant nutrients. These include potassium, fiber, vitamin C and folic acid. Diets high in potassium help to maintain lower blood pressure.

Anthocyanidins are also abundant in blueberries, grapes and grape seeds, apples, beans, cranberries, peaches, plums, raspberries, rhubarb, strawberries and pine bark (pycnogenol). They are potent antioxidants, which neutralize free radicals and block cancer initiators and promoters. These anti-inflammatory agents also are neuroprotective, antiaging and anticancer.

Beneficial carbs are essential to our diets. You and your body will notice when you replace refined carbs with healthy food by your increased energy, mental dexterity, gut health, spirit for life and reduced body fat.

Fats: the Good, the Bad and the Ugly

Like carbs, fats often get a bad rap. Because many eat harmful fats and refined carbs, health-conscious people seeking a better diet sometimes conclude wrongly that all fats are bad.

That's not the case. We just need to know which fats to eat—and which to avoid. When I'm working with patients, I refer to what I call the "Good, Bad and Ugly" of fats in our diet. Here's a look.

The Good: Polyunsaturated, Omegas and Monosaturated

Polyunsaturated fat is found mostly in nuts, seeds, fish, seed oils and oysters. The omegas include three particular sets of polyunsaturated fatty acids. Omega-3s come from fish oil and plants such as algae, pigweed, nuts and seeds. It includes EPA (eicosapentaenoic acid) and DHA (docosahexaenoic acid) from fish, and ALA (alpha-linoleic acid) from nuts and seeds. Conversely, omega-6s, 7's and -9s derive from seeds and nuts. All omega fatty acids need to be balanced for appropriate cell membrane function. Many of our functional medicine tests now measure omegas and report on their balance.

Omega-3 is called an "essential fat" because the body can't produce it naturally. EPA helps reduce inflammation and reduces symptoms of depression, schizophrenia and bipolar disorder, and also reduces the risk of psychotic behavior in those at risk. It can also reduce cognitive decline and improve inflammation or arthritis, autoimmune diseases, and cardiovascular function. It increases our good cholesterol (HDL) and DHA, crucial for brain development and function; DHA makes up 8 percent of our brain's weight. Omega-3 comes from converting ALA from nut and seed plants, which changes into EPA and DHA that the body uses for energy. ALA is a fatty acid. Omega-3 also reduces low-density lipoprotein (LDL), which transports cholesterol through the body. This can improve the cardiovascular system by decreasing blood pressure and reducing the formation of plaque in vessels.

In addition to reducing inflammation, EPA can support brain development along with DHA, promote bone health and reduce asthmatic symptoms.

The Western diet is a poor source of omega-3s. It does, however, have a predominant amount of omega-6 fatty acids, primarily a source of energy. The most common is linoleic acid. They can also be converted to arachidonic acid, which is pro-inflammatory, especially if too much is consumed. The recommended intake ratio of omega-6 to omega-3 is 4:1. Unfortunately, in the standard American diet, the ratio is closer to 10:1, which creates a pro-inflammatory diet.

Just to make it more interesting, gamma-linoleic acid, or GLA, is a "good" omega-6 fatty acid, drawn from primrose or borage oil. The body converts it into dihomo-gamma-linoleic acid (DGLA), which is anti-inflammatory and reduces arthritis symptoms.

The body can produce omega-9 fatty acids. Oleic acid is the most common monosaturated fatty acid in our diet. It comes from olive, coconut, avocado, macadamia and other non-inflammatory nut oils. Omega-9s are also sourced from nuts and seeds, as well as our own bodies.

In general, it is best to focus on a balance of omega-3s, -6s and -9s. Use proportions of 4:1:1. But limit the intake of unhealthy omega-6s from refined vegetable oils and fried foods. Refined vegetable oils, the cooking staple of fried fast food, often use hexane, which is both a carcinogen and neurotoxin. Fried foods often emerge from overheated oils, which result in advanced glycation end products that lead to heart disease, colon and stomach cancer, and diabetes. Omega-9s do not need to be supplemented, because the body makes its own, and they are abundant in meat (animal fat) and refined vegetable oil.

Monounsaturated fats are the only fats that cannot be made into an inflammatory molecule; they are extremely beneficial. They can be found in olive oil and avocados. Coconut and palm oil also are good sources, primarily because of their antioxidant qualities. (Unfortunately, palm oil's healthy qualities are offset by the environmental devastation caused by how it's farmed. Millions of acres of rainforest have been cleared for palm farms, damaging the ecosystem.)

We need a certain amount of good fat for production of good cholesterol (HDL), hormone production and to keep the inflammation-causing levels of prostaglandin type 2 at bay.

The Bad: Saturated and Trans Fats

Saturated fat and trans fat pertain to fatty acid chains that have a predominantly single chain of hydrogen molecules. Some of you might remember your grandmother cooking with Crisco or lard. Remember how the fat stayed solid until it was heated? If it doesn't melt on a hot day on Grandma's counter, what do you think is going to happen when it enters our stomachs and bloodstreams? These artery-clogging fats form when vegetable oils are hardened into margarine or shortening. The hydrogenated, man-made fats result from raising the temperature to over 700 degrees and bubbling hydrogen through to add hydrogen molecules, which changes the molecular form of the fat.

Trans fats are made through a chemical process called hydrogenation: hydrogen molecules are added to all the carbon sites in the molecule. Many food companies use it instead of oil because it reduces cost, extends the storage life of products, and can improve flavor and texture. However, hydrogenation solidifies the fat and makes it so unhealthy that, in 2018, the FDA required trans fats to be removed from foods, the same year the World Health Organization called for a global ban. However, they still exist in pizza crusts, baked goods and other foods as a preservative, so read your labels.

Most animal fats are saturated, as opposed to fats in plants and fish, which are generally unsaturated. Saturated fats tend to have a higher melting point, making them solid at room temperature. These nonorganic animal fats are inflammatory. And carcinogenic.

The health issues associated with trans fats are numerous. They are known to increase blood levels of low-density lipoprotein (LDL), or "bad" cholesterol, while lowering levels of high-density lipoprotein (HDL), known as "good" cholesterol. They can also cause major clogging of arteries, type 2 diabetes, and increase the risk of cardiovascular and all inflammatory diseases.

Read the ingredient label and look for shortening, hydrogenated fat or oil, or partially hydrogenated oil. The higher up on the list these ingredients appear, the more trans fat you will find in the food. You can also add up the broken-down list of fat on the label. (Note: fat designations are a relatively new labeling requirement.) If they don't match up, the difference is likely the trans fat slipped inside, especially if partially hydrogenated oil is listed as one of the first ingredients.

The Ugly: Omega-6 Vegetable Oils, Sugars

The intake of omega-6s, particularly through soybean oil, began to increase in the USA in the early 2000s, when butter and lard began to decline. This caused a more than two-fold increase in the intake of linoleic acid, the main omega-6 polyunsaturated fat found in refined vegetable oils. Our cell membranes use linoleic acid to synthesize prostaglandins, which helps the body build muscle and reduce fat. Natural sources include flax seeds, rapeseeds, soybeans, pumpkin seeds, tofu and walnuts.

Unfortunately, linoleic acid from refined vegetable oil is associated with an increase in heart disease, as well as cognitive decline. In a country dealing with serious cardiovascular and cognitive issues, we need to be really mindful of the balance of omega-3s-6s-9s. Remember the 2:1:1 ratio I mentioned earlier.

Harmful Sugars: Food Supply Enemy #1

Now we get to "Public Enemy Number One" in our food supply—harmful sugars. Sugar is one of the biggest contributors to illness in our country. How bad is it? Functional medicine expert Dr. Mark Hyman, author of *The Food Fix*, minces no words. He calls sugar a "recreational drug."[37] Sugar lights up our nucleus acumens, or addiction center of the basal ganglia in the hypothalamus of our brains. Some studies have shown that it's harder to kick a sugar addiction than it is heroin, alcohol, nicotine or even opioids.

I believe we were born with a sugar addiction, though while human beings were evolving, sugar in its purified form did not exist. Our hunter-gatherer ancestors found a small amount of sugar available in overripe fruit, a flower or honey. That small amount became a survival advantage because of the energy it provided. Their bodies responded, and the mechanism that drives our sugar cravings evolved. This innate craving was passed down to us, and it seems stronger than ever. So strong that today, it's not a survival gene but an *anti-survival* one.

Sugar causes imbalance in our bodies. Within our digestive tract, our guts grow unhealthy organisms under the influence of excess refined carbs and sugar, and our metabolisms shift because of the excessive glycemic load. This causes weight gain, leaky gut and inflammation. It also weakens our immune system and disrupts our gut-brain axis. Inflammation is particularly concerning, since it is the common denominator of all chronic disease: heart disease, cognitive decline, arthritis, autoimmune disease, diabetes, asthma, cancer and others. Sugar also feeds anxiety and depression, and makes us emotionally unstable, possibly through the imbalance of the gut-brain axis.

The best thing you can do to promote longevity and health is to cut out overt sugar and refined carbs. Get your body back in line. See your doctor and make sure your hemoglobin A1C (HbA1C) is normal. HbA1C, or glycated hemoglobin, is a blood test that can measure the amount of sugar or glucose attached to hemoglobin in our red cells. It can estimate the average blood sugar level over the last three months.

The next item to look at critically, and consider stopping, is refined carbs. Once you are stable and free from symptoms like aching, bloating, gas, diarrhea, excess weight and constipation, you can make refined carbs a "sometimes food" or treat, like a piece of cake or ice cream on your birthday or a cookie at Christmas.

Ideal Sources for Meat Products

Now let's go back to our meat products and their sourcing. We've already discussed the importance of sourcing pasture-raised free-range meat. Honestly, when it comes to meat products, they really need to be *organic* pasture-raised free-range, because the collected herbicides, pesticides and fungicides within animal fat makes it dangerous, inflammatory and cancerous. If the animals are not happy, which the majority of livestock *is not*, I call it "eating our own misery." Miserable DNA alone would be enough to damage us. However, it comes with a highly toxic frosting of carcinogenic (cancer-causing) chemicals.

The best way to source meats for those that want to eat it is to work with a regenerative farm (see below). Animals on regenerative farms are happy because they live in a natural environment, which has been copied from nature using biomimicry. However, most of the meat industry does not follow suit. It's as industrial as can be. If you've ever had to hold your nose while driving by noxious feedlots, you've seen and smelled it for yourself. All the animals are crowded together and given growth hormones and antibiotics, in addition to the chemical-laden foods they are fed. *When you eat meat, you eat what they ate.*

The Future of Food: Regenerative Agriculture

If meat is something you still feel you need, there's a growing source of pasture-raised meat, with no growth hormones or other harmful chemicals. They are known as regenerative ranches and can be found online. These are among several new biosustainable models for the future growth of food; a few great resources for future farming are Blue Nest Beef, Primal Pastures and Kiss the Ground. Kiss the Ground produced a great documentary which, in my opinion, should be part of health class curriculum in schools.

Also of note is a new kind of nontoxic indoor farming. OnePointOne Willo vertical farming, for which I served as board member. VertiFarm, as the vertical farming movement is known, is quite big in Europe and making an impression in the US.

What exactly is regenerative ranching? It is a pasture-raised form that mimics the predator/prey relationship, known as biomimicry. All of the animals we sang about in "Old McDonald's Farm" as schoolkids—cows, chickens, pigs, sheep, ducks—are all together on an open piece of land. The animals feel respected and happy. By restoring farms to their natural states, and by moving the animals from area to area on a farm, they also restore the grasslands, which not only produces organic products, but also replenishes oxygen and draws down carbon dioxide. Additionally, they grow fruits, vegetables, grains and other crops in exactly the same way. The best part? *No pesticides, herbicides, growth hormones or other byproducts are used.*

While this probably seems radical and new to farmers and others today, it is the way *all farmers* raised crops, livestock, farm animals and their own vegetables for the first 160 years of our nation's history. When agribusiness emerged after World War II, everything changed.

Regenerative farming of crops and animals can slow carbon emissions and even hold in place carbon dioxide, the primary greenhouse gas. It sequesters carbon within the soil and plants. Tilled soil releases carbon into the atmosphere, which combines with oxygen to make carbon dioxide. Instead, these farmers use composting to minimize tilling, along with cover crops and crop rotation, hedges and windbreaks to reduce carbon loss. When you put it all together, crop yields increase markedly—in volume *and* in healthiness—and livestock health improves. The restoration of native grasslands and wetlands on the property creates greater resistance to drought, reduces erosion and flooding, and improves water retention in the soil. This gives farmers the ability to stop using synthetic fertilizers and grow more diverse crops, far more than the obligatory beans, corn and wheat, the government-subsidized crops.

Over time, these practices reduce costs and possibly the need for federal subsidies, saving taxpayers money—and giving farmers more freedom to manage their farms without the watchful eye of the US Department of Agriculture, which is tight with top chemical, pesticide and herbicide manufacturers in a way that does not result in healthier food for us.

To learn more about this, I spoke with Kentucky-based regenerative farm pioneer Timothy Kercheville. I was so moved by his efforts that I invited him on my *Soul Stories* podcast. Timothy went beyond merely restoring farms to their natural states, even incorporating what's good about regular industrialized farming.[38] For starters, he looked at the economics. Today, few farmers truly make money from taking animals, milk, grain or produce to market. They make a living because the government subsidizes them. In 2018, the farm bill passed by Congress totaled $428 billion, much of that subsidies.

Timothy persuaded some local governments to support regenerative farms for the people of Kentucky. "Grow local, buy local" is the healthiest philosophy we can adapt to buy truly organic and nutritious meat and produce, because the product goes from farm to table, without trucks, warehouses and age-preservatives wearing down the nutritional value.

Timothy taught me the regenerative agriculture movement has mostly focused on techniques that promote soil health and biodiversity in farm contexts. This brings up the number one problem in agriculture today, the very problem preventing the regenerative agriculture movement from spreading broadly across the US: the overproduction of commodities.

Regenerative agriculture will have much more room to flourish when we control production of the major commodities. Overproduction is an enormous waste of food and money in a world increasingly starving. Overproduction drops the price of commodities and encourages planting even larger acreage, with subsidies and crop insurance guaranteed. Worse, it squeezes out the family farms that grew America and many of its values. That presents insurmountable obstacles to young and beginning farmers, creating a graying industry (the median age of today's farmer is nearly 60).

With his approach, Timothy and other regenerative farmers may hold a key to saving our planet. He is slowly transforming farming in Kentucky while restoring the grasslands and forests through agroforestry. He has become a transformational coach for farmers changing over. Tim reported on Facebook that his company Festina Lente Farms keeps getting hired to design, install and help manage farms and gardens further south into Tennessee. Kentucky and Tennessee are becoming regional (and, hopefully soon, national) agricultural models, regional exporters of whole foods, sustainable fiber and fuel economy in both rural and urban contexts. Truly groundbreaking! This is the wave of the future. It warms my heart to watch this movement grow rapidly. There are many small regenerative farms rising up around California as well, which is very encouraging.

Recently I had the great opportunity and privilege of talking to and working with Charles Dowding.[39] He was one of the first and most respected regenerative "no-dig" farmers/gardeners in the world apart from the ancients. Inspired by his choice to be organic vegetarian and desire for fresh food, he began this type of farming in the 60s. Since he began his efforts in Somerset, not 10 miles from where he grew up on a dairy farm, he has studied the best ways to grow plant-based food. Although he specializes in lettuce, he grows every kind of vegetable you can imagine.

I am impressed by his dedication to research. One of his takeaways is that the less you interfere with nature's processes, the better your garden grows. For instance, plants love friends. When you plant them close together and allow them to network their roots, it increases the yield. It also increases the soil health and results in more microbe-rich soil. While he has some suggested rules to follow, in most cases, less is more. This supports the notion of the "milpa" gardens from the ancients in South and Central America. They took seeds of all types of vegetables and fruits and dispersed them randomly without digging or tilling, allowing them to grow where they wanted. This technique gave greater yields than the more labor-intensive method of digging rows. That process actually injures the soil, which takes time to heal before growth occurs. It yields more bounty when you do less. He has also studied the carbon release from soil, backed up by larger studies which measured atmospheric carbon and showed that dig methods release carbon, adding to the carbon debt, and no-dig methods preserve it in the soil. He uses compost which also likes to be undisturbed for the highest number of microbes and nutrients.

I loved the story about his lettuce. First, don't cut them—gently tear or break them from the mother plant. One restaurant owner told him Charles's lettuce was superior because "the leaves could stand the dressing," meaning they were stronger and crisper, indicating health.

His passion for growing food is evident. He calls his three-acre farm Home Acres and emphasizes that you don't need a vast amount of land to be successful. Charles has several books and is currently working on one for children, *No Dig for Kids.* You can find his online courses and his YouTube channel at charlesdowding.co.uk.

For a deeper understanding of the regenerative farmer/gardener and their passion for the land, the planet, food production and consumption, and regenerative lifestyles check out the *Soul Stories* podcasts for both Timothy Kercheville and Charles Dowding.

There is no one perfect diet for everyone. However, I feel the whole-food plant-based Mediterranean-like diet is the best for our bodies, and makes the best use of the planet's resources while also reducing greenhouse gases. For the highest degree of health, we need organic, locally grown, plant-based fresh whole foods. Building muscle and strength is really about getting the right amino acids. The adage that you have to eat meat to make meat is simply not true. You need to eat the appropriate amount of amino acids (protein) for your body size and activity. What is good for the planet is good for us.

CHAPTER 15
A Word about Vitamins and Supplements

Our diets and food choices provide us with enough vitamins and minerals to keep us healthy and solid without taking a multivitamin/mineral or supplement . . . right?

Food should be plentiful in vitamins and minerals, and it certainly used to be the case. But not anymore. The Organic Consumers Association, University of Texas Department of Chemistry and Biochemistry, and a number of European studies show that soil mineral content has depleted by 60 to 80 percent since 1930—right before industrialized farming entered our food supply along with World War II.[40] Consequently, other studies show up to 50 percent fewer vitamins and nutrients in our food compared to the pre-war supply—and much higher for crops like carrots and tomatoes. Not only have we lost 20 percent of the topsoil we had in 1930, but an additional 40 percent of fields are no longer arable; they cannot grow food. In 1950, Congress even sounded the alarm on mineral depletion in our topsoil, and how it would hurt our food supply.

It's gotten much worse—which is why we need to supplement.

Compare food to gas, and vitamins to the spark plugs in your car. If you always keep your car full of gas but are missing a spark plug or two, it will either sputter or not run at all. The car has nothing to be able to convert the fuel to energy effectively. Your body is much more intricate than a car, but likewise, it needs its "spark plugs"—vitamins and minerals—since many vitamins act as cofactors in enzymatic reactions that drive your metabolism.

More and more people are turning to organic food, which is a great thing. Organically grown food has more nutrients and is helping to reestablish the balance in our bodies and on the planet, but it still may not be meeting our requirements for maintaining optimal or balanced health.

Because of this, everyone needs a good multivitamin. It should be taken once or twice a day, depending on your need, with food. It metabolizes better this way. Powders in capsules, or powders alone, are more readily absorbable than most tablets. Plus, unlike tablets, they do not have extra additives (binders) to hold them together. Sometimes, the binders work too well, and the vitamins do not dissolve inside our digestive tract.

I'd like to remind you of something else: vitamin manufacturers sell products. They *work for us*. Without us, they have nothing. Every time we buy a product, of any type, we cast our vote. We also have the right to contact them, ask to speak to a technician, and find out if they have done absorbability studies with their product. Ask to see the data. If they don't have it or won't talk to you, then choose a different company.

There are too many supplements, herbs and health products to talk about individually in this book. However, there are a few I consider vital and essential to health management. I'd like to elaborate on those:

1. A high-quality, high-potency multivitamin with B vitamins and minerals. It is difficult even for the most dedicated to meet our ideal nutritional needs every day. We can't make DNA out of RNA without B vitamins and minerals. They are crucial for healing—and for energy. With all the physical demands and stresses of modern life, we chew up nutrients faster than ever. A good multivitamin acts like a safety net; think of it as the base of our metabolic pyramid. We want to stay at the top.

2. Omega-3s are vitally important, for many reasons. The standard American diet (SAD) has a disproportionate amount of omega-6s to omega-3s in our diets; it should measure less than a ratio of 4:1, omega-6s to omega-3s. I wrote extensively about this in Chapter 13 and 14.

3. Vitamin D is another essential vitamin. It still astounds me how many sun dwellers, surfers, lifeguards and other sun-splashed people in Southern California, where I live, register low vitamin D levels. Some could be due to genetic reasons. Sunscreen use could be a factor, as it blocks the UVB radiation from the sun, necessary for vitamin D synthesis in the skin epidermis. Of note, almost all patients admitted to the hospital with COVID-19 had low vitamin D levels.
    Vitamin D is crucial for the absorption of calcium, magnesium and phosphorus. It reduces cancer risk by up 16 percent, along with further benefits such as reducing inflammation, macular degeneration, depression, inflammation and Alzheimer's. It also helps fight infections, pneumonia, colds, flu and tuberculosis, and has been credited with helping seizure control in epileptics. A

couple of foods naturally provide vitamin D, including fatty fish, milks and vitamin-fortified cereals.

Take vitamin K2 with vitamin D. At Randall Wellness, we include K2 in our vitamin D supplement because it prevents vitamin D toxicity and excessive calcification in arteries. K2 directs the calcium where it is supposed to go—your bones and teeth. As mentioned above, deficiency can be present in anyone, even sun lovers, but it is generally more prevalent in people of color and those living in northern areas.

4. CoQ10 is a powerful antioxidant that promotes energy production and detoxification. It also supports mitochondrial function and strong, stable blood pressure. CoQ10 has been shown to increase athletic performance and decrease inflammation. The body's ability to produce CoQ10 declines with age, so supplementation should be considered to prevent cardiovascular disease and cognitive decline.

5. Natural food sources for CoQ10 include soybeans, lentils, peanuts, spinach, cauliflower, broccoli, oranges and strawberries, along with meat and eggs.

6. N-acetylcysteine (NAC), when converted to glutathione or S-acetylglutathione (or liposomal glutathione) is very beneficial. (Other forms are not absorbed or broken down in the stomach.) Glutathione is the number one nutrient for energy production and detoxification in the mitochondria, the powerful, energy-converting substance in our cells. The most vital molecule for every cell and organ in our bodies, glutathione is known as the "master antioxidant." It prevents oxidative damage, improves skin health, fights infections, reduces type 2 diabetes, improves heart health and protects the immune system. It helps mitigate degenerative disorders, such as Parkinson's and Alzheimer's, and benefits treatment of mental health issues like PTSD and depression. Glutathione recycles other antioxidants throughout your system, like vitamins C and E, CoQ10, and alpha-lipoic acid. Liposomal glutathione is said to have the highest absorption.

7. Foods that contain glutathione include mostly meats, eggs and animal organs. Whey protein powder also provides the amino acids your body needs to make glutathione, while selenium plays a role in maintaining glutathione levels. For vegans, try asparagus, almonds, spinach, broccoli, walnuts, garlic and tomatoes.

If glutathione is the fuel source, then NAC is the power plant.

It boosts glutathione production in the body. It can be used to support the liver and combat liver toxicity. Take either glutathione or NAC; you don't need both. However, we live in such a toxic world that the antioxidant power of these supplements will improve your health and performance.

8. Curcumin is my favorite supplement, due to its antioxidant and anti-inflammatory effects. It is such a beautiful root herb and can be taken and used in several forms. Curcumin derives from turmeric, used for thousands of years as an Ayurvedic medicine and in cooking. The curcuminoids from turmeric inhibit inflammation and help with chronic inflammatory conditions, along with digestion, especially concerning gut inflammation.

9. The most important quality is free curcuminoids. Water-soluble curcumin provides the highest bioavailable curcuminoids in the blood system. This makes it more effective for systemic inflammation, such as arthritis, vascular disease or inflammation-based neurodegenerative disease. Its native root, turmeric, is fat soluble when ingested as a tea or in food. Most of it remains in the gut, making it ideal for treating gut issues. Adding black pepper or BioPerine makes curcumin even more absorbable.

A final note: if you are a vegan, you may consider further supplementing this list with Vitamin B12, as well as alpha-lipoic acid. Among our food sources, these vital substances are typically found in meat. But they are critical to our long-term health.

More on Antioxidants

I want to dive a little further into antioxidants, which has been a buzzword in the vitamin and supplement world during the past 25 years. Antioxidants counteract free radicals. There have always been free radicals in our environment, but because of pollutants, far more of these damaging, often cancer-causing agents exist. Free radicals are highly reactive molecules that damage cells throughout the body. They contribute to cardiovascular disease, cancer, neurological disorders, cataracts, arthritis, cognitive decline and aging in general.

That changes when antioxidants enter the body. They quench, counteract and cancel out the damaging effects of free radicals, thus slowing down, delaying or even preventing chronic degenerative diseases. They can extend the quality of life, and maybe even life span. According to the American College of Cardiology, more doctors take and administer antioxidants than aspirin to help prevent cardiovascular disease and heart attacks.[41] Antioxidants may also reduce the risk for Alzheimer's disease by preventing buildup of toxic protein in the brain (amyloid plaques).

This effect is important for men and women, but women may be more susceptible to the oxidative stress of free radicals, according to some studies. Oxidative effects of aging include arthritis, wrinkled dry skin and atherosclerotic vascular disease.

Explosive Growth in the Vitamin and Supplement Market

Interest in vitamins and supplements began skyrocketing in the 1980s, but it has accelerated since. In 1998, US consumers spent $2 billion on vitamins, immunity and herbal supplements combined, according to *Nutrition Business Journal.* [42]In 2020, according to industry research analyst IBISWorld, that figure was *$35.7 billion* in the United States alone and almost $150 billion worldwide.[43] MarketWatch estimates that, by 2026, total sales will reach $349.4 billion.[44]

This increased interest and awareness is a good thing. Along with it comes the necessity of educating ourselves about the pitfalls of supplements, how to distinguish beneficial supplements and how to individualize choices.

How do we pick the right supplement? First, we need to know if it truly contains what the label claims. Also, does it break down properly in the body so its ingredients can be effectively absorbed and utilized? Is it free of impurities and toxins? Does it truly give us something we cannot supplement through a healthy diet? Know that neither the US government, nor any federal or state agency, is responsible for routinely testing multivitamins or other dietary supplements for their content or quality.

Faced with these questions, how do we determine quality? One way is to work with an experienced functional medicine practitioner such as myself, who has spent more than 40 years going the extra mile to study supplements, make site visits, and investigate sourcing and absorption studies and the efficiency of each recommended supplement.

Let's start with sourcing—where our supplements come from. This is only now *somewhat* effective, since up until recently, labeling regulations for supplements have been lax. Where does the manufacturing company source their ingredients? *Is it the cheapest available or the highest quality?* We need to know. Some companies can help give you good guidelines like ConsumerLabs and Labdoor. There are general principles outlined below.

Checking the Ingredients

Ingredients are listed in descending order of how much is in the product. Often, lesser quality supplements do not list ingredients, nor do they warn about ingredients to which people might be allergic, such as wheat, tree nuts, soy or rice. The FDA requires certain ingredients add up to 80 percent or more of the amount listed on the label: vitamins, protein, minerals, carbohydrates, dietary fiber, and polyunsaturated and monosaturated fat. In other words, supplements may contain 20 percent less product than the label states. They can also contain toxins such as mercury or lead.

Dietary supplements should list the active and inactive ingredients, the amount per serving (dose) and how many servings per bottle. Good supplements must follow the GMPs (good manufacturing practices) to ensure quality, strength and composition. Still, they are only required to include 80 percent of the product volume as listed on the label.

How can this happen? Well, supplement companies are not required to tell us the complete truth. Their only obligation is to follow the "truth in advertising" law, which allows them to place 20 percent less product in the container than stated on the package label—and also to not include untruthful health claims. Reports of some supplements have actually shown worse results. There is a company, Consumer Labs, that tests supplements for ingredients and validates whether the label matches the contents. The problem? Companies pay Consumer Labs to have their products tested, which implies a possible bias in the reported results.

Ingredients can present one quality control problem. Another concerns poor supplement absorption. It's pretty simple, really: if your body doesn't absorb the supplement and receive positive results, it doesn't matter how much product is in the bottle. You won't benefit. A perfect example is magnesium, one of our most important minerals. Magnesium drives more than 300 metabolic reactions in our bodies, but it must be absorbable to be effective. When you combine magnesium with another substance, it may or may not absorb well. The difference can be a factor in your health. For instance, magnesium oxide is not well absorbed, making it a good laxative. Magnesium citrate falls in the same boat. To choose a more absorbable, metabolically active magnesium, find a chelated product, attached to an amino acid. Magnesium glycinate, magnesium taurate and magnesium aspartate are all chelated products. Magnesium L-threonate is also well absorbed and helps brain function, because it crosses the blood/brain barrier. Magnesium malate is good for fibromyalgia, as it is well absorbed and relaxes muscle and fascia (the covering for muscles).

There are many different forms of magnesium. We need to be aware of what we are buying and why. And that is just one nutrient. Besides absorption, labeling and ingredient accuracy, we also need to be aware of toxins or allergens (incipients) not listed on the label, additional colors, fillers and allergens, along with poor sourcing and low manufacturing standards.

Now imagine moving through this careful process, and multiplying it by hundreds of different brands to choose from, whether in stores, functional practitioner offices, or online sales campaigns. How do we select the best supplements? It is difficult, to be sure. If you know what to look for on a label, which I've just broken down, then you should be able to gauge the better brands from those distributing poor-quality supplements.

CHAPTER 16
Be Your Own Blue Zone

Do you know there are societies and places where the people practice optimally healthy lifestyles without suffering the effects of poor eating, pressure and stress—and as a result, enjoy tremendously long and healthy lives? Have you heard of blue zones?

I first heard about blue zones in a November 2005 *National Geographic* story, "The Secrets of a Long Life." In the article, they identified five blue zones associated with people that live 90 to 100 years, and sometimes up to 150 years.[45] (The average life expectancy in the United States is 76 years for men and 82 years for women.) These "superagers" reside in small, isolated societies in Okinawa, Japan; Sardinia, Italy; Nicoya Peninsula, Costa Rica; Icaria, Greece; and the United States' one known blue zone, a community of 9,000 Seventh-day Adventists in Loma Linda, California, near Los Angeles.

There are two more blue zones I want to bring into this discussion (and, I'm sure, there are even more). One is the Caucasus Mountains, which intersect Europe and Asia between the Caspian and Black Seas. The Abkhasian ethnic group thrives there. The other hot spot of longevity, especially among men, is the Italian mountain village of Seulo, south of Sardinia. In the tiny community, more than 20 centenarians were thriving from 1996 to 2016.

So then we begin to inquire: what is it about these areas? What do they have in common, geographically? What do the people in them have in common? Is it their lifestyles? The food they eat? The water or some medicinal herb?

The most interesting thing to me as a practitioner concerns what they have in common. First, the people in all blue zones are regular practitioners of their religions, or their spirituality, and they are dedicated to family and spiritual lives above all else. They are also very community-centric. While being socially active, they balance themselves by regularly taking quality alone time to contemplate and regenerate. They don't smoke. They engage in moderate physical activity. They don't need to go to the gym; they are constantly moving, working, exercising outdoors. Another thing the blue zones have in common is empowered women. Women work alongside the men, but no one allows work chores to overrun their lives. Balance is a part of everyday life.

In his book *Blue Zones: 9 Lessons for Living Longer from People Who've Lived the Longest*, Dan Buettner writes about a few more common characteristics: the people hold strong life purpose, and they don't overstress—and in fact practice stress reduction just by their daily routines.[46] Having a life purpose, what the Japanese call *ikigai*, is critical. It means a reason for being. One's life feels and becomes more important when we operate with purpose. The blue zone inhabitants also feel no sense of urgency, which I have always considered a major contributing factor to our country's healthcare crisis. Stress and stress chemicals are very detrimental to health, and especially to the brain.

Even the blue zoners' interaction amongst each other is something, I believe, we should adopt more in our lives. They practice many forms of physical contact, from holding hands to locking arms, and often put their arms around each other as they go for walks. It might have to do with being in a relationship, but often, it does not. They are very touchy-feely, and that is seen to be part of their secret to longevity. Within their marriages, a deep relationship and sex seem to be very important for a person's stability. Studies have shown that married couples have longer survival rates—especially men. They don't suffer from as much cardiovascular disease as unmarried men. While not new, I find it interesting that all of this is common practice in blue zones, and they're the outliers we need to be learning from.

What about the blue zoners' diets? They are mostly plant-based, with plentiful portions of whole grains, legumes, seeds and nuts, and olive oil. They don't eat much red meat. In terms of animal protein, they eat mostly fish, and some poultry. Their food is locally grown and organic and contains the protective polyphenols I described in Chapter 13. They also have a modest caloric intake. Unlike the standard American diet (SAD), which falls between 2,000 and 2,500 calories a day, including many empty calories, blue zone populations typically don't exceed 1,800 calories per day. They don't starve themselves; they eat whatever they want. But here's the key: *they don't overeat*. There is a Japanese phrase, *hara hachi bu*, which roughly means "eating until you're 80 percent full" or satisfied. Well, 1,800 calories turn out to be 75 percent of 2,500 calories. They naturally know not to eat until they're stuffed. Also, they typically imbibe in small but never excessive amounts of alcohol, with wine being a favorite.

Virtually all of these superagers tend to either personal or communal gardens; all of the blue zones are located in sunny climates. The gardeners have healthier microbiomes as well as pure food sources. They also utilize native wild plants, picking herbs for medicinal, food and healing properties, or have specific herbs or plants with life-prolonging properties. Researchers even tried to find herbs in common that offered a magic "fountain of youth" effect. However, they did not find anything definitive. Lifestyle choice and practice seems to produce the most health benefits in these blue zones.

Some might be surprised to see "alcohol" and "wine" mentioned. Don't be. We know red wine has particular benefits from the resveratrol it contains; resveratrol is a potent antioxidant and also lengthens telomeres (the ends of your chromosomes), associated with long healthy lives. Research has shown that a small amount of drinkable alcohol of any type is associated with a decrease in cardiac disease and cardiovascular and cognitive diseases.

Finally, let's look at the locations of the blue zone societies. They live in the mountains, on islands or in isolated parts of peninsulas. Because of their locales, they are less exposed to social pressure and the "hurry-up" urgent anxiety that is a daily part of life in our society. And deadly, I might add, if we don't address it with a good attitude and practices.

That's why staying present in the moment is so very important. We have to find ways to remove ourselves from the sense of urgency. *I'm going to get there when I get there.* That is the blue zoners' approach, and it clearly is a much better way to live. One's purpose and one's function in life is important, but not to let function overrun existence. And I think that's very interesting too, not to let life's chores or work chores overrun their existence. They stay in the now. A very healthy regenerative lifestyle pattern.

How to Be Your Own Blue Zone

Now that I've taken you on a tour of the blue zones and we've "visited" their superagers to learn their secrets, what can *you* do to become your own blue zone? What does all of this look like in our lives? How does it change our quality of life, and our life span itself?

First, we know that attention to body, mind, spirit and soul are all key. We also know that finding lasting meaning, purpose and connection with the Source in our lives and activities is highly important, and that maintaining physical health and getting exercise matters. What is good for us is good for the planet—and what is good for the planet is good for us.

What do we need to live long and healthy? First, if you don't have a meaning and purpose, a spiritual connection, belief in a higher power, or something that you know that you're here to do, you're going to have a more difficult time. If these key qualities do exist in your everyday life, you are likely to have a happier and more fulfilling life for a longer period of time. I have shared these qualities several times on my Instagram TV show.

But not everyone believes in quality aging—not to mention superagers. Dr. Ezekiel Emmanuel wrote an article in The Atlantic that really shocked me. "Once I live to 75, I'm not going to do anything to end my life, but I'm not going to do anything to prolong it anymore, because after 75, more than one half of people get cognitive decline and biologically disintegrate . . . I've never seen anyone after the age of 75 do anything positive."[47]

When I read that, I threw up my arms and said, "Wait, just a minute!"

That is not my experience, nor what I believe—and certainly not what I teach. Maybe he is looking at people in the United States that eat mostly the SAD diet, or maybe he's basing it on people in other countries that don't eat anti-inflammatory diets. What is true from his statement is this: for people with a daily and long-held diet of conventionally raised meat, high amounts of sugary starchy foods and refined carbohydrates, they may well decline by the age of 75. This is reflected in the US health crisis, with rising incidences of diabetes, heart disease, obesity and cognitive decline. These foods are slowly poisoning your system. They are very slowly disintegrating your brain, mostly from inflammation and toxins. Inflammation is the final common denominator of chronic disease. That's what those on the SAD diet are slowly dying from, day after day . . . but we don't have to. We can choose organic regenerative food and grass-fed meats and poultry.

But I would suggest the far better regenerative practice is to put a lot of attention on what we put in our minds, our hearts, our souls, *as well as our bodies*. It's not just what we eat. Rather, the question should be, *what is eating us?* Where do we want to point our sacred arrows? What is our spiritual intention?

Now back to Dr. Emmanuel's comments. First of all, I have an issue with anyone claiming that you cannot have life purpose or be a contributor after age 75. Or 80. Or 85. What about Michelangelo? Benjamin Franklin? Wolfgang von Goethe? Thomas Edison? Or the wonderful George Burns? Or Betty White, Ruth Bader Ginsberg and Maya Angelou, to name three influential long-living women who recently passed at advanced ages? All of these brilliant people continued their world-changing work well past age

75. The data shows that if you live to 80, and you still have your full cognitive faculties and reasonable physical conditioning, your chances of living to 90 without serious illness or cognitive decline is nearly 100 percent.

What about being 100 years old and still making a difference, like the elders among the blue zone populations? In 2021, I featured two such centenarians on my *Soul Stories* podcast. The first was Dr. Gladys McGarey, the mother of holistic medicine in the United States, who is still going strong at age 101. She is charging ahead with a new literary contract to her next book, working title *One Hundred Is for Quitters*. She knows she is here for a purpose, which is to form the Foundation of Living Medicine, and she eats and lives a healthy lifestyle and has a large supportive family.[48]

Gladys and others are living proof that the longer you continuously live a healthy, productive, happy and purposeful life, the longer you will live. Her example offers a perfect reason as to why we need to look to outliers for our longevity answers, those centenarians on the right end of the bell-shaped curve that continue doing fantastically well. They are strong, smart, clear in their heads and focused on what they are doing. These people can show us how to live very long healthy lives. We're not going to find answers among the left side of bell-shaped curve or people not doing well.

Right? All these people that aren't exercising or taking care of themselves and saying, *That's the way it's going to be. I'm not going to take care of myself anymore.* That makes no sense. No sense. OK. So let us look at these superagers and see what they're doing.

I remember being inspired by a Henry David Thoreau passage, where he talks about "sucking the marrow out of life." That's what we should be doing, though I've reframed it to state, "getting every drop of goodness out of life." If you can have that kind of attitude and stop worrying about "am I going to make it to 70 years?" then you will sprint past 70 and likely enjoy many more fulfilling years. For my part, I *am* 70, and I think I'm in really good physical shape. And I also continue to be in a phase of cognitive and spiritual *expansion*, rather than decline.

Now that doesn't mean my path, or anyone else's, has been easy. Quite the opposite. Life throws some pretty difficult things at us. I recently endured yet another bout of cancer requiring surgery. Many would been debilitated, or possibly even died from this. If you can overcome stressful situations and challenges with the same positive "I belong here and I have a purpose" attitude I used to overcome cancer, you find the gift in it and become stronger because of it. It actually strengthens your resilience. I am stronger because I knew I could overcome my situation using all of my practices and skills and then help others as well, because life is also about service.

The other centenarian I featured on my podcast was Mamie Kirkland. I attended the documentary about her life, *One Hundred Years from Mississippi*. She and her family fled Mississippi when she was seven years old, and she experienced the chaotic and sometimes violent events that shaped the demographics of Black people throughout the country. She returned to Mississippi at the age of 107 to make peace with the violence and lynchings that caused her family to flee a century before. She lived to be 111, a truly transcendent being and living proof that forgiveness and embracing the diversity of all peoples can make us "One." And that having the purpose of sharing her story, and struggle, contributes directly to longevity.

A very important part of life is being of service. We are all here to serve other souls. If you can find a way to be of service, then it is going to help you as well as the person(s) you serve. It is important to be of service. Even if it's opening the door for a little old lady, picking up trash on the beach, dog sitting or setting up a nonprofit for orphans, like my friend Caroline Boudreaux, innovator of the Miracle Foundation. There are so many things you can do, whether small or large. Or both.

Being of service will also feed your body directly in a way that might surprise you. Research shows that when you participate in a random act of kindness or serve someone else out of compassion and generosity, that action raises your T cells. As a reminder, T cells are your *immunity cells*. That's what we all need right now. T cells and B cells bolster our long-term immunity.

Gratitude also promotes and increases the quality of life. The more we express it, the more life force energy we seem to receive. The yogis call it *prana*. Give thanks every day for what you have. Look at your life, bank account and possessions as a half-full glass (or better), no matter what. Move away from the "glass half empty" mindset. It's been shown that people who retrain their mindsets and attitudes this way change positively— resulting in better mental, physical and spiritual health.

You can do everything right: right diet, right exercise, even consistent meditation. However, if you don't have a positive attitude and are not thankful every day for what you have, then you're not going to be as healthy as you can optimally be.

Family, Friends, Community: Key to All of Our Blue Zones

The other key ingredients to good health and longevity are community, friends and family. They provide the feeling of being valued, while always valuing others. Exchanging information, being social and part of a group is crucial. That has been proven difficult during COVID-19, but you can still do it. Try the phone or Zoom. You can do it in other ways, even if you feel safer physical distancing in these times. Simply sit outside or go for a walk with friends, and take precautions.

Compassion is also an important part of health. It is equally important to be as compassionate to others *as to yourself.* Be kind—to yourself as well. I know there's a lot of fierceness and scariness and low-density energy in the world right now, but the best way to combat it is by putting out the opposite energy. Shine your light, be compassionate, be kind. Also be smart: there are people who take advantage.

What do the blue zone societies suggest about our future quality of life? The *Encyclopedia Britannica* refers to "quality of life" as the degree to which an individual is healthy, comfortable and able to participate or enjoy life. The World Health Organization says it's an individual's *perception* of their life. Perception is the key word. So, if you perceive yourself to be successful, a lot of people may want to see the physical manifestation of success, like "where's the car or the house?" But success to another person may be measured by how kind you are, or how well you love—or are loved by others.

Blue zone populations are an ideal blueprint for practicing a regenerative lifestyle. What we need to do is go back to nature, to what we know is healthy. Look at what these populations of superagers do. Learn from the people who have proved their longevity for many centuries.

CHAPTER 17
Happy Gut, Happy Life

During the 2017 Christmas season, my wonderful exterminator told me that mold was growing underneath my house. I was shocked, because there was no mold according to the meticulous inspector when I bought the house, nor did I have any plumbing problems or leaks. We attempted to figure out the problem, only to learn I was sitting on the tip of a large, scary iceberg.

After battling with my home insurance company, which led me nowhere, I hired contractors to redo my bathroom and remediate the mold beneath it. They told me "back pressure" was causing a slow leak between the subfloor and main floor, which made it unnoticeable from inside or beneath the house until the mold appeared. Not good. The insurance company usually claims that if you have mold, you have ignored an existing problem. Not so here, as my exterminator visits under the house every two weeks.

Because of the bathroom situation, my family and I decided to celebrate Christmas at my son's house. We had a great holiday, with a lot of love, hugs, good eats and presents.

The next day, I walked into a house completely flooded with sewage. Every bathtub, toilet and sink were flooded, and it overflowed onto my wood floor. The grounds manager determined the problem through endoscopy. How ironic, as I was part of the team that invented video endoscopy. Now, it was being used to show me an obstruction in the park's sewage line that caused the destruction of my house. "See that?" he asked, pointing at the screen. "It's a large root ball. We'll have to break it up and get it to move down the line. This large root ball lodged in the main sewage pipe for your area. And for some reason all the backup came into your house."

This was a catastrophic event for my life, my house—and my health.

The park sent someone to analyze the damage, which turned out to be more to serve their purposes than mine, as I learned later, when they refused to release the results to me. Appalled, I had to get my own remediation, and fast! Not easy on the day after Christmas. Turned out I chose well, as Moises and his band of superheroes at Dry Down not only began remediation, but helped me move my things into the house across the street. I talked the owner into renting to me because I noticed the previous renter had moved out and I was in great need. I got out in four days, which I thought was pretty fast. But not fast enough. I was promised help by the park, which never materialized. It was left to me to rebuild the entire interior of my house, a huge undertaking.

By some fluke or intuition, I had decided to move everything away from the bathroom that was being worked on shortly before Christmas. I moved my bed and furniture away from the bathroom in the master bedroom suite. That saved most of my furniture, but I lost a lot of belongings that day. Despite really good insurance and being able to secure a house across the street while I reconstructed mine, I suffered greatly. I didn't complain and continued to work and exercise.

The next year, 2018, wildfires came to Malibu and devastated much of it, creeping dangerously close to my home. It was our worst fire experience ever. People would ask, "Did you lose your house? Are you OK?" They all held focus groups in financial and psychological support. I told them I already lost my house and had no one to help me.

A Serious Gut Problem

Sewage aerosolizes and can contaminate those who breathe it. The men who came to remediate my house wore full face masks, gloves and hazmat suits. Since I didn't have such a suit, I was contaminated and developed dysentery of the worst kind. While trying to maintain a full work schedule, I suffered through 20 bowel movements a day. Many times, I could not hold it, to the point where I took extra pants to work. It was humiliating. Trying to maintain my weight, health and energy proved difficult.

When I went to my Western doctors, none could find or do anything other than prescribe strong antibiotics like Levaquin, which only made things worse by wiping out my good bacteria and making me sicker by poisoning my mitochondria. I took multiple blood and stool tests; nothing was found. I was already a fabulous gut doctor and gastroenterologist, but I initially sought Western care like most, because I was frightened. I had lost 35 pounds and most of my muscle, and no longer held any control over my bowel movements. Even some of my non-Western stool testing let me down.

After that, I went about finding a better way to test stool and treat dysentery. I found a few companies that do RNA testing on the stool. That's what I needed! The results confirmed I had *Shigella*, *Salmonella*, *Entamoeba histolytica* and a number of other really bad dysbiotic bacteria. In other words, the worst developing world type of dysentery, all from poop in affluent Malibu. Talk about ironic.

My other trouble was simply functioning. I would almost pass out on my way to the kitchen when I tried to rehydrate every morning. I knew how to help myself, but my dysentery was so severe that I suffered for seven months despite my knowledge. The reason? When the gut blows, the immunity goes. Since 70 percent of our immune system resides in our gut, there's no guard at the door when it collapses.

Slowly but surely, through a pristine plant-based diet with no refined carbohydrates, strong bactericidal herbals and a gut healing program with synbiotics, collagen and glutamine (among others), I cured my gut problem and put on 25 pounds, primarily muscle. Pretty good for a woman in the second half of her 60s. Then the next challenge hit when cancers broke out all over my body, the effect of the dysentery suppressing my immunity. I found everything I could do to cure myself, but cancer presented a whole new challenge. I had a lesion on my leg all the way down to the bone, and one on my mouth that required surgical removal of my entire lip and part of my chin—and then building a new one. In addition, huge chunks of my scalp were impacted. Assorted areas of my upper legs, shoulder, wrist and chest were involved.

"Wow, your immune system must have taken a real beating for these all to come out so quickly and for them all to be so invasive," my doctor said.

"Yes it did, Doc," I replied through my tears. "Yes it did."

During the process, it occurred to me to go into a barometric chamber, because cancer hates oxygen. That led me to create a list of the things cancer hates: oxygen, potassium, an alkaline environment, anything stress-relieving and calm, a vegan diet, and a plethora of herbal remedies. I also eliminated a list of things that feed cancer, like sugar, salt, heavy metals, stress, alcohol and toxins of any sort. I put myself on an intense program.

At the same time, I realized this same list can be applied to things that strengthen and weaken our gut, and by extension, our immune system.

From all this *heal thyself* work, I received a couple of gifts. First, I learned how to diagnose and cure any kind of gut problems, even the worst kind. I used functional medicine to heal my gut and strengthen my immune system. I've always been good at gut medicine, but this experience made me much better. Now, I know how to help people with cancer more than ever.

I share these programs, in part or completely, with patients suffering from similar ailments.

I received another huge gift after the fires. Unfortunately, everyone in my neighborhood whose homes still stood, as well as most residents of Malibu, the surrounding areas and the western San Fernando Valley, had to remediate for smoke. I had to rebuild my house from the earth up: new floors, new walls, new windows, new everything, except for the layout. Three weeks after the fire drove me out, I returned to a pristine home. The replaced windows were tight. I put in an electric fireplace, which eliminated any smoke coming down the chimney. The moldings on the doors and windows were tight and well made. My floor was rebuilt all the way to the subfloor, so there really was no smoke damage at all. I also installed a top-of-the-line air filter from Canada. Out of this disaster arose my beautiful, environmentally controlled house.

I learned and realized many things through the sewer backup, dysentery, fires and healing. I learned how critical our gut is to our ability to live happy, healthy and vibrant lives. From this, I coined the phrase, "happy gut, happy life." Almost all disease begins in the gut, and can be traced back to an imbalance there. Most diseases can be treated and cured through investigating and treating the gut.

Microbes and Neurotransmitters: the Passengers Inside Us

We all have passengers inside of us. It's a funny thought, but true. There are 100,000 times more microbes in your gut than there are people on earth, and 30,000 times more microbes than total body cells. Moreover, we have a symbiotic relationship with these passenger bacteria living inside our bowel. They need us and we need them.

The normal human gastrointestinal tract contains hundreds of different species of harmless bacteria, or intestinal flora. When the balance of these bacteria is disturbed by poor diet and lifestyle, illness, stress or antibiotic treatment, common effects are diarrhea and/or constipation, gas, bloating and abdominal pain. Our immunity suffers. The resulting imbalance also leads to overgrowth of unfriendly bacteria, also possibly candida or yeast. Without correction, it can contribute to arthritis, irritable or leaky bowel syndrome, immune suppression, maldigestion, indigestion, gas, and chronic diseases. These can be diagnosed easily with RNA stool testing and treated with probiotics, diet and herbs.

Healthy bacteria are central to a healthy gut. But there's more—the immune and neuroendocrine functions of the gut. This can be traced to the thymus. Humans are the only mammals born with a thymus that involutes, or "goes away," by the time we're pre-adolescent. It leaves behind T cells, responsible for fighting viruses and fungi and other immune functions for the rest of our lives. How is that, if the host organ goes away?

Welcome to the miracles of the human body. When the thymus involutes, those crucial T cell warriors resettle in the gut, where they set up Peyer's patches, a string of intestinal "camps" or "villages." They also move into our bone marrow. Right now, you have an enormous number of immune cells and lymph nodes in your intestinal tract, all of which play a role in your immunity.

Your gut and brain are also connected through chemicals called neurotransmitters. Serotonin calms you and helps with sleep. Your gut bacteria produce a gamma-aminobutyric acid (GABA), which helps control fear and anxiety. Neuroendocrine cells play into the fight-or-flight reaction by producing norepinephrine and epinephrine. Your gut and brain communicate through myriad neuroenteric and neurotransmitter messages, along with the vagus nerve.

The enteric nervous system uses more than 30 neurotransmitters, similar to the brain. About 95 percent of the body's serotonin comes from the gut, which may be how the gut, or "second brain," influences well-being or mood. In a February 12, 2010, article in *Scientific American*, Dr. Michael Gershon, chairman of the Department of Anatomy at New York Presbyterian Hospital and author of *The Second Brain*, wrote, "The second brain doesn't help with the great thought processes . . . religion, philosophy and poetry are left to the brain in the head."[49]

Emeran Mayer, author of *The Mind-Gut Connection* and a colleague of mine at UCLA since the early 1990s, talks about an intricate, complex communication system between gut and mind, involving abundant endocrine cells in what amounts to the body's largest endocrine organ, the gut's immune system. They are capable of producing cytokines (inflammatory molecules). These immune cells are outside the gut space and alongside dendrite cells, which may extend into the gut and interact with the microbiome. This means they always have their "eye" on what is happening inside the gut. Cytokines can enter the bloodstream by crossing the gut lining and getting to the brain. Endocrine cells signal the brain through these dendrites and eventually the vagus nerve.

Our food choices are also critical in how our gut works. Sadly, industrialized farming has changed the American diet from largely organic to one filled with processed foods high in sugar and fat, low in fiber, and chemically contaminated. This has altered our gut mitochondria, causing a multitude of diseases and symptoms—diabetes, neurologic diseases like Alzheimer's and Parkinson's, obesity, inflammatory bowel syndrome and other inflammation-based ailments, diarrhea, constipation, arthritis, auto-immune diseases, digestive disorders, depression, anxiety, food sensitivities, allergies, fatigue, and several forms of cancer. Many seemingly unrelated diseases and symptoms are triggered by gut problems, imbalanced micro-biota and consequent malfunctioning gut lining. Gut health literally affects your entire body.

The gut houses three pounds of bacteria and up to 500 species of micro-biota. These have been shown to have an effect on the brain. Imbalanced and affected gut microbiota are associated with symptoms such as brain fog, fatigue, achy joints and the diseases noted above.

Getting Clear on Probiotics and Antibiotics

Two other crucial terms connected with gut health and the immune system are *probiotics* and *antibiotics*. We've heard a lot about probiotics over the past 15 years, when they went mainstream and found their way into your grocery store, health food store or pharmacy of choice. Probiotics are sup-plements of the normal bacteria found in the bowel. Contrary to popular opinion, they do not colonize the gut. However, they do result in a more robust population of flora, mostly in the large intestine, and they discour-age the disease-causing bacteria, restoring balance to the intestinal flora. They may also produce substances that inhibit pathogenic bacteria, com-pete with them for nutrients, stimulate the body's own immune system, and prevent unhealthful immune reactions to unfriendly bacteria and yeast.

Probiotic supplements are available in varied forms such as yogurt, fer-mented foods, capsules, gummies, tablets, beverages, teas (such as kombu-cha tea) and powders. *Probiotics* should not be confused with *prebiotics*, which are complex sugars (such as inulin from soluble fibers in most plants, and fructo-oligosaccharides) ingested as fuel for bacteria already present in the gastrointestinal tract. Sometimes, prebiotics and probiotics are com-bined and termed *synbiotics*.

Meanwhile, antibiotics are primarily prescription medications used to treat specific ailments. Most of us have been prescribed them at one point or another. Unfortunately, while eliminating their intended targets, antibi-otics often lower the number of beneficial bacteria in the body and can lead to leaky gut, colitis and other side effects. So act preventively when taking them. Try not to eat sugar. And alternate your taking of probiotics with the times you take antibiotics, if prescribed. Don't take them at the same time.

Probiotics can help balance the missing or low beneficial bacteria and lessen the negative side effects of antibiotics. *Saccharomyces boulardii*, *Enterococcus faecium* and *Lactobacillus* are clinically proven to prevent antibiotic-caused diarrhea. Successful clinical trials have also been conducted using *Lactobacillus* to treat *H. pylori* infection and *Lactobacillus plantarum* to treat irritable bowel syndrome. *Lactobacillus GG* (a strain of *L. rhamnosus*) and *Lactobacillus reuteri* have been shown to reduce the duration of diarrhea due to certain infections in infants and young children.

When you shop for probiotics, head for the refrigerated supplements section in your store. *Lactobacillus acidophilus* and *Bifidobacter* are the most important bacteria to find on the label, although there may be others. *Lactobacillus acidophilus* (*L. acidophilus*) is important for the small bowel, and *Bifidobacter* or *Bifidus* for the large bowel. A typical dose should supply at least 3 to 5 billion live organisms per capsule; 50 billion flora per capsule is ideal. Take the product right after eating, when the acid in the stomach is lowest. However, the dose should be individualized to the patient and condition.

Balancing Your Microbiome

The balanced gut microbiome from our diet, self-care and probiotic use is essential for optimal digestion, absorption and integration of nutrients, and elimination. It supports a healthy inflammatory response and keeps our immune system strong, while also supporting our emotions by balancing our neurotransmitters. A few food choices can keep your microbiome balanced:

- Asparagus—prebiotic
- Sauerkraut or kimchi—good source of probiotics and fiber
- Garlic—prebiotic; discourages growth of dysbiotic bacteria
- Onion—prebiotic and antioxidant
- Apple cider vinegar—stimulates digestive juices, helps break down foods
- Ginger—relaxes stomach, assists digestion treats nausea, increases warmth (Chi)
- Dandelion greens or cilantro—anti-inflammatory, cleansing, detoxifying, chelates toxins

We've focused so far on our *in*vironment, how our gut health and immunity work from the inside. What about the relationship with our outside *en*vironment? No matter how dedicated we are to gut health, we must deal with a largely unhealthy environment—and likely to get worse before it gets better. The latest pollution or climate change news reminds us of that every day.

Unfortunately, we have to put foods through these unnatural processes because our environment has been contaminated by chemicals and pollutants. In a cynical twist, agribusiness regulations, poor soil conditions and weak plant seeds force many farmers to use highly toxic pesticides and fertilizers to grow our food! There are also new super viruses and parasites that we cannot risk ingesting or transmitting; our colossal battle with the coronavirus is a perfect example.

Another is SIBO (small intestinal bacterial overgrowth), first described in 2004 by Dr. Mark Pimentel at Cedar-Sinai.[50] He and his team found that methane and/or hydrogen gases produced by bacteria alter the motility of the intestine and cause constipation, bloating, pain and sometimes diarrhea. In the healthy gut, most bacteria stay in the colon. Sometimes there is too much or reduced motility, and they move up into the small bowel. High methane levels cause abdominal pain, bloating and constipation. High hydrogen levels are usually associated with diarrhea. Breath testing for SIBO uses lactulose, a poorly absorbed carbohydrate. This has been the gold standard for SIBO diagnosis, although it is not perfect. After ingestion, collected breath samples are tested for hydrogen and methane. An organism called Archaea produces methane and another causes hydrogen. Hydrogen-associated SIBO usually causes diarrhea, whereas methane-related SIBO causes constipation. The antibiotic rifaximin treats SIBO without resulting in antibiotic-associated diarrhea. It may need repeating, as SIBO often recurs. Reducing intake of indigestible fibers (legumes, cruciferous veggies) broken down by gut bacteria can help SIBO patients with gas production and discomfort. I often treat simultaneously with bactericidal herbals and promotility herbs, which helps resolution.

The cause of SIBO is unknown, but it is believed to be related to diet, previous antibiotic therapy, motility and other illnesses. There is evidence to suggest the sweep effect of the migrating motor complex is lost in some people with SIBO, most likely from a previous food poisoning event. This results in the accumulation of too many bacteria in the small bowel. Dr. Pimentel says that the subset of SIBO is secondary to a preexisting food poisoning event. This can be found by doing ibs-smart, an antibody test. I offer them in the office. Patients have antibodies to vinculin, part of the migrating motor complex of the bowel. Thus some SIBO is a motility problem. That's why bacteria move north! Chinese medicine calls it reverse stomach Chi. Treatments for this, herbs and acupuncture, can often help.

Dr. Pimentel advocates restricting yourself to an elemental diet for two to three weeks, which reduces methane producers by 80 percent. (Rifaximin only reduces it 50 percent.) It helps but is difficult for patients to stick to. Treatment with motility activators and herbal bactericidal agents, and following an elemental diet, can help resolve this problem. This can also be accomplished holistically. Western doctors use an erythromycin pediatric solution of about 50 milligrams per day to start. I use herbs like artichoke and ginger, which are promotility agents.

Lately, more patients have been coming into my office with SIBO. My experience tells me that there are other causes for this. One is stress, which alters gut immunity and kills off good bacteria. Another is antibacterial soaps, which make us *too* clean. Others are chlorinated water and the presence of microplastics in foods.

I perform dozens of stool tests on patients every week; our findings are borne out by the test results. Many results by accurate RNA stool testing show increased numbers of good bacteria, as well as increased dysbiotic or bad bacteria. Diagnosis is by breath tests, but not always accurate, and taking a culture by small bowel endoscopy is expensive. I have found that the combination of clinical presentation, stool and breath tests are the most helpful for diagnosis. I've also found that a reduced fiber and refined carbohydrate, low FODMAP (fermentable oligosaccharides, disaccharides, monosaccharides, polyols—short chain, poorly absorbed carbohydrates) diet during the treatment phase help symptoms.

Often, we are able to resolve SIBO with natural medicines. If we do resort to antibiotics (rifaximin), we follow up with berberine active intensified with milk thistle and high-dose, enteric-coated oregano. SIBO tends to recur but can be controlled with diet, natural therapies that improve gut immunity, and emollients like licorice, marshmallow or slippery elm.

If you have these symptoms, you may want to contact a functional medicine doctor experienced in gastroenterology to help you.

Your Gut Depends on How You Eat and Live

What you eat and how you live can affect your immunity and emotional balance through your gut. Eat a plant-based, low refined carbohydrate diet. Avoid vital wheat gluten, an industrialized gluten added to many foods, even packaged meats and vegetable products. This is in contrast to pure gluten in the ancient version of semolina durum wheat, which has its own anti-gluten molecule. The gluten portion of the seeds grown in the United States is two-thirds larger than the original seed, and, sadly, contains glyphosates and other chemicals. Not beneficial. The vast majority of my patients who remove gluten from their diets experience fewer symptoms of what ails them, and their gut health improves markedly. Some are gluten sensitive or intolerant and can be diagnosed by stool or blood tests.

In summary, how do we balance our gut and care for our microbiome? First of all, we need to remove all the foods that have been developed since 1970 thanks to industrialized farming—refined sugars, refined fructose, animal fat, and mass-produced, processed food. Choose organic, locally grown whole food, mostly plant-based. Plants contain the valuable pre-biotics on which microbiomes live, in the form of soluble fiber and inulin.

Optimize your microbiome by eating and taking naturally fermented foods and probiotics. The jury is still out on which probiotic organisms are the best; it may vary according to the individual and condition. However, we do know we need a mix of *Lactobacillus* and *Bifidobacteria*. If yeast is involved, then *Saccharomyces boulardii* can be helpful. I won't get into genetic subtypes here as there are too many to cover. That said, *Lactobacillus GG* seems to be more helpful for colitis patients.

Stool testing is also the approach recommended by Dr. Emeran Mayer in *The Mind-Gut Connection*. "A gut microbial analysis from a simple stool sample [through an RNA or MAP test] could become one of the most powerful screening tools in health care," he wrote.[51] That's exactly what I have been practicing, in one way or another, for more than 20 years.

Dr. Mayer also recommends using mindfulness meditation to tune into messages from the gut. "By becoming more aware of these gut feelings, those associated with good and bad gut reactions, you can better regulate your own emotions."

I believe emotions can begin in the gut, and then be sent to the brain through the complex communication system I've described. It is only then that the brain decides what to make of them.

CHAPTER 18
Dream Doctoring

I was invited to Glasgow, Scotland, to speak at a prestigious conference in mid-July 2002. After a particularly hot and dry year in Arizona's Sonoran Desert, plus a terrible drought and fire season, the idea of spending time in the moist, lush, rainy green-ness of Scotland sounded delicious.

Whenever I tried to make travel arrangements, though, the most unusual feeling came over me. It was a block, an obstacle of some kind. On the night of June 1, before falling asleep, I asked for guidance. I really wanted to make the trip, and am usually a decisive person. But something told me to hold off on a decision until I received the guidance I sought.

Overnight, I had the following dream:

I am making a huge platter of food for a circle of women, an artistic arrangement of fruits and vegetables around a golden roasted wild turkey. The women are circled in a room that offers a 270-degree view of the ocean and setting sun (like my house does today!). I point out a cloud formation over the water. It assumes the shape of a deep magenta-toned rainbow bridge, similar in shape to bridges I have seen in Europe, and rises above a smooth flowing river with several arch-like structures. I cross the bridge into a large auditorium, where I am speaking to a capacity crowd. I'm in another country, but not in Europe.

After my presentation, a Latino gentleman greets me. He is clearly the guardian of this place, and he graciously arranges for my every need to be met. He introduces me to a beautiful grandmother. I know her to be of the earth, a being of great power, wisdom and endless kindness. I place my hands on her heart and she places her hands on mine. A tremendous healing exchange occurs. A gentle, constant rain begins to fall, blanketing the parched land around us.

The dream told me what I need to know, and what to do next. I called the organizers of the Scotland conference and told them I would not be attending. My inner voice and this dream told me to stay home and gather the members of my dream circle for a meeting. On July 15, six weeks after the dream, I held the circle, and presented my dream. Each woman responded similarly. The dream stone made its way around the circle counterclockwise. Each woman spoke her heartfelt soul impressions of the dream.

"It's some kind of prophecy," Julie said as she held the aquamarine stone to her heart with her left hand. "That's what I'm getting. Whoever this Grandmother is—she's going to come into your life and together you will create the energy for some sort of healing to take place. Whew—powerful."

The stone was passed to Sharon. "I agree, and also I feel you are going to be leaving us. As much as I don't want that, I feel that you are being called to another level of work." When Val had the stone, she added, "It's some sort of celebration, because of the healing and the work. You are moving into another realm with this powerful Grandmother."

Afterward, there was a feast of fruits, vegetables and organic turkey, as in my dream. (The turkey is symbolic of peace and unity.)

Within a week, I received a call from Deborah Szekely, founder of the Rancho La Puerta fitness and health resort in Tecate, Mexico. She was introduced to me by a dear friend, the world-renowned pianist Mona Golabek, a longtime guest of the ranch. Deborah invited me to meet her and give a lecture to the guests. During my visit, Deborah and Jose Manuel Jasso, the general manager and partner, began recruiting me to become part of the Rancho La Puerta family. Soon, I was welcomed in as the new executive director of guest services.

Choosing not to go to Scotland became a life-changing event that my soul knew was part of my destiny. Also, the figures in the dream became apparent: Deborah, a Taurus like me, was the Earth-Grandmother. Jose Manuel was the noble Latino guardian.

"As We Dream, So Becomes the World"

Heather Valencia (Onamwashatina) used to say, "As we dream, so becomes the world." Heather was one of my dreaming teachers; she is a medicine woman and the author of *Queen of Dreams*.

This phrase summarizes the powerful notion that dreams literally shape our existence. We dream as a collective. What each of us dreams touches all people and becomes a part of the great dream weave, which affects the reality of all people and the planet. When we are dreaming, Great Spirit is dreaming us. Beyond the collective is a higher awareness, from where we source our dreaming. It is usually altruistic, as the soul, or Higher Self, naturally knows the inter-connectedness of all things and the "right path."

Dreaming has been a part of my life since childhood. While a young girl, I had three friends who would come at night to guard and keep me comfortable. One was a huge male black panther that would pad down the hall once the house was quiet and lay by my bed until the sun rose. Another was a rainbow snake made of light. She would circle clockwise around the ceiling, then move counterclockwise to keep me still and entertained until I fell asleep. A third friend, my favorite, would appear when I ran into the neighboring cornfields and lay between the rows to watch the dancing white clouds and corn swaying in the breeze. She was beautiful and kind, with white hair and blue-green eyes. She would talk to me in a low, sweet voice and watch over me while I lay there. She told me of the importance of plants and how healing they were. She always reassured me that everything would work out all right. She said, "Lay there, see the blue sky and feel the beautiful energy from the earth, sky and plants." It felt divine.

I felt so blessed and happy to have my dream friends.

I would also regularly dream-fly over the neighborhood and see my horse friends, the school and houses laid out. Years later, I learned to fly small airplanes. When I flew over this area of Omaha, I was astounded to see how accurate my dream flight memories were.

Dreaming for Personal and Planetary Healing

When I met my first Native teachers on the Lakota reservation, my grand-parents, they spoke of the sacred nature of dreams. They taught me that dreams were messages from the ancestors, the planet or the Great Mystery, about our path or purpose on the planet right now.

Since the beginning of time, indigenous peoples have maintained secret dreaming communities to bring in guidance for the greater community to function. Women especially give birth to the future through collective dreaming and moon lodge ceremonies. Some of my Native teachers shared this while opening their boundaries to not only me, but other races and cultures. Their purpose: to keep the dream and the planet alive.

Personal and planetary healing go hand in hand—and dreaming is a big part of it. The time of remembering is now heavy upon us. Every single person on this planet is being asked to wake up, remember who they are, and become part of the cosmic consciousness to assist humanity and help the planet return to a balanced place.

Types of Dreams

Connie Kaplan, my teacher and author of *The Woman's Book of Dreams*, says it best about dreaming: "Truth presents itself in dreaming and later exposes itself in form. The dreamer must simply learn to read and track the energy.

Dreaming can only be spoken indirectly in metaphor. Nothing is precise about dreaming, yet to be a dreamer, one must be extraordinarily precise in living the dream."[52]

Connie teaches 13 types of dreams. My approach is a little more inclusive. My work includes most types that she describes, including:

- In **Psychological Dreams**, we process things going on in our lives, unresolved issues, things that impressed us or that are unfinished. We are trying to resolve them in the dream.
- **Recurring Dreams** are the same dream, replayed over and over. They are often somewhat unpleasant. The dreaming circles say this is your soul giving you the same information, repeatedly, until you get it. Recognize the issue and resolve it. Or get onto the path it is showing. Once we follow the message presented, the dream will not recur again.
- **Healing Dreams** can be of several types. First is the dream for the healer personally—self-healing. Something in the dream, whether a situation, person or animal, comes with a healing message, self-empowering tools or healing energy. In the second type, the dreamer is healing another person, or a group. Lastly is a dream where the collective is healing each other, or the planet as a whole. This is very powerful dreaming, needed more now than ever.
- **Phenomenal Dreams** are among my favorites. The dreamer moves through a high-vibrational dream that ultimately changes ordinary reality in a profound, beneficial way. Within a short period of time, the changed ordinary reality tumbles into existence. I love that!
- **Prophetic Dreams** are also personal favorites. These powerful dreams leave a deep impression on the dreamer. Such a dream usually involves a global perspective or a group of people, resulting in a beneficial change. The key difference between a prophetic and psychic dream is that the prophetic dream usually occurs well before it manifests physically, often several or even many years or decades prior. Like the Sundance vision I had about this book.
- **Psychic Dreams** are like prophetic dreams, but more immediate and less collective in nature. For instance, I may dream about a patient I've never met, and then they come in to see me the next day or week.

- **Daydreams** aren't always true dreams. Studies show we spend 70 to 120 minutes per day daydreaming. When we let the imagination run wild, we lose general awareness and get lost in our own fantasy. Still, when we receive a message or vision, it can be a guide or call to action so be mindful.
- With **Lucid Dreaming**, we gain awareness in the dream and use our willpower to change its course. The problem? We are usually the best version of ourselves in the dream already, we "know" exactly what to do and our actions are perfect. When we become lucid, we allow our everyday ego to enter the dream. I suppose some are so evolved that they can do this and create great results. I personally trust my soul, unaccompanied by my ego, to make my dreamtime choices. Still, I find it a fun experience to dream lucidly.
- **Nightmares** can be disturbing. Often in my dream circle, we say, "There is no such thing as nightmares," because once a dream is presented to the circle, it immediately changes the energy. When you understand the meaning, the dream is no longer scary. It only becomes a nightmare when you allow your ego to respond to it in a concrete way.

  For instance, getting shot or stabbed sounds horrific, but it could mean you are processing karma. Any metal entering the body is karmic, and usually nothing further happens in the dream. This is different from a *night terror*, very real and usually the result of a major trauma or PTSD. Night terrors are a symptom of a psychological imbalance and should be addressed as such.
- **Epic Dreams** take us on a journey. They are usually long, involving many aspects and different people or situations. In "structure," they resemble the twists and turns of a long story or novel. They can either review your past, summarizing and showing the meaning, or present the path before you, showing the way to your purpose.
- **Ecstatic Dreams** are so huge and moving, they may not be explainable in ordinary terms. They may appear as colors and symbols. One thing for sure: they leave you with a wonderful sense of happiness and expansive knowledge. While many dreams can be life-changing, these surely are.

How Dreaming Works

How does dreaming work? A number of sources speak of high-frequency brain waves in REM and non-REM sleep operating from a posterior "hot zone" of the cortex. Science often describes dreams as a simple phenomenon of electrical activity. Those of us that practice spirituality through dreaming know dreams to be much more than simple electrical brain activity.

Many of us who practice dreaming know the dream to be an opening for soul energy to enter for a personal and/or collective reason. Or healing. If we pay attention to our dreams and begin to track the energy, certain patterns appear. Dreams carry messages. As mentioned, if you're having a recurring dream, it is trying to get you to pay attention to something you may need to clean up energetically, perhaps an aspect of your life. These messages are nothing less than seeds from your soul on where to direct your attention.

Dreams are a major part of my soul doctoring practice, and something I continuously remind my patients to study, keep a journal and heed as they work toward greater self-awareness and self-care. I also remind them to awaken to our role in joining the cosmic consciousness, to remember we are part of this greater consciousness and that our collective role is to serve as guardians of the planet.

I've been fortunate to either know and work with, or know of, many great dream teachers—all of whom I recommend. In addition to Connie Kaplan's *The Woman's Book of Dreams,* authors such as Jayne Gackenbach and Jane Bosveld, *Control Your Dreams,* describe how conscious intent can guide our unconscious dreaming into higher states of awareness. In *Welcome Home: Following Your Soul's Journey Home,* Sandra Ingerman describes her own healing experience through the dream, along with practicing thera-peutic dreaming intervention with her clients.

The work of psychologist Patricia Garfield also promotes healing through dreams. In *The Healing Power of Dreams,* she describes dreams that demonstrate all phases of healing, from diagnosis to cure.[53] She also teaches how to program our dreams to heal ourselves or others, using creative visu-alization and lucid dreaming. There are prophetic dreams that foretell the future, such as the one that opened this chapter and led me to Deborah Szekely and Rancho La Puerta. Dreams also guide me in my daily work as a physician-healer, as I was reminded of in a seemingly terrible dream about Mark, a patient:

I was responsible for an ER; it was entirely full. People were intoxicated, had draining wounds, infections oozing pus and were bleeding. Many needed surgery. It was complete chaos!

I kept trying to dial the phone, looking for my girls and my team members, Rhonda and Toni. They were not there. I tried my best, but it was difficult. The most moving part was when a dark-haired boy came up to my right side and looked at me, his eyes wide. "Don't give up!" he said.

The following morning, my first patient was a dark-haired young man, an ER doctor. Very bright and versed in functional medicine, he had originally presented unusual physical symptoms. I found him to be remarkably improved from his last visit. After dealing with his physical issues, I asked him if he was frustrated. "Yes. I don't think I belong in the ER profession for the rest of my life," he said.

I assured him he was well on his way to being healed and that his path would become clear. I looked into his dark eyes. "Don't give up."

His face and shoulders relaxed. "No, Dr. Randall, I won't. Thanks. I needed to hear that."

How Long Have We Worked with Dreams? Forever

Dreams have guided and informed us from the time our hunter-gatherer ancestors sought out interpretation from their shaman. Dreams became a central guidepost to how people, communities and societies conducted their lives, as well as being sources of healing information.

Five thousand years ago, in ancient Mesopotamia (Iraq), Sumerians practiced dream incubation. There is strong evidence that they used it systematically to gain knowledge about the future. The same held true further east-southeast, with the Vedic scholars and masters of ancient India. The practice spread to the great civilizations of Egypt, Troy, Greece, and Rome. All of these ancients sought guidance and healing in the dreamtime. They camped and slept in sacred places and temples, and asked for dreams to guide them.

Early Greeks also practiced dream incubation for the express purpose of healing. They practiced at temples dedicated to the healer-turned-god Aesculapius (Asclepius) during the sixth and seventh century BC. The practice was transplanted to Rome in 293 BC when, guided by a dream, Epidaurus sent a great snake (purportedly Aesculapius, taking that form) to heal an outbreak of the plague. It subsided.

The largest and most complete ancient compilation of dream information is *The Oneirocritica* ("The Interpretation of Dreams"). The author, second-century BC Greek Artemidorus of Dladis, focused primarily on divining the future.

Today, sadly, dream divining and doctoring is not a regular part of our social fabric. Nor do Western doctors typically pay much attention to dreams. However, dreams are as powerful in healing us, foretelling our futures, and guiding us into or out of major decisions as they ever were—and it behooves us to incorporate dream work into our growing awareness of our lives and emphasis on self-care and planetary balance.

Conscious Intent: Working with Sam and Irene

A patient of mine, Sam, became ill about a week after he returned from Mexico. He put himself under my care for severe abdominal pains, bloody diarrhea and high fevers. We diagnosed intestinal parasites, and he underwent appropriate medical therapy, but was not improving.

Before falling asleep one night, I prayed and asked for a healing for Sam. The following dream happened next:

I find myself in Sam's bedroom, a place I've never seen before. While floating or levitating above his bed, I watch him sleep. I see the red heat congested in his bowel. With my intent, I guide the heat out and replace it with a beautiful turquoise blue. Sweat pours from his body. He awakens with a sigh of relief and the distinct feeling that something unwanted has left his body.

The next morning, I called to check on him. "Thanks for last night," he said.

"What?" I knew what he was referring to, but was still surprised by his matter-of-fact attitude. "Did you feel that?"

"Oh yeah! I saw you hovering over my bed in a white flowing dress working on my energy."

Sam enjoyed a quick and uneventful recovery. I never cease to be amazed at the mysterious and powerful ways in which the universal forces work through us.

On another occasion, I had the following dream:

I stand next to a patient in a metal hospital bed. She is young and beautiful with long curly dark red hair. Her kidneys are failing. I also know that if they perform a scheduled test (intravenous pyelogram), her life will be in danger. I take her by the hand and lead her out of the hospital. I prepare electrolyte solutions for her to drink and flush her kidneys. I also illuminate her kidneys with orange light, followed by green light.

Six months later, I met Irene, a woman with long curly dark red hair who endured a near-death experience from kidney failure. "I would have died if I had gone through with that dye test of my kidneys the doctors tried to get me to take," she said. "But something or somebody told me not to do it."

If intravenous dyes are given to people with failing or stressed kidneys, renal failure can result. Irene said her "angel guides" told her that her doctor was a woman with an office by the ocean, near where she lived. (I was practicing in Malibu.) When we finally met, I carried out the color healing on her kidneys I was shown in the dream. I also gave her some kidney cleansers and a protomorphogenic (cell-specific proteins) supplements for the kidney (PMG). After a few weeks, we checked her kidney function; it was normal.

Another prophetic healing dream happened in the early morning of May 13, 1998, a dream both personal and collective:

I am performing "angelic-like work," moving among many people in geographic areas throughout the planet. When the subject of my work is encountered, I enter the scene. Although these people are unconsciously aware of my input, they cannot see or hear me as they would another human. I telepathically send them a thought given to me, which registers to them as an idea or inspiration they believe has come from within themselves.

I'm working on a personal level with a middle-aged woman dealing with suicidal thoughts. She wears thick glasses and is overweight. She lives alone in an inner-city apartment. She's never been married, and has no children of her own. She feels alone and worthless. I put my hand on her shoulder and remind her of her friendship with the eight-year-old boy next door. He came from an unstable home. His father abandoned the family, and his mother worked all night as a waitress and drank too much. I send a vision of the boy into her mind and heart. Her spirits lift. She feels purposeful and whole again.

The scene shifts to Ireland, where I am working with the leaders of the IRA and British government in charge of Northern Ireland. They cannot see or hear me. I whisper into their ears that they should consider setting up a series of meetings. They agree among each other that three negotiation meetings be arranged. In the first, they agree to disagree. In the second, they set up committees to see what the two groups hold in common. In the third, I suggest they hand out pieces of blank paper to everyone. I propose an exercise in which one group pretends to live by the other group's belief system, then write down the redeeming qualities of that belief system.

Within a few days, I saw a report in the *Los Angeles Times* that peace negotiations were being held in Ireland. In no way am I claiming any credit for what occurred in Ireland. Nor has their age-old, historic strife been my focus in conscious reality. However, this dream emphasizes that we all have the potential to work together to manifest planetary healing and collective wholeness. We are all connected and part of the same dream wave.

The late, great Swiss psychotherapist and author Carl Jung said that much of the world's mythology and folklore represents manifestations from the collective unconsciousness—our inheritance of the collective experience of humankind. It is a storehouse of all of humanity's experiences, archetypes or prototypes that subconsciously predispose us to organize our personal and social structures in a certain way. This helps explain the similarities or overlays between the world's great religions and philosophies. It also explains how dreams can occur in metaphors and archetypes, even for those uneducated in interpreting these symbols. Furthermore, Jung said that when we sleep, a part of our brain connects to that storehouse and can download information in the form of archetype dream images.

That would explain my dream about Northern Ireland—and countless other dreams we have. The key is to recognize the archetypes, symbols and metaphors. Rather than take them literally, *interpret* what they mean or symbolize in our own lives.

Brenda: Dream Healing Self

The most common type of dream healing occurs when a patient dream-heals herself or himself. This happened to Brenda, who first came to my office for what she felt was a fairly routine visit. My intuition suggested otherwise; we would walk some fiery paths together. Brenda lived with a well-differentiated lymphoma (slow-growing and less life-threatening form of cancer). It was "in remission." I knew her hematologist (blood doctor) from UCLA, a well-trained and astute physician. Brenda visited me for complementary therapy to augment her Western medicine treatment. I put her on a regimen that combined an organic foods diet, nutritional supplements, herbal remedies and intravenous vitamin infusions.

A year later, Brenda returned for a complete evaluation. She was disturbed. "The swelling in my right arm is worse than it ever has been," she said.

When I examined her arm, I could see and feel fluid accumulating under her skin, from her armpit to her wrist. "You better go see your hematologist and see if she wants to get another CAT scan and do some blood tests," I suggested.

During the time between visits, Brenda's lymphoma had transformed into a poorly differentiated lymphoma (rapidly growing, life-threatening). She underwent several rounds of chemotherapy to control it. After the final round of chemo, she was again declared "in remission."

A few months later, Brenda returned to my office, with the same look I saw when her arm was swollen. "What is it?" I asked.

"I don't know. All I know is I don't feel good. I felt better when I was on the chemotherapy than I do now."

Brenda was very attuned to her body and spirit. She practiced Buddhism and was sensitive to her energetic system. I watched her eyes, distracted by something else that didn't look right. "What are those bumps in front of your ear?" I asked.

"My hematologist checked those last week. She said it's normal for them to come and go, and she doesn't want to see me for a month."

"Perhaps. But I'd feel more comfortable if you went back as soon as you can get in."

I called her hematologist's office. They gave her an appointment for two weeks later, since they'd just seen her. However, Brenda's body had another plan. The next morning, she called me. "Dr. Randall, I have black stool and I am so dizzy I can hardly walk."

"Don't try to walk," I told her. "Call nine-one-one and go immediately to the hospital, and I will call ahead. I'll also call your hematologist."

Brenda was diagnosed with a gastric ulcer. During her hospital stay, it was also found that her lymphoma had recurred, worse than before. While in the hospital, she called me. "Let's plan a healing ceremony, OK?" she asked.

"OK. First, let's see what hematology and the gastroenterologists have to say. Then we will ask in the dreamtime for your healing, and perform a ceremony when the time is right." We agreed to speak again in a week, when we had more information about her condition and she was feeling better.

That night, I prayed for the best possible outcome. I asked that the elements of earth and the heavens come forward to assist with Brenda's healing process, whatever that might be. After my prayers and just before going to bed, I was moved to sing the stones in my bedroom circle, the medicine wheels around the house, all of the stones and mineral *people* (as American Indians call them) on the property, and in the mountain on which we lived.

What followed was this dream:

I sit in an ancient stone temple, engraved with wisdom from times gone by. My role is to teach people what "they already know"—to access the inner knowing we all possess in order to heal. I was shown the bones of the body and told they are like the stones of the earth. Bones and stones carry the most memory. In humans, memory stores in crystallized form in the bones and cells, in progenitor DNA form. This memory can be activated by golden divine energies that look like tiny space shuttles, or angels with four wings. Activating this energy gives the potential to change DNA, to accelerate evolution or bring healing. In the case of the stones, other energetic phenomena occur, such as heat. Perhaps this was how Frank Fools Crow, the famous Lakota shaman and medicine man, heated the stones for his sweat lodge without the use of fire.

I'm taking a class in this temple setting. A woman in the class asks if I want her to show me the goals for our class. "Sure," I reply.

The woman is Brenda. She takes me to a wooden box with symbols carved in the top and gives me a wooden block. It is key to selecting the appropriate symbol atop the box. I place the key over the upper right corner symbol, and line up the two symbols. A hole opens, and golden light floods through it. When I look through the hole, I see the same golden divine energies I was shown before.

A priest appears at my side, offering to show something to our class. He looks exactly like Pope John Paul II (who reigned from 1978 until his death in 2005). He points the way through the forest and tells us to follow the stream. Brenda takes a much harder route, but I follow essentially the same path and keep up with her pace. Before we reach this square stone building, the Pope-like priest hands us nine stones of incredible beauty. He conveys to us telepathically that they will assist with waking up memory in the bones and transferring it to the stem cells. After he leaves, we walk together toward the stone building.

Miles away in the hospital, Brenda had the following dream, which she later recounted to me:

"I was under the water, but I could breathe. It seemed as though we all lived in the underwater world. A group of eight women came around me in a circle, with me in the center. My body began to glow, and I saw myself grow young and healthy again. I was with my lover in a tree house. Then my body lifted out of itself and I floated brilliantly like a star up into the sky, with the Dalai Lama at my side."

After she was released from the hospital, Brenda came into the office. Her lymphoma had grown even more aggressive, and her hematologist wanted her to undergo a stem cell transplant. In this procedure, doctors remove your bone marrow cells and treat them so they will grow new bone marrow and blood-producing cells when returned to your body. They preserve the stem cells while putting your body through a process of chemotherapy and radiation therapy that kills virtually all blood cells and other rapidly producing cells in your body. You must stay in isolation, because you have no immunity to fight off infections.

The letter I received from Brenda's hematologist stated she had a 10 percent chance of survival without the stem cell transplant, and a 40 to 50 percent chance if she underwent the procedure.

Brenda chose to live. She went ahead with the transplant.

One week later, Brenda called to arrange the ceremony that revealed itself in her dream. We brought together eight healers and performed a medicine wheel healing, with Brenda in the center. Her resulting stem cell transplant proved successful, giving her vital additional time with her lover and son. She never would've had this time without the transplant.

Unfortunately, her lymphoma recurred several months later. She passed away in her tree house–like home, her mate at her side, in alignment with her traditional Buddhist practices. As she passed, prayers were said for her in the Dalai Lama's temple in Dharamsala, India, and the temple of Venerable Van Geshe Gyeltsen, spiritual leader of Thubten Dhargye Ling, a Buddhist center in Long Beach, California, named by the Dalai Lama himself. Van Geshe Gyeltsen had fled Tibet for India during the Chinese insurrection in 1959, at the same time as his dear friend and leader.

Van Geshe Gyeltsen was a venerated monk, one of the Dalai Lama's highest-level monks in the world—and also Brenda's lover and the father of her son. (Monks in some Buddhist sects can marry.) He was called to return to the Dalai Lama's seat for this part of his life service, and was able to give Brenda this final honor and tribute. A few years later, in 2009, he passed as well.

Try This at Home

Let's try an exercise to establish your work in the dreamtime. We need to call into being a dream, vital if you're going to focus on dream work for yourself. You can use a dream catcher or a bowl to symbolize receiving the dream seed. The bowl, or spiral symbol, also emphasizes the feminine energy.

The best protection for conscious dreaming is to clear yourself of any attachments or excess energy to which you might be clinging before bedtime. Smudging with sage, or taking an Epsom salt bath, can clean your spiritual and emotional energy and allow you to attract your highest dream seed. Traditionally, if you place a dream catcher beside or above your bed, it will not only catch the good dreams, but allow non-beneficial dreams to pass through the hole in the center. You may also want to adorn your dream catcher with certain totems, feathers or medicine items that are special to you.

Keep a dream journal by your bed to remind you to pull back the energy of the dream when you awaken. If you do not have time to journal the full dream, just make a few notes; you can come back to it during normal waking hours and pull it back. Journaling allows you to track the energy of your dreams. It is fascinating to later look and see how the dreams paint the story of your life. They can assist you in making the right choices for your best future.

CHAPTER 19
Miracles Happen

The mystical law of transformation is to release all judgment and expectation. There is no room to hang on that which we think we know or old scripts. We must release them to make room for new knowledge from which true healing and wisdom may unfold. We need to be in that place of childlike innocence and become completely teachable.

Reports of miraculous or spontaneous cures have become popular during the 21st century, especially through the works of physician-writers including Andrew Weil, Joan Borysenko, Eben Alexander, Dean Ornish, Deepak Chopra and Larry Dossey. Miracles big and small also happen daily, despite the claims of errant belief systems that they haven't happened in 2,000 years. That simply is not true; we all have that innate inner power to transform lives and manifest great moments and events into our own. Marianne Williamson created *A Course in Miracles*, one of the most important works of the past 50 years, to strongly remind and empower each student of this power, and to participate in their own miracles.

While the dynamics of a miracle seem impossible for Western science to explain, they are described quite scientifically in the Indian Vedas, Kabbalah, Egyptian and Aramaic texts, and other ancient sources. Rather than dismiss miracles as occurrences of a past millennium, accidents or "random events," it's time to embrace them as rays of hope and invitations to open our hearts and souls to receive them in our own lives. We need to study these events and see what environmental factors they have in common.

As one who has experienced, witnessed and participated in miraculous healings, I also suggest that they speak strongly to the power behind the process of healing. That includes addressing spirit and being open to higher intervention. Cases of miraculous healing need to stand as beacons for doctors, rather than being thrown out as wacky, inexplicable freaks of nature or mistaken diagnoses. We as doctors need to encourage deeper looks to guide our patients and provide additional hope for those with long-term or terminal illnesses. We mustn't discount the medical facts and statistics, but neither should we discount the power of spiritual healing, meaning and purpose for patients with severe disease.

Being open to miracles is one of the greatest gifts you can give yourself. This opens you up to the inexhaustible and eternal source of the energy, light and breath that gives you life.

Miracles in Action

In 2002, while presenting a workshop at a future-thinking spiritual and social conference, I participated in a wonderful experience of miracles in action with my dear friends at the Sierra Dove Healing Center.[54] Sierra Dove lay at the base of a native Mescalero Apache power spot in southeastern New Mexico, the quartz-covered Sierra Blanca mountain range (once North America's southernmost glacier).

There, I was introduced to Doug, a man in his late 50s suffering from severe adult-onset diabetes. Doug and a friend drove to Sierra Dove from Florida in a last-ditch effort to save his life. He didn't necessarily believe that the treatment we planned in New Mexico would help him; in fact, several friends had to persuade him for months to head west. Quickly, we realized his physical condition was so bad that he needed nothing less than a medical miracle to stay on the planet.

In New Mexico he was given a place to stay in a small house atop a mountain ridge at 8,000 feet. The "backyard" was an eagle's eye view of Sierra Blanca, eight miles due west. On an average warm day, 10 to 20 eagles flew overhead. Since Doug had never been above 4,000 feet in his life, his spirit immediately soared—step one in healing thyself. A lifelong folk, bluegrass and rock musician who performed on more than 50 albums and produced many others, he played for hours against this backdrop.

Each morning, a hummingbird hovered outside Doug's bedroom window, unwilling to budge until he arose and the hummer saw that he was all right. On the native medicine wheel, the hummingbird is the archetype of clarity and vision. It asks those receiving its medicine to see the truth and make the most of a new situation. (Being atop a mountain in a strange place, facing death and needing to change almost everything in his lifestyle would qualify as a "new situation.") Also, to stop longing for the past and to focus on the benefits of the present (a chance to heal and grow).

For the past 30 years, Doug had given himself daily insulin shots; by now, he was up to an alarming 200 units. He was also 100 pounds overweight. When Julia Price, the Sierra Dove director, first read his energy field, she described it as "almost totally shut down. Looks like he's getting ready to go." Then she sat down with Doug to present a treatment plan involving Sierra Dove's fine healing team (myself included). It included major dietary changes, herbs, supplements, pranic healing, the use of color and sound therapy, exercise, enzymatic solutions, reflexology, ceremony, plus meditation and visualization.

Not surprisingly, he balked. For the rest of that first day, he seriously considered driving back to Florida. However, Doug's soul overrode his head, and he hung in there.

The spirit of the place and people, their loving concern for him, and the effect on his soul and heart pushed him forward. Julia also adjusted the treatment plan to a more doable level for him to start.

Doug spent the week with a variety of practitioners. One was psychologist and medical herbalist Dr. Gerald St. Clair, who became his best friend for the last fifteen years of their respective lives. In Albuquerque, as a tribute to me, Doug played guitar in a sacred Indian kirtan (devotional chanting) while Gerald played a native drum—where he, my editor and others sang to my soul while I was undergoing cancer surgery in Tucson.

Doug stood outside in the lightning and driving rain, absorbing the electric prana of his first-ever high-mountain thunderstorm, and made many new friends. For the first time in many years, he also exercised, beginning with breathless walks of 100 yards. He already was up to comfortable strolls of nearly a mile—at an altitude of 8,000 feet, not the easiest place to breathe—by the time he went back to Florida two weeks later.

When he got home and went to the doctor, Doug learned he was a walking miracle. His 200 units of insulin had plummeted to just 30 units daily—a decrease of *85 percent* from the "permanent dosage." He lost 30 pounds, meditated daily, ate almost entirely organic, wholesome foods, and experienced his greatest burst of musical creativity since his prime studio recording years. His wife, Ellie, could not contain her amazement. She continually referred to Doug's time with us as "the miracle that brought my husband back."

When we met Doug, he had maybe a year to live. As it turned out, he created music and joy for Ellie and others for another 15 years, until he left his body in 2018 at age 74.

Keys to Miraculous Healing

There is no quick fix or "miracle formula" that will work for all patients. Everyone responds differently, from the medicines they take to the ways they connect with the soul. Through my observation, though, there are similarities among cases of miraculous healing, such as Doug's. Four key similarities are:

1. A sincere desire on the part of the patient to return to wellness;
2. A certain surrender or trust to the process of the illness and healing, which leads the patient to a greater unique sense of inner knowing (where the illness acts as a life teacher);
3. Doctors, specialists or healers who can see past the physical person, understand how energy works, and also how to unblock and let flow healing energy; and
4. Loving support from family, friends and self.

If you look at Doug's story, you'll see that all four factors were in place.

The most difficult task in participating in our own healing is obtaining inner knowing or insight from an illness that seems to be sucking our lives away. How can we concentrate on the deeper, core reasons for being sick when we're fighting off the pain and discomfort every day? Also, we often are afraid to face what has contributed to making us sick in the first place. Our initial impulse is to do something to fix it. Most often, we look outside ourselves for that fix. We want to take a pill or cut out a tumor to cure the disease. We rarely set our focus within, where we can access our inner wisdom to find the answer.

These are difficult and sensitive issues. Each person's way of dealing may be slightly different. Some may meet the issues head-on and put everything on the table, like my younger brother demonstrated in his passing. By confronting and dealing with his issues, he healed not only spiritually, but physically, really part of the same thing. That's the beauty of it! He still died, but with dignity and full quality of life. Others may deal with these issues inwardly and only need our support. In this work, physicians need to be sensitive to the uniqueness of each patient and honor his or her specific needs and belief systems. In this way, we can best facilitate a return to their healing path, whether or not they choose to live.

Healing My Mother

My mother, Helen, experienced a truly miraculous healing. Just one and a half years after the passing of my brother, her youngest son, she underwent a routine chest X-ray prior to a cervical disc operation for an entrapped nerve. After the neck operation, the doctors told her they'd found a golf ball–sized mass in her upper right lung. My first reaction was an overwhelming feeling of dread; she'd just buried my brother! Casey was my mother's youngest child, and she had never reconciled his loss. My mother had also cared for my father before he died in 1986 after a grueling years-long battle with Alzheimer's disease. I knew in my heart that the cancer was her body's way of dealing with her tremendous sense of loss and grief.

The biopsies of my mother's tumor proved malignant, and the doctors recommended surgery. I arranged coverage in my busy practice and professorship at UCLA and flew to Omaha to be at my mother's side. She was going to be 75; the risk of surgery was considerable. We discussed potential risks and benefits with her and the family. She chose surgery.

My mother was old school, raised Irish Catholic and educated by the Jesuits through college. She later changed her place of worship to the Protestant church and retained her deep religious convictions. While honoring her beliefs, I asked her to work with me on a very personal level. We talked about my brother, my father and other losses she felt in her life. I told her that in some kinds of medicine (Chinese, for example) the lungs are the organ of grief. This broke into the public eye in 2004, when actor Christopher Reeve (*Superman*) died, followed a year later by his wife, who died of lung cancer—despite never smoking a cigarette in her life. Her grief consumed her.

Likewise, my mother's disease implied that she had unresolved issues in that area. With my guidance and support, she worked in her own inward way to clear any unresolved issues regarding my brother, father, and other losses. We used gentle guided meditation and prayer. She found these methods acceptable. She also allowed me to perform hands-on healing sessions (pranic healing), to which she would respond, "Oh! Are you giving me another one of those heat treatments? That feels good." She took anti-cancer herbs such as astragalus and maitake and other tonic mushrooms, and antioxidant teas I made for her both before and after surgery.

After weeks of work, the day of her surgery arrived. I sat with my older sister and brother in a small, windowless waiting room for what seemed like an eternity. Finally, the surgeon arrived. My mother had done well, he said, although there were some surprises. She would be on a ventilator and, because her good lung collapsed in the recovery room, tubes would remain in her chest for some time in order to keep her lung expanded. "We'll know more when we get the pathology report," he said.

Then he added something I'll never forget: "Oh, also the tumor underwent necrosis or something. We had a hard time finding it. It was just a hole about the size of a golf ball."

In other words, the tumor mass was gone when they went in to remove it!

How did that happen? Well, it was a convergence of healing agents and treatments, Mom's belief, prayer and meditation, and my work with the subtler energies of her body and the tumor itself. When you bring together treatment, belief, prayer and/or meditation, and conscious awareness of how energy works at deeper levels, you step into the elemental world of miraculous healing.

The sun was down by the time the nurses allowed us to visit Mother, who was settled in her ICU bed. I could see the panic in the eyes of my brother and sister when they saw her with tubes in every part of her body, dependent on a ventilator to breathe for her. The nurses made it clear that we were to visit for 10 minutes, one at a time. There would be absolutely no visitors before 8 a.m. or after 8 p.m. The fact that I was a doctor from UCLA had no bearing on their rules. After we were certain she was comfortable and aware of our presence, it was nearly 8 p.m. We left.

I drove to my mother's house and sat in the backyard. I made offerings in the four directions around a huge tree in her backyard. I was deep in prayer, giving thanks that my mother passed through her surgery and the immediate threat to her life. I prayed that she would receive all that she needed to become whole, so she could return to her path.

Then I heard the rattling of someone or something on the chain-link fence. *Oh! Must be one of those raccoons she told me about. What a blessing it would be to see a raccoon in the middle of town like this.*

Astonishment washed through me when a red fox walked directly to the great tree and moved to each of the four directions—as if reading my prayers from the offerings I left there! It turned and looked directly into my eyes, the yellow-green gleam of its own entering my soul, comforting me. Once its message was transmitted, the fox turned and walked away, as unhurried as it had come.

Did that really just happen? I knew the Lakota meaning: the fox represents family unity and love. I understood the teaching and the message.

I resolved to return to the ICU. How could I make myself invisible in the wee hours so I could sit with my mother? I brought along a piece of jasper, a stone that is supposed to impart invisibility to the wearer. I stuck it deep into my pocket and drove to the hospital. When you're nearly six feet tall with long white hair, as I am, being invisible is a real challenge, jasper or not. Knowing the workings of the ICU, I waited until my mother's nurse went to the back for a break.

I made my move. I walked like the fox, deliberately and directly, to my mother's room and sat in a chair in the corner. I sat until 6 a.m. Nurses and respiratory therapists came in and out of the room, but never so much as looked at me. I left before the next shift began, knowing my brother Gary would be there at 8 a.m. sharp. This way, Mom received almost constant in-person loving from her family.

Finally, the day of reckoning arrived: the pathology report. As the surgeon told us, it showed the tumor had almost entirely disappeared from the space it had occupied. However, tumor cells were spotted near and inside a medium-sized blood vessel and lymph vessel. In Western medicine, this is often considered a death sentence, as it predicts a spread of the cancer to two of the body's primary transport vehicles—the bloodstream and the lymphatic system. Based on this finding, her doctors recommended chemotherapy. When Mother refused chemotherapy and radiation, the doctors said the cancer would likely recur within six months. We finally got her home, and continued the herbal, prayer, love and energetic therapies we had started before the surgery.

It was time for me to fly back to LA. On the way to the airport, my brother drove us through Elmwood Park, located in the middle of Omaha. I saw a family of red foxes by the stream. I had never seen them before, nor since. I felt blessed the fox family came to assure me our family stood unified and strong. After I got home, my sister, brother and loving aunt helped Mother continue her therapies.

In 2004, nearly a decade later, four generations came together for Helen Casey Randall's 85th birthday. Mother would go on to live until she was 93, a miracle in and of itself, considering how close she came to dying two decades before.

Several years later, after I moved my practice from UCLA to an integrative wellness clinic overlooking the ocean in Malibu, a sudden illness overtook me at work. It was early May, on a day I came to find out later was the full moon of Buddha. A few months prior to this event, I had the following dream:

I am lying on a sandy beach, clothed in brown smock-like clothes. There is a ceremony of some type. I am there to help some people, but too weak to get up. I look down and see a trail of blood coming from between my legs, making a small stream running down the beach and into the water. I try to get up. Instead of standing, I lift out of my body into a grouping of beautiful pastel lights.

That day was a rarity. My partner in the practice, Jesse Hanley, and I hardly ever worked at our office on the same day. We decided to share lunch together. As we arrived at the restaurant, which was only down the stairs from our office, something began to overtake me. I felt horribly weak and put my head down on the table at the restaurant. I had to leave her in the restaurant. It took every ounce of my strength to walk back up to the office. There, I collapsed on the examining table and began to have violent, uncontrollable chills, shaking, and severe abdominal pain.

When Jesse returned, I was barely conscious, but heard her say, "Your blood pressure is barely measurable and your pulse is thready."

My pain was so severe I would have screamed, but I was too weak. I was sinking and falling—until suddenly I felt better. I felt myself out of body, watching from above, as Jesse started intravenous lines, took blood samples and poured in fluids. It was only later that we found out: I was suffering from a large ovarian cyst that had ruptured suddenly.

My interest drifted. I looked up to see beautiful, brilliant colors swirling about—golds, pinks, peaches, all of an unearthly sharpness and clarity. There was no pain. I thought, *I felt so free and ecstatic.* The colors seemed to speak to me so kindly. *"Go back now. Turn around. You are needed and must complete your purpose."*

I felt a deep sense of recognition. *The kind ones*, I thought. *The kind ones* from my birth.

Some would call this a chemical reaction to hypotension. However, this same experience is known to many who have had near-death experiences, or NDEs. I have no doubt; I was out of the body, looking down at my physical form, falling into the absorbing colors and comfort beyond the physical plane. Today, many years later, I am thankful for the experience giving me a glimpse of the soul's journey after this life. I'm also thankful to Jesse Hanley for saving my life and making it possible to finish my work on earth with renewed purpose—the core of *the kind ones'* message to *go back now. Turn around. Finish your work.*

CHAPTER 20
Healthy Brain

Today, an increasing number of patients of all ages, including my own patients and those of other doctors, are presenting with varying degrees of cognitive decline. What is different in our environment, food or lifestyle that could be causing this increase? And what does it look like?

Let's answer some of those questions with a look at Chris, my patient of more than a decade. Chris is a brilliant lawyer with a measurable IQ of 180 who initially came to me with unusual medical problems, including severe rashes and allergic reactions. Turned out he was overconsuming aspartame (a known toxin) through eight diet sodas a day and using a Teflon pan to cook his food on a daily basis. He also had a yeast infection that resulted in esophagitis. I was thinking he must be so toxic, with an inflammatory component because of the infections. It took me about four years to persuade him to change his diet by removing toxins, refined carbs (bread, pasta and sweets), and taking supplements for reducing inflammation and eliminating yeast.

One day, he came in for a follow-up and gave me the same speech I'd heard for the past two or three years. "I'm seventy-eight years old," he said. "I can still play and win at bridge, I earn lots of money in the online stock market, but I can't do something as simple as remember names or sometimes where I park my car."

I looked at him, ready to ask the same question I'd asked before: "OK, so that is not acceptable right?"

"Right" he said.

"So are you ready to make a few changes?" I paused to let that sink in. "You really need to exercise. It is key for the brain. It increases the production of brain-derived neurotrophic factor (BDNF), which is central to remembering and growing new brain cells. All I'm asking for is thirty to forty minutes of walking, three times a week."

Chris pondered that for a moment. "OK, OK," he said. "I'll do it."

"Also, there are a few supplements I'd like you to try." He was listening, so I proceeded. "Coffee fruit increases your BDNF. Ginkgo biloba increases the microcirculation in your brain and the rest of your body. A complex formulation with rosemary and sage also helps BDNF and memory."

I had wrestled with Chris over supplements for years. This time, he agreed to take them. *He must really be suffering*, I thought.

I circled back to a previous medical issue which was almost certainly playing a role in his declining cognitive function. "And, since you had that bad shingles episode on your face a few years ago, I would love for you to take a strong natural antiviral herbal complex, particularly effective against herpes [shingles is caused by the herpes virus], since that can affect your brain." Studies have shown amyloid brain plaques (hallmarks of Alzheimer's disease) located right next to or inside a viral inclusion (abnormal structures in the nucleus of the host cell), indicating that chronic viruses like herpes are a cause of some cognitive issues.

Also, I asked him to start fasting intermittently and to skip breakfast. That was a huge sacrifice, since he took his wife out to breakfast five days a week.

Much to my surprise, he returned to see me just two months later. "I wanted to tell you those things you gave me are really helping," he said. "I still forget stuff sometimes, but I can feel the difference."

"That's great. Are you exercising?"

He flashed a particular smile . . . *No.* "I still take my wife to breakfast but I just have coffee and a salad."

"What kind of salad?" I asked.

"A Caesar salad with extra dressing."

"Can we go to the next level?" I asked. "You know the things I'm suggesting are working. Let's try it."

"OK."

Next, we agreed on dietary changes, replacing his Caesar salads with dark lettuce with olive oil and balsamic vinegar. We discussed earlier that olive oil also reduces inflammation if full of polyphenol antioxidants.

Two months later, Chris came back, declaring himself improved. This time, he wanted something else from me—a date.

"That's a little out of my area, Chris," I said, fighting off a chuckle, "but I am sure you can handle that on your own."

"If you say so." he said with that flirty twinkle in his eyes.

Cognitive Decline: a Growing Challenge

When we think of brain health today, we tend to focus on cognitive decline and the terrible toll degenerative illnesses like Alzheimer's and other forms of dementia take on the affected person plus family and friends. Others focus on anxiety-involved disorders that can crop up at the earliest age. Never have we seen so much cognitive decline or anxiety in our culture—or disorders such as anxiety, OCD, autism spectrum disorders, dissociative disorder, depression, bipolar syndrome, PTSD, ADD/ADHD, or variations of these. In the 19 years between the releases of two editions of the *Diagnostic and Statistical Manual of Mental Disorders, DSM-IV* (1994) and *DSM-V* (2013), the number of named and defined mental health issues *doubled.*

Without a doubt, cognitive decline is a serious public health problem in the US. As of 2022, there are more than five million people with Alzheimer's and other forms of dementia in the US. Those are just clinically recorded cases. By 2050, that number is expected to grow to 16 million.[55] In addition, there are more than a billion people worldwide suffering with chronic diseases. These often lead to cognitive decline; the brain can only do so much without clean food and healthy exercise before it wears down.

All of this is directly related to the highly stressful, busy lives we lead, a society filled with toxins and distractions, and the race to make money or have "success" that seems to keep getting harder and faster. It's also related to the large disconnect of many from deep, purposeful and spiritual lives, and the price we pay for not eating brain foods, exercising, stretching our minds "outside the box," or getting outdoors enough for exercise and fresh air.

While much of this chapter addresses the alarming rise of cognitive decline issues, it speaks to the importance of all of us doing everything we can to feed, nurture, love, exercise and protect our brains. The nutritional, medical and lifestyle solutions I describe in this chapter are for all of us; I consider them vital. And never more so than for those suffering from cognitive issues.

The most important place to start is with our mindset. Ask yourself: Am I mostly positive? What is my purpose in life—and do I focus on it enough? Is there prayer, meditation, journaling or some other form of introspection and reflection in my life? Am I compassionate toward others? Empathetic when something happens? And do these attitudes and behaviors accompany me in (nearly) everything I say or do? If you or a friend or loved one is experiencing cognitive decline, this mindset is even more crucial.

Six Main Causes of Cognitive Decline

According to international neurodegenerative disease expert Dr. Dale Bredesen, cognitive decline and the impending onset of Alzheimer's and dementia occur due to six major causations:

1. Inflammatory or Hot—Infectious, autoimmune, gut related
2. Glycotoxic—Insulin resistance, hyperglycemia, diabetes
3. Atrophic or Cold—Hormone and/or nutrient depletion
4. Toxic or Vile Toxins—Heavy metals, other toxins
5. Vascular—Decreased microvascular supply, strokes
6. Traumatic—PTSD, head trauma[56]

One of the largest risks for Alzheimer's, especially if coupled with poor lifestyle, is genetic—the presence of a gene called ApoE4. When activated, it increases the number of "suicide" messages sent to the brain cells. The gene allows amyloid plaque to build up; ApoE4 also presents a cardiovascular risk with increased cholesterol plaques in coronary arteries.

"Suicide messages" kill cells and outstrip the brain's ability to create new ones. Poor lifestyle choices increase their frequency. If there are signs of cognitive disease, then genetic, biochemical and nutrition analysis can be helpful to root out contributory causes that, when addressed, can reverse and slow down disease. The general consensus is that drugs do not work for Alzheimer's, is mostly because there are too many factors that play into its development and expression, and the drugs' range of actions are too small.

In *The End of Alzheimer's Disease: The First Program to Prevent and Reverse Cognitive Decline*, Dr. Bredesen also describes three main types of Alzheimer's:

Type 1: Inflammatory or hot. This is a genetic form of Alzheimer's. In addition to ApoE4, there is ApoE3, with a 9 percent risk, and ApoE2, which carries a very small risk of Alzheimer's. Almost 25 percent of all Americans have one copy of the gene, while seven million people have two copies.

Type 2: Atrophic or cold. ApoE4 gene carriers express this type. This typically appears about 10 years later in life than Type 1. There's also a "Type 1.5," which is glycotoxic or sweet, made worse by high blood sugar, HbA1C, insulin resistance and diabetes.

Type 3: Toxic or vile. While more common in ApoE3 genetic carriers, it is not usually inherited. It is due to exposure to toxins, such as in Chris's case. Other toxins associated with it are glyphosates in products like the Roundup weed killer, and organophosphates from pesticides used in industrial farming. Younger people, often between 40 and 60 years old, express this type, which can be induced by great stress. It is quick and destructive, and apparently does not respond well to Dr. Bredesen's ReCODE protocol, a nutraceutical approach with a multivitamin, probiotics and multi-mineral. This type of cognitive decline is also associated with heavy metal toxins in the brain and body, such as mercury and tin. It seems as though lifestyle and supplements aimed at detoxification of these chemicals and heavy metals will help.

Now for the good news: While a huge issue, cognitive decline is almost entirely preventable and treatable with diet, exercise and lifestyle changes such as eliminating toxins, smoking and alcohol, as well as a healthy plant-based organic diet and supplements individualized to the person. The healthier the lifestyle, the better our chances of not experiencing cognitive decline or, if we are dealing with it, to either mitigate or eliminate the symptoms and debilitating effects.

From Shock Diagnosis to Cognitive Recovery

My longtime friend, Hayden, has enjoyed an active life as an award-winning author, marathon runner, sports coach, ocean sports enthusiast, yoga and meditation practitioner, and much more. He's been a professional journalist since he was 16, a straight-A student in both high school and college. Despite long hours and deadline stress, typically a combination ripe for a fast-food appetite, he has followed a largely meat-free plant-based diet since the late 1980s. I say "largely," because his appetite for snack foods was less than desirable—with ice cream, chips and cookies leading the way.

Imagine Hayden's shock when, in his late 50s, he realized his brain had stopped working properly. He couldn't focus. He would "space out," his stare vacant, his brain seeming to jump offline, first for minutes, then hours. Sometimes, it would take him a few *weeks* to get back into his regular life flow. Worse, this loving, considerate person stopped caring about his relationships, work and spiritual life. He withdrew from his friends. Most out of character, he stopped running after 20 years of high-level racing, and spent entire weekends in bed, binge-watching reruns after years of hardly watching TV.

More than once, Hayden wished that when he closed his eyes, they would not reopen. He stopped going to the beach and mountains, his most central connections with nature. He even stopped journaling, after 40 years of keeping journals. Thoughts would come . . . and they would go. He was clinically depressed, which often accompanies cognitive decline.

Desperate, Hayden sought out the neurological center that treated him for a small series of TBIs, or so-called "mini-strokes," he'd suffered in 2014–15. They diagnosed him with frontotemporal dementia, a nasty group of uncommon brain disorders that affects personality, behavior and language as the brain slowly dies. The lobes controlling these three functions atrophy. According to the Mayo Clinic, some experience dramatic changes to their personality and become socially inappropriate, impulsive or emotionally different. Others lose the ability to use language properly. Most stop caring, or have trouble caring, about things that always mattered greatly to them. Hayden had experiences with all of these behaviors.

A PET scan of Hayden's brain showed poorly metabolized nutrients in that crucial area, a result of degeneration, as well as a small but concerning amount of brain plaque. He received three injections of Solanezumab, a drug in late-stage FDA trials that, in some, reduces brain plaque. Doctors also wanted to prescribe him both an antidepressant and antipsychotic, but being a stubborn anti-pharmaceutical man with a "heal thyself" attitude, he refused. He'd endured a terrible adolescent experience with both antidepressants and doctors. It wouldn't be easy talking him into any treatment.

A few months later, Hayden called me up. He had been further spooked by a *60 Minutes* piece that spelled out the *incurability* and awful symptoms of this particular form of dementia. When we spoke, I presented something quite different. "Hayden, in my experience, early-stage dementia *is* entirely treatable and often curable with diet, lifestyle, exercise, and the use of natural medicines and supplements focused on the brain and nervous system and other root cause etiologies of reduced cognitive function," I told him.

He stayed quiet. It was the first time he'd heard the words "curable" or "treatable." "While I certainly don't claim to have the cure for everyone, I do know how to treat cognitive decline and have really excellent results even in older people," I continued.

Then Hayden brought up his livelihood; you can't write or edit books if you can't think or focus. "I have to work, Dr. Randall," he said with a sense of urgency.

"I know, Hayden . . . trust we can do this!"

We got right to work. I insisted he stop eating all refined carbs and go totally organic to remove the toxins from his brain and body, and to do some active daily cleansing with dark intense leafy greens in a smoothie, as he was a fish lover. I shared with him the green drink and color teachings from my Randall's Rainbow Detox Program. I also asked that he focus more on high-protein, low-carb, good-fat "brain foods" such as blueberries, avocado, olive oil, cruciferous vegetables, dark chocolate, green tea, turmeric, celery, pumpkin, sunflower and pumpkin seeds, beets, spinach, leafy greens, oranges, legumes, almonds, sage, rosemary, and tomatoes. Finally, I advised he drink lots of water—half his body weight per day, measured in ounces, as I mentioned before. For this 175-pound man, that meant 88 ounces, or almost three quarts.

The hard part was getting him onto a robust supplement and natural medicine regimen, and helping him to overcome some negative self-messaging. He's always taken supplements, and believes fully in their effectiveness. However, telling this man "You'll need to stick to this regimen from now on, with some adjustments later" is like telling a 50-foot granite boulder, "Move on down the road. Now."

I knew how to turn him around. "Hayden, I understand your resistance, but you know I am not just any doctor. I am your friend and healer of many years."

He heard that message, but more importantly, he understood what he was facing this time—that self-diagnosing and self-care would not be enough. Having me as his longtime trusted friend, and knowing my background, made all the difference. Instead of fighting and blocking me like he had other doctors, he put himself in my care with complete trust. I cannot emphasize how vital that was to the healing that has occurred since.

"We are going to get your brain into a healthy place," I said. "We are not only getting you through this, but *over and past this.*"

I put Hayden on a course of natural medicines to reduce inflammation, increase microcirculation, treat several different brain functions, boost his BDNF and more. I also advised him to return to his active lifestyle, mingle with people, answer the phone when it rang, and reenter the world. He needed to adjust his attitude to be more positive and stop looking for the pitfalls. I knew his high level of receptivity to spiritual healing, so I stayed attuned with him as he set out on a road to recovery he thought impossible.

Within nine months, Hayden felt like a new man. He was again razor-sharp and happy, able to again write entire books and keep their storylines in his head. He eventually began running again regularly, and his natural tendency to care for and serve others was back, as shown when he paced a friend on a 100-mile ultramarathon in 2021. In a truly gratifying moment, he put his newly healed brain to work and cared for his 40-year-old stepdaughter when COVID-19 hit her hard. He called me up, we consulted on caregiving steps, and I sent strong natural medicines, immune system builders and antivirals. Within three weeks, she was 100 percent recovered. While I provided the medical care, Hayden's stepdaughter benefitted greatly from his positive "you-will-heal" attitude.

Hayden also realized a few things. First, he'd been living for years in a depressed state, of which he was largely unaware. "It's really weird; I didn't think I was depressed, but feeling the way I do now, I feel like I just emerged from a giant black cloud," he said. "And every day, that cloud feels further and further away." When we back traced his recent history, we realized he had been working at diminished capacity for about five years. Imagine *five years* of not being at 100 percent—and not realizing it. Most of all, he remembered a saying that added to his care package: "Movement is the enemy of depression," which he learned from author and educator Susan Dermond, a colleague from when they taught college together.

Now, instead of watching the clock and wondering how long it will be until his brain fades out completely, Hayden makes his moments count. He looks forward to many more years of dynamic living and writing, racing again, and enjoying "having my brain back," as he puts it.

Tools to Restore Healthy Brains

When I work with patients suffering from cognitive decline, my tools are a nutrient evaluation with Genova Diagnostics' NutrEval or Spectracell. If not possible, I order B12, folate and homocysteine levels through regular lab testing, in addition to levels of mercury and other heavy metals, vitamin D3, and hormones (free and total testosterone for men; estradiol, progesterone, FSH and testosterone for women). Also, I order a thyroid panel for both men and women—high-sensitivity TSH, free T3 and free T4, and TPO antibodies—as well as FBS and HbA1C tests to check blood glucose level. High blood sugar and insulin levels are very damaging to the brain, heart and microcirculation throughout the body. This is key; a lot of people don't understand that excess insulin as a result of high blood sugar causes amyloid plaques to build up, because it deactivates the enzymes that degrade amyloid.

I have a testing system that can sort this out and help improve memory and stress symptoms. I began using Sanesco InternationalTM neurotransmitter endocrine testing and therapy intensely in the early 90s when we took holistic functional integrative medicine into the addiction recovery world and helped change the conversation in addiction therapy. We showed that holistic testing and treatments improved patients' outcomes and reduced symptoms like memory loss, insomnia, cravings, anxiety, depression, fatigue and even relapse rate. We looked at levels of neurotransmitters (serotonin, GABA, dopamine, norepinephrine, epinephrine, glutamate, cortisol, DHEA). I continue to use this system in my clinic. It literally changes people's lives!

A physician I know in a large British hospital was born without adrenal glands. After finding extremely low levels of all her neurotransmitters and adrenal hormones (not surprising, without adrenals), she feels better than ever. Her neurotransmitters are actually normal after taking Sanesco NeuroSupport—targeted amino acids and nutrients by Sanesco. People ask her, "What have you done!? You look amazing."

Once we find out the pattern of imbalance, we pick from the formulas Sanesco has to treat imbalances using biomimicry, targeted amino acid and nutrient therapy. We know what nutrients and amino acids feed the chemical pathways for each neurotransmitter. We correlate the patient's symptoms and history with the pattern on their tests. It is a great window into the patient's hypothalamus, pituitary, adrenal axis and neurochemical endocrine balance. It takes a few months of NeuroSupport. Then when a patient's symptoms are relieved and long-term health has been restored, annual or semi-annual testing can be done to maintain the patient's health and prevent recurrence. I also include a stress reduction program along with treatment, since most imbalances stem from stress. This is the most common reason for presenting to medical care.

The diet I recommend for ideal brain health and to deal with cognitive decline is very similar to Dr. Bredesen's protocol. It consists of whole, organic plant-based foods. He recommends mild ketosis. This occurs naturally with intermittent fasting, 12–14 hours without food from your evening meal to your first meal the next day (see Chapter 17). I also recommend healthy fats, olive oil and other monosaturated fats, along with avocados, nuts and seeds. Along with this comes low-glycemic fruits such as berries, 4 to 5 servings of vegetables per day (Bredesen says 10 to 15), and protein from legumes.

Meanwhile, it is very important for optimal brain health that we avoid refined carbohydrates, cookies, crackers (except for pressed seed crackers), bread, pasta, cakes, pastries, pizza, sugar, white rice, and all artificial sweeteners except stevia and xylitol. Also avoid gluten, and any processed food packaged in plastic, or packaged frozen.

The Power of Positive Thinking, Attitude—and Nature

What Dr. Bredesen does not include in his cognitive health regimen is something just as vitally important as nutrients—*positive thinking and attitude, empathy, and compassion.* Getting out and connecting to nature. Having a spiritual practice. Recall my approach with Hayden: I told him immediately, in a deeply empathetic way, we were not just getting him through his cognitive issue, but we were getting him *over and past it.* That statement inspired and motivated him; he thought about it every day.

In their book *Brain Wash*, David Perlmutter and his son, Austin, talk about the importance of empathy to deal with the cognitively affected.[57] This not only goes for the person affected, but for practitioner, family and friends. Austin Perlmutter also stated part of my approach well when he wrote, "Spending time in nature is one of the easiest things you can do to stay healthy and happy—you just need to step outside."

We seek nature when we need balance or to release stress. It relaxes our brain, our mind, our soul, and provides the prana, the life force, that naturally opens our brains to their fullest, healthiest forms. Nature is the greatest healer of all, whether through exercise, medicine, supplement, food, meditation or perspective. It, along with all aerobic exercise, is the greatest drive for increasing our brain-derived neurotrophic factor (BDNF) and neurogenesis—increasing the brain's ability to change and grow, to create new memories and connections.

BDNF is one of the most crucial elements in healthy brain function and neuroplasticity. Turns out that coffee fruit, the fruit of coffee around the bean or seed we modern people have been tossing aside as garbage for centuries, can increase our BDNF by 143 percent! BDNF is a protein that works with the brain synapses, tiny spaces where nerves and cells build up to pass along communication through neural messages. The plasticity of our brain, its ability to form and adapt synergistic connections, is totally dependent on our lifestyle and the quality of our thoughts. Positive thoughts and healthy lifestyle, good diet, and exercise increase BDNF.

It has been shown that high BDNF is associated with mental clarity and neuroplasticity. Exercise, sage and rosemary have also been shown to dramatically increase BDNF. Even if people have anatomical signs of brain plaques or neurofibrillary tangles, they do not express cognitive decline with high levels of BDNF. BDNF causes the brain to increase its neuroplasticity, which enables us to make new memories and create new things. This is monumental!

Anything that increases microcirculation, like exercise or ginkgo, protects brain function and brain stem cells. Turmeric is recommended by most experts to be the number one protectant for the brain because many cognitive issues are, at their root, inflammatory. Magnesium is the most prevalent cofactor throughout the metabolism, and magnesium threonate crosses the blood–brain barrier and assists brain function. The brain is mostly composed of fatty tissue, so fish oil and lecithin also support healthy function.

Another cognitive issue our brains face today is so-called "brain fog." Medically speaking, brain fog is an increased blood–brain barrier permeability traced back to dysbiosis and gut imbalance, caused by the overgrowth of "bad bacteria," yeast or parasites. Toxins such as alcohol, BPA, glyphosates, diesel exhaust and other petroleum products, mercury and lead are known causes. So are neuroinflammation food intolerances related to leaky gut, oxidative stress from poor diet, lack of antioxidants, and autoimmune diseases often related to gut imbalances and certain bacteria, such as *Prevotella* and *Klebsiella* which are autoimmune triggers.

Leaky gut can result in inflammation in the body systemically, which can eventually cause "leaky brain," with an incompetent blood–brain barrier. With this, the brain becomes inflamed, leading to plaques and neurofibrillary tangles.

This type of plaque buildup can also be related to poor clearance of toxins for a genetic reason, for example, a methylation defect or other genetic SNP's (single nucleotide polypeptice defect), low glutathione, and weak mitochondria. These are all fixable. On top of that, we're dealing with the effects of stress, which causes its own internal toxins, including leaky gut, poor glucose control and high insulin. High blood glucose and insulin levels are probably the most damaging to the brain.

Other issues associated with brain fog include reduced blood flow and circulatory deficiency due to poor sleep (the brain naturally detoxifies at night), and vascular disease, which can be reversed with a plant-based diet. It is also a result of not enough exercise (low brain-derived neurotrophic factor) or nutrients in foods, as well as hormonal imbalances.

The main thing is to live well, eat well, exercise regularly, sleep and keep stress to a minimum. Keep a positive attitude and spiritual practice, along with a consistent meditation and/or daily breathing practice.

A Brain Exercise for You

Speaking of exercise and meditation, I would like to offer an exercise that feeds the brain and expands our consciousness, while further awakening our empathy and compassion. It is useful for any situation:

1. Go to your power spot or a place where you can be quiet and meditate for approximately 10 minutes.
2. Get into a comfortable position, align your spine by drawing a line like a string from the top of your head to the bottom of your spine.
3. Breathe deeply in and out through your nose, quieting the mind.
4. When you feel quiet, you will allow your mind's screen to visualize your appearance and your behavior from three different perspectives, one at a time.
5. Visualize yourself from the position of the observer—like an outsider looking in from a window.
6. First look at yourself the way you normally do, using your personality. If you normally have critical comments about your appearance or your behavior, allow yourself to see an image of yourself including those perceived imperfections.
7. Allow your consciousness to move down from your mental space to your heart space. Get in touch with the love that exists in your heart.
8. Then visualize yourself through your loving heart. See your body and behavior with the eyes of a lover. See the imperfections melt away and understand how everything about you is perfect in its own way. Be thankful to your body for being there for you and for being your best friend.
9. Allow pure consciousness to move deep into your soul. Tap into the knowing of the ages. Visualize your body and behavior with the knowingness of the soul connection. See the beauty of learning in action. Have compassion for your soul's path and see how you may best express that walk in your current life situation.
10. Allow yourself to return slowly to ordinary reality.
11. Make notes in your journal about your impressions and insights.

CHAPTER 21
Challenges to the Unfolding Soul

"The God in me is the best part of me. The God in me is who I strive to be. The God in me is the best version of me."

—Morgan Freeman, *The Story of God* Netflix series

I first saw Jacob for joint pain. He was concerned about Lyme disease after suffering a few tick bites, leaving many of his joints swollen and painful. While waiting for blood tests to confirm or rule out Lyme's, we put him on a regimen of acupuncture treatments, a diet that restricted refined carbohydrates and sugar, and anti-inflammatory supplements that included curcumin, boswellia, and specialized pro-resolving mediators (SPM Active), which supports the resolution of inflammation by activating macrophages to mobilize and eat up dead and dying neutrophils, which are a huge source of inflammatory cytokines. We also started him on omega-3 fatty acids and antioxidants.

After only three weeks, Jacob's widespread pain was limited to a sore left elbow and a stiff lower back. However, he was concerned about his kidneys. We performed a comprehensive metabolic panel to test his organs. His kidneys were functioning normally.

I thought about the distribution of his pain, how it affected his joints most, and then receded to his elbow and back after initial treatment. This suggested something might be amiss in his emotional body. The left elbow pain runs along the heart meridian, and the back suggests a heavy emotional burden.

Finally, I asked him straight out: "Are you upset about something, maybe a girlfriend? Jason, are you heartbroken?"

"Yes, I'm very sad." He looked at me, a bit surprised by my bold but accurate question, but then relieved for the opening. "I am separating from a woman I have been with for seven years."

"That's tough."

Tears formed in his deep blue eyes. "Yes, it is."

Jacob was a beautiful man. Many thought his appearance quite striking, but what made him shine so brightly was an enormous heart, the depth of his soul, and his unassuming, generous nature. He was unaware of this gift and did not see himself clearly, because emotional wounds from early childhood left him feeling unwanted and unworthy. His wounds had always directly conflicted with his deep soul, but now, they were manifesting on the physical plane in a sharp, direct way. When pain announces itself like a person shouting, "Time to deal with this!" into a bullhorn, then it's time to act. Unless we move forward, we cannot heal, unfold and grow into our potential as laid out by our soul purpose.

I considered his emotional wounds. Childhood wounds often leave us feeling unworthy. If we're not strong and careful, we allow ourselves to be abused, either by another or ourselves (through self-medicating with drugs, alcohol or other means). We feel unloved and do not love ourselves; as a result, we place ourselves in relationships to receive such punishment. We repeat the abuse pattern from our childhood because it is familiar and we feel we deserve it.

Most of us spend the better part of our adult lives shaking off some sort of childhood trauma. This is the first and greatest challenge to the unfolding soul. These traumas, and wounds, modify our behavior profoundly and change the course of our lives. We will do absolutely anything to protect them from being exposed, and to keep anyone from seeing or touching us there. We continue to feel their lingering pain. As we discussed before, we need to uncover and expose them to the light of truth, and shine the light of understanding love and compassion upon them. When we do, our greater creative and spiritual potential awakens, and we begin to heal and integrate our wounds.

We all have wounds. They only vary in how we suffer them and allow them to affect our current behavior. We will develop whole behaviors just to hide these wounds, letting them affect our present reality, control us, and cause us to lie to others and ourselves to stay hidden. If we can become aware and acknowledge them, we can then send them to the past, where they belong. They are not really applicable to our present reality and evolving soul. They only belong to us because we hold onto them.

We can choose differently, to not believe the poisonous thoughts that come from the old wounds. We can choose not to carry the neurotoxins of fear, anger, lack of purpose, sense of unworthiness and dismal self-esteem that arise from them. We can choose healing. When we heal our emotional bodies and old wounds in this way, our bodies will follow.

My thoughts turned to Jacob's girlfriend. "How have you two come to this break up?" I asked.

"She is a beautiful lady. She's just mean." His answer was brief, his voice a guard barring the gate.

I pressed him lightly. "How is she mean?"

"She is verbally abusive. I don't understand how someone who used to say 'I love you' now can't stand you. She doesn't like my stuff around. Everything I do annoys her. She withholds her emotional support, intimacy and love from me. She's only nice when she wants something from me. She shouts at me and calls me terrible names for no reason."

I shook my head. "Oh, that's sad. She likes to control you, and you don't love yourself enough to know that you don't deserve it."

His eyes softened, becoming limpid as the sea. His shoulders relaxed a bit. "I never looked at it like that," he said.

"We can give you treatments, medicines and supplements to help you with your pain and balance your energy. But it's really up to you to do the work of true healing."

"I understand. I want to be free. Help me."

His body language and relaxing spirit confirmed he was ready to receive truth, a vital aspect of soul doctoring. Direct honesty is vital for both doctor and patient.

"The awareness of the truth can set you free; it gives you choices," I said. "Only if you learn to love yourself very strongly will you be free. You have to make the choice instead of letting someone else or some past belief system choose for you. Choose someone you like and who likes you the way you are."

Jacob considered my comment. "Rejection is hard to take," he said.

I nodded. Indeed, rejection can lead to tailspins for even the strongest people. For those with deep wounds? It can be tragic if we attach ourselves to the rejection, or it connects to old feelings or experiences of being rejected.

"It's better to find out straight away than spend seven years with someone who is mean to you," I said. "What is it about rejection that is so hard? Sounds like you are buying into some message from the past."

He nodded as his eyes fell to the floor. "Yeah, I was the invisible kid."

"I think I know what you mean, because I was that kid." I certainly understood his struggle. "Can you share with me?"

"I was the middle kid and only eighteen months from my sister. I have an older brother and a younger sister. They just didn't have time or energy for me. I was on my own."

"How did that make you feel?"

My own past experience gave me a sense of the answer to expect. "Like I was 'less than,' or not as loved as the other kids," he said.

"What did you do?"

"I became very involved in sports and was a track and field champion. Mostly high jumping. But my parents didn't have time to come to my meets. Anyway, I made friends and had some sense of accomplishment," Jacob said.

"Great! You can use that initiative to evolve and heal yourself now." I decided to share a bit of my story with him. "I had a real similar situation as a kid. I swam and rode horses. My parents wouldn't pay for any of it or my school, despite paying for the other kids. So I paid for myself all the way through medical school."

Jacob flashed an astonished grin. "That's amazing. I too paid for myself to go to college."

"My feeling was, my experience made me stronger," I said.

"I guess you're right. It really did. I just never got over the personal feeling of not being enough."

"Because you learned not to love yourself, because you felt your parents didn't love you," I told Jacob softly. "They were just overwhelmed. It doesn't matter now. *You* need to love you! Look inside and find the love that is you. That's where it comes from—someone else can never fill that. Once you fill your own empty space, you will be whole and happy. Then someday, you'll find the one for you. If you treat yourself well, others will, too."

Relationship Controls—and Their Problems

Unfortunately in a relationship, there is often one who controls to avoid being wounded, and one who allows control for the same reason. Neither works effectively. A good relationship happens when each person takes care of their own half—themselves—then works out any common issues with the other person.

For that and many other reasons, it's important to choose someone who likes you for exactly who and what you are—physically, emotionally, mentally and spiritually. For that to happen, you must like yourself in the same way. You must also like the other person for exactly who they are. Never expect to change another, or to mold or shape them into some idealized version you might envision. That will create *your* delusion of falling in love with an imagined version of the other person. At the same time, the other person not only has no idea what's going through your mind, but they will never be able to live up to your conception of them. Sadly, these relationships end typically with horrible breakups, permanent loss of contact, great emotional damage and, in extreme cases, domestic violence. Or worse.

As your soul unfolds, and you learn to love yourself, you will clear these wounds. For some, it will be a huge challenge, but you must ask yourself: *Do I want to live the greatest expression of my soul, my greater purpose, and share that with someone who loves me for it?*

We can only know and be responsible for our own actions, reactions and responses. That is the extent of our control in a healthy relationship. Our reactions determine the course of our lives. Only when you have control over them can you join in a relationship and begin to share the same dream or common goals with another. But first, open your invisible shield and allow the light of love to shine. Know you are enough.

Facing Trials to a New Path

Jacob and I continued our work together. After a few more sessions, he told me of his plans to return to Arkansas, finish building his house, then sell it and move. Separating a relationship and a household was enough of a challenge. However, sometimes the Great Mystery tests us even further, to the deepest core of our soul. Jacob's challenge? To determine if he really loved himself enough to carry through with his plan.

When he arrived in Arkansas, Jacob learned his brother had fallen suddenly and terminally ill in North Dakota. He headed north to see his brother, who was a father figure to him. A few weeks later, he passed. Emotionally reeling, Jacob returned to Arkansas to carry out his obligations—only to face a severe tornado that swept through the state and caused the evacuation of his entire town. On top of the emotional turmoil, Jacob's sweet hound dog, Sammy, started fighting stray animals. In the darkness of the country night, Jacob fired his rifle, the bullet meant for the stray dogs. Instead, it hit a tree, and a piece of shrapnel spiraled into the shoulder of his dear little Sammy.

With a relationship break up, splitting of a household, death of his beloved brother and serious injury to his precious canine friend, the tornado literally touched down inside of Jacob's heart.

He called me after the ordeal.

"Believe it will get better and better from here. But you're going to need a little time," I said.

"It can't get any worse. I just don't understand. There are so many people barely alive. Mean people, too. Why would someone so good, like my brother, be taken?"

I felt every bit of his pain. It would have been easy to shake my head, but this afforded me an opportunity to talk directly to his soul. "That's one thing we don't get to know," I replied. "We can give healing. But when someone actually passes, that's between that soul and God. Your brother was finished—he was good."

"Yes, I know, I just miss him."

"You are strong, Jacob. The Great Mystery has given you a lot to endure. The light will return. Remember, you always have a friend here. And you are your own friend and God is always with you. So you are never alone."

"Thank you, that means a lot."

Jacob called six weeks later with some welcome news. "I finished the work on the house I promised, and I'm packing up my stuff and moving to Utah where my family is," he said.

I was impressed by the strength of his soul. Would my soul have endured as well as his? I wondered about that. I've been through the breakup of a long-term relationship, loss of a brother and a dog, a sudden move and even a tornado, but not in the course of a few months! Thoughts of those emotional impacts plummeted into the pit of my stomach, causing an aching pain. I wanted to fall to my knees.

Not knowing exactly what to say, I asked, "How is Sammy?"

"Oh, just fine. He is healing fast—and hardly limping now."

"Thank God." I breathed a huge sigh of relief. "How are your arms?"

"Good. No more pain."

What a pleasant surprise. "Really?"

"Yes. Better than before. And my back is fine, too."

"That's great!" Now Jacob was lifting *my* spirit. The improvement in his physical pain told me he was also healing emotionally. "Your heart is better."

"Yeah, it is. I'm not carrying around all that negative energy and lack of self-worth and self-love."

"That's fantastic! I'm really proud of you."

I was deeply thankful he acknowledged, opened up to and received the true gift of love—from himself. His healing heart and recovering body were telling an increasingly happy story and foretold of a good future.

Developing Our Spiritual Body

In my many years of practicing medicine, I have found a *balanced* and nourished spiritual body is essential to attain the fullest measure of health. When we develop our spiritual body, we feel greater meaning, purpose and belonging—which contributes most to longevity, according to research. A developed spiritual body lets us know we are not alone, that we are here for a reason. Frank Fools Crow described the resulting spiritual power that animates our life in this way:

"Sometimes it feels like energy or electricity, when it is moving in and through us. But spiritual power is a distinctive kind of knowledge that is like the key that opens the door, or the switch that starts the energy moving. It is that special insight that we need to break up a log jam of knowledge. Other people may have gathered up the same amount of information we have, but they can't get it moving. They go nowhere because they have not called in the power and have not been given the key or switch to turn it on.

The primary challenges in reaching this point are often lodged in our behavior from early childhood wounds. These unhealed wounds carry into adulthood and result in low-vibration emotions such as fear, anger, doubt, jealousy, envy, unworthiness and the willingness to be controlled—or control others. Like Jacob, we will do anything to keep our wounds safe and hidden, even allowing ourselves to be controlled and/or abused. We also will try and control others, manipulating them through their wounds so they don't do it to us.

Despite his tumultuous relationship breakup and incredible run of personal tragedy around it, Jacob got in touch with his own love for himself and made a change. He easily could have caved to the stress of his circumstances. Instead, he methodically pushed through the fog and woke up to his own healing path.

Another type of relationship presents challenges to our growing, evolving souls: the relationship with ourselves. When we fear we are not "enough," we project a persona other than who we are authentically, in order to compensate and "protect" ourselves. Thanks to our brain's amazing neuroplasticity, its ability to adapt to and rewire to any situation, we can re-form our personalities around wounds we are trying to hide.

These may not be beneficial changes. Jealousy and envy stem from fearing we are not enough. If we are satisfied with our authentic, essential selves, there is no reason to feel jealous or envious. We are good, strong, talented, smart, beautiful and capable. We know we are enough! When we are balanced and see someone who appears (or actually is) more beautiful,

245

graceful or intelligent, then our own beauty, grace and intelligence shines ever brighter. We're happy to be around them, and our own gifts resonate with theirs.

Fear and constriction of the soul can also result from the judgments of others—and/or our judgments about ourselves. When someone judges you, they express part of *their* reality and insecurity, not yours. By remembering that, you will not be hurt often. We have no control over others' judgments. But we can react in the most impeccable way possible. If another has a different opinion, so be it. What if someone walks up to you in the grocery store and says, "You are a bad person?" They are expressing *their* issue, an aspect of themselves, like looking in a mirror. How will you react?

Your choice will make all the difference. You can internalize and believe their words, allowing them to reinforce an old wound. You can also reject the comment with anger, growing indignant and losing your emotional balance over someone who would dare call you bad. Or, you can realize their remark has *nothing* to do with you. You know who you are. Don't take it personally.

We have choices about how we react to situations. We may not be able to control what happens around us, but we can control our own reactions. Let's go back to the person who called you bad. Be present and aware in the moment, and say to yourself, "This really has nothing to do with me. Perhaps that person's shoes are too tight or they have a headache." By reacting and responding positively to any given situation, it liberates the soul to evolve.

Ego Central

In today's culture, the ego often gets a bad rap. We say, "That guy has a big ego," or "It was her ego that made her" respond in a certain way. This implies that the ego is a selfish child or devilish quality of our personality that needs to be controlled. On social media, people remind us constantly of something great they did, that they or their families are "the best ever," narrating their life stories daily with higher degrees of hype than we've ever seen. Our leaders tend to act far more from their egos than the greater cause of public service.

With these negative expressions of ego flying around, it's very easy for any spiritual or truly service-oriented person to blame the ego as the enemy that must be conquered and subjugated at all costs.

But here's the thing: in philosophy and higher religions, the ego is considered the *seat of consciousness*. In psychology, the ego combines all conscious acts and states. In the Freudian sense, ego is the response to our physical and social environment, the superficial consciousness, while id is the subconscious part of the personality. Metaphysicians may describe ego as a permanent real being to which all conscious states and attributes belong. All of these definitions would imply our conscious behavior really needs our ego. This is how we survive without getting run over by cars or falling off ladders. The right use of will and ego determines our success in society, giving us the power to make appropriate decisions and carry them through to completion.

This is a different expression of ego than an egotist would have. An egotist is so consumed by self-importance, belief that she/he has all the answers, and that everyone else in the world is inferior by comparison. Noted 19th-century author and poet Ambrose Bierce defined ego(t)ist as "a person more interested in himself than in me."

We talk a lot in spiritual work and psychology about "not letting your ego get in the way." What does this really mean? To me, it involves letting the truth flow through us without trying to control or *will* it to align with our expectations. What we need is an accurate, authentic picture of self to shape a *healthy ego*, not try to take it away. My dreaming teacher Connie Kaplan says, "It is arrogant to believe you are greater than you authentically are. However, it is just as arrogant to believe you are less than you are." If we can function from that basis, the ego realigns to its natural, vital role as a transmitter of the soul's wishes. Or, as Indian yoga master Paramhansa Yogananda (1893–1952) put it, "The soul is the boat and the ego the rudder."

In working with our sense of wholeness, or that of others, it is important to develop a mature ego aligned to the soul and master the right use of will. This requires complete acceptance of self to stop judging others. Many belief systems agree that the Creator gave us free will to be guardians of this planet and to have the potential of God-like expression. It is a very special gift to express our life force in any way we choose. However, when we use that force for selfish gain or to manipulate, rather than liberate others, we are not in alignment with the right use of will.

We must surrender, to a degree, to arrive at mature ego and right use of will. For instance, if we feel victimized or restricted by our life situation, we are giving ourselves permission to stay stuck. We often turn our angered will onto those around us, holding them back as well, so we are not alone in our misery. That's a deeply negative misuse of ego. However, if we can find the gift and wisdom within those restrictive experiences, we surrender our will to that source greater than ourselves, thus liberating self and others. By going with the flow, we often find ourselves ahead of where we imagined.

The Healing Relationship

This same mechanism takes place in the healing relationship. When the healer sits in acceptance and releases all judgment, he or she surrenders personal will. The resulting flow of healing energy is strong, directed and unhindered. With the personal ego out of the way, true healing energy can flow. Healers must also recognize when a patient is struggling with sense of self, as well as when a patient is manipulating them. It is the healer's job to help people strike the delicate balance between ego and will in order to liberate the flow of their own healing power.

I experienced this struggle with Gary, a 52-year-old who underwent three heart surgeries in as many years for a severe irregular heartbeat. A very successful businessman, Gary succeeded in any venture to which he set his mind. When he was diagnosed with a heart irregularity, doctors told him he would need to take medication for the rest of his life. The medication came with undesirable side effects that this highly athletic man could not tolerate, such as weakness and fatigue. It decreased his physical activity and sexual performance.

Gary set out to solve that problem in the same way he handled business challenges. He located several heart arrhythmia specialists and underwent extensive testing to delineate the problem and search for a solution. He underwent two unsuccessful attempts at intra-cardiac laser ablation of the excitable focus, causing the irregular heartbeat. He kept pushing. After visiting several heart specialists around the country, he finally found one that performed a rare type of open-heart surgery for removing the excitable focus from the heart. This operation required hours of heart-lung support to literally lift the heart out of chest, open it, turn it inside out to ablate the excitable focus and several months of recovery. Intense to say the least. I tried to advise him against it—he was determined.

Three months after that surgery, Gary came to my office. For the first time in three months, his heart was beating regularly. The operation had been successful. His complaint and reason for seeing me concerned his sternum, where they opened up his chest to operate. "There is a clicking sound in my sternum when I move my chest in a certain way, especially during workouts," he said.

Upon exam, I noticed some degree of instability. After reviewing his situation and volumes of charts and X-rays, I discussed my conclusions.

"Gary, my recommendation is to support your healing with some nutritional supplements designed to provide the catalysts you need to promote and heal the bone and cartilage completely," I explained. "I would also suggest energetic modalities like acupuncture, meditation and physical therapy to encourage cartilage formation bone healing. But most of all, give it a little time. It really hasn't been that long since you've had a major surgery." Surgeons typically recommend six months of recovery to completely heal from surgeries such as Gary's.

Two months later, Gary grew impatient and returned to his heart surgeon for an opinion. A CAT scan showed a two-centimeter separation of his sternum, as well as a lot of new bone and cartilage where it was trying to heal. The cardiac surgeon felt that the repair of the sternum was good and progressing. However, Gary visited at least one other thoracic surgeon, who agreed to surgical repair.

Gary met with me two more times before that surgery. He wanted a spiritual ceremony. He arranged to work with a medicine person he knew in New Mexico and invited me to join them. The medicine person made sweat lodge, and after the lodge doused Gary in cold water from a nearby stream. He laid Gary on a blanket, and we sang and prayed over him beneath the stars for most of the night. Before dawn, we walked Gary to his bed. The medicine man told him to ask for a dream vision to guide him.

Later in the morning, we put on some coffee and checked on Gary. The medicine man asked if he had any dreams.

"It was unbelievable!" Gary exclaimed. "I don't remember ever having such a vivid dream. I was camping in the forest. It was so peaceful and green. I decided to leave camp and walk down the path and see what was there. A huge, fierce bear came lunging out of the trees. The bear was furious and rose up on its hind legs snarling, roaring and pawing at me. The bear came down jaws first and sank his teeth right into the center of my chest."

The medicine man's eyes widened. I was just as stunned. He thought Gary's dream may be related to his recent operation, but also suggested an association with the course he'd chosen for his next surgery. He advised Gary to reconsider his choice. Gary liked his dream vision but was not the least bit interested in exploring the option of declining a surgical repair of his sternum.

Gary returned to my office a few weeks later. He hadn't yet undergone the surgery. "I am feeling so good, I almost hesitate to have the surgery," he said. Even at that, he wanted to "be perfect again" so he could hunt, scuba dive and return to the other activities he enjoyed. I examined his chest and found it to be more stable and solid than before. Despite the known findings on the CAT scan, I suggested he consider giving it a little more time. His clinical situation had definitely and obviously improved.

Gary responded like a well-schooled arbitrator. He used his will to manipulate the second surgeon. He wanted to be perfect. Furthermore, he attempted to enroll me in his "ruling," his decision to have the surgery. "I will support you in whatever you choose to do," I said. "However, since you feel better and clinically you *are* better, I suggest giving it more time to heal. I know *I* have to listen to my visions, or get my butt kicked. Gary, what is it going to hurt to wait a few more months?"

He chose to have his chest repaired. Ten days after the surgery, he developed a highly dangerous infection in his newly repaired sternum, one that can lead to life-threatening osteonecrosis and sepsis. He was taken to emergency surgery, where surgeons removed his entire sternum and the ends of his ribs on either side of his chest. The message of the bear was apparent.

Gary made another remarkable recovery. Most importantly, he now is able to reflect upon his experience and see where his personal, ego-driven will thwarted his progress. A year later, we had a conversation. He told me, "One thing for sure, I learned a lot of humility last year."

He sure did. He also learned that the same use of willpower that made him a successful businessman nearly took his life. Sometimes, in both the soul *and* everyday life, the right use of will means surrendering to something greater.

CHAPTER 22
The Finer Art of Healing Thyself

Have you ever received a diagnosis that shocked you, made you fearful or put a spell on you? The beautiful actress Olivia Hussey Eisley offers an example of how a frightening diagnosis can drive an illness further into us—and how we can turn it around into a shining example of healing ourselves.

Nearly 50 years after her star-making, Golden Globe–winning portrayal of Juliet in Franco Zeffirelli's *Romeo & Juliet*, Olivia came to see me after undergoing intense chemo and radiation therapy for metastatic breast cancer. Her eyes shone with fear, and for good reason: she had a large estrogen positive-receptor mass near her heart. After telling me her story breathlessly, her words falling out like gravel over a cliff, she circled back to her trauma and illness, making me know they were attached. "Dr. Randall, I just can't do chemotherapy anymore. They won't stop. It's killing me."

Her husband, David, was with her. He nodded vigorously in agreement and blurted, "It was just awful. Inhumane!"

I tried to dispel their fears. "It is your choice, Olivia," I said. "You don't *have* to do it anymore if you don't want to. We can design another program for you. Many have healed using it, including myself."

She relaxed a little, not realizing she was the one really in charge. "How do we know if it comes back or if it still there?"

"We will watch you very closely, and we can always go back if we need to. In the meantime, let me hold the burden of your fear."

She relaxed further. Within her, the light of hope began to grow brighter.

"I love you, Olivia, and I'll be with you every step of the way. Along with God's help and the devotion of your beautiful family. You mean everything to your husband and India. And your amazing healer, Howard Wills, will continue to play a big part, too."

She settled into a safe place within herself. "Yes, yes, you are right."

"We can do everything possible naturally to treat an estrogen receptor-positive tumor and monitor you closely," I explained. "As long as you continue to improve, we know things are good." I reminded her of her wide circle of support, the many people pouring heartfelt love and energy into her, both at home and from around the world. "You have our support, the support of your lovely family, community and God. Your husband and daughter are so devoted. You mean everything to them.

"Everyone gets healed, Olivia, and some people get miraculously cured," I pointed out.

Olivia and David allowed their trust to fill in the space where fear from the diagnosis once existed. This helped them begin to heal the trauma they had experienced even before the cancer, a trauma that could have easily broken her forever. Her strong spirit and loving nature brought her to a place where I could help her.

Olivia's Program

We put together her program. It consisted of a vegan diet, exercise, prayers, meditation and an herbal regimen. Recent studies have shown that practicing a strictly vegan diet for as little as three months can reverse cancer genes. If it could work for study subjects, I told Olivia, it could work for her. We gave her herbs to reduce the estrogen in her body and removed high-phytoestrogen foods such as soy from her diet. I also added many supplements, working from the premise that all cancers are inflammatory—a crucial fact often overlooked in Western oncologists' offices.

Next, we turned to the most important ingredient of her program: healing herself. We needed to dispel (*de-spell*) her diagnosis, removing the spells cast by her trauma, past treatment and the term "metastatic cancer." We would then fill in the spaces with love, compassion and generosity, resulting in hope and healing.

A healer has many purposes, but often our biggest role is to shed a different light or perspective on a patient's problem or illness. By changing perspective of their illness, we change their relationship to it almost magically. This activates a higher consciousness, which opens a portal that can return wholeness to the body.

Two years later, in July 2019, I asked Olivia to repeat an imaging study. I read the images with the radiologist. Not only had the mass *not* grown, but the scan showed primarily chronic scarring. What about the tumor? It was either very small or gone. Our program was working! I can't tell you how great a blessing it was to share the good news with Olivia and her family later that day at Randall Wellness. We all laughed, cried happy tears and hugged for a long time. We will always remember that wonderful day.

It has now been over four years and no signs of disease. A truly deserved miracle for this extremely talented actress and compassionate being of light.

Going Beyond the Physical Symptoms

In Western medicine, we usually start treating disease only after it has manifested into a physical form. We biopsy a lump. Patients see us with active coughs and fevers, flu, or bronchial infections. We prescribe insulin and/or strict diets for diabetics after blood tests reveal the disease has taken root. Yet, upon a deeper dive, and looking at it from an Ayurvedic medicine point of view, the physical manifestation of disease is the fifth and final stage of an evolution that begins with a seed, whether it be swimming in a polluted river or exposure to another harmful environmental influence, exposure to a sick person, or impure thinking, grief, fears, trauma or negative attitudes.

When we talk about healing our patients or ourselves, we need to go beyond the physical symptoms, into the subtler levels that gestate disease. Recognizing these deeper causes in our own bodies and minds is one of the best ways we can heal ourselves. When we see how our attitudes, beliefs, actions or lexicon of fears feed into the bad cells of a cancer, blood sugar level, intestinal ailment or flu, we can sometimes reverse the course of the disease on the spot.

What does that vital moment of authentic self-recognition look and feel like?

Jen was a picture of health when she came to my offices, a bright-eyed, tall, thin 40-year-old woman. A ballet dancer in her younger years, she had become a proficient fitness trainer and health coach. Beneath that shining exterior, though, she had been undergoing chemotherapy treatments for breast cancer for six months following a mastectomy. She was bracing herself for the next phase—radiation. She saw me for an alternative view, a second opinion. She increasingly feared her future and whether she would be able to keep up her energy, appearance, performance and satisfy her clients. She stopped going out and socializing with clients and friends, which had been one of her favorite activities.

"Jen, you look great and feel pretty good right now, don't you?" I asked.

"Yes," she said tentatively. "I'm just afraid of what is to come and I'm getting ready. I can't have a glass of wine anymore; they have me on Lupron [a strong anti-estrogen that results in menopause]. That's not fun and I do feel a little frazzled and fatigued. What do I do when it gets worse?"

"You are pretty tough on yourself, aren't you?"

"Yes, I guess so," she admitted. She needed to reverse this thinking and to treat herself more kindly so she could heal.

It was time for me to help facilitate that. "So tell me, Jen. If you had a friend or even a client with the same thing, would you judge them during their healing process? And not want to interact with them?" I asked.

"No, of course not. Dr. Randall, what if my body is deformed? What if I can't keep my muscle mass and strength?" She was tossing her fears into the future, and they were boomeranging on her like a tsunami.

Recognizing her courage, I told it to her straight. I began with my cancer journey. "I really think people and your friends will respect you more for the journey you are completing," I said. "Look how great you look and how well you are doing now, even after a mastectomy, chemotherapy and the devastation of chemically induced menopause. You are doing great! I can see that others will see that, too. Why do you hold so much judgment for yourself when you would not give it to another in your situation? You need to let it go. And who cares about a glass of wine? It's really about the company of your friends and the activity, isn't it?"

Jen looked down, then looked back up. Tears welled up in her eyes. "Yes," she said softly.

She realized she could overcome her fear of not being enough by getting back in tune with the same courage she used through ballet and fitness training. "I am going to trust my life again and use this cancer episode as a gift, like you did," she said.

What followed the next day was truly beautiful. Jen celebrated her major step with a six-mile run on the beach, her longest run since before the chemo started. She spent the next two months using her courage to reach out to friends and clients to break her isolation and shake off the self-judgment and fear that had paralyzed her. She took on the responsibility of healing herself, and very soon found herself living a full, rich life again. She also carried the greater gifts of learning the lessons cancer had brought to her and how courageous and worthy she is.

Every Meaningful Change Begins from Within

As I've stated throughout this book, every meaningful change begins from within—or must go within early in the process. I suggest we look at our own paths, our own journeys. What can we do in our own lives that will positively impact our health, our happiness, and our purpose on this planet as a whole? Most recently, COVID-19 has forced our hand, sentencing us to our own homes until we figure it out. As practitioners, what can we do to create better treatments and outcomes for our patients, our medicine and our people as a whole? How do we keep our balance?

In the midst of an exploding health-care crisis, global pandemics, widespread public debate over health issues from hormones, genetic manipulation, slow viruses, the latest trendy carbohydrate or protein-heavy diets, and environment- and animal-borne diseases, the timing of this discussion could not be better. Consider the pair of catastrophes that hit in the winter of 2019–20: the "super flu" that hit 15 million Americans; and the coronavirus pandemic that shut down the US and world—including killing more in the US in six weeks than the super flu did in a year. That number is now above 1.1 million and continuing to climb, as of this writing.

Against this challenge, we practitioners and physicians are asking ourselves, *How do we perform the work we entered this field to do? How do we continue to serve more people in less time and keep our promises to those we dedicated our lives to help? Is there a better way?*

We can be leaders again by using a few simple tools from our own lives to make our careers and social and family lives sustainable. We can be the first bricks in the wall of a new sustainable medicine. Every change begins within.

The Wise Woman's Journey

I spend a great deal of time with women patients, and as a woman on a spiritual and wisdom path my whole life, I pay particular attention to the "wise woman's journey." It contains seven points of focus: balance, intention, goodness, compassion, awareness, love and mindfulness. Here is an acronym to remember these seven: BIG CALM. Each tool represents a merger of science and ancient philosophy. We all have access to these seven tools and can begin using them right here, right now. (And, I might add, men benefit greatly from these tools as well!)

Let's go deeper into these seven points of focus:

Balance: A primary goal of healing thyself to balance our medicine with ourselves, and work from that state. As the Dalai Lama wrote, "With the ever-growing impact of science on our lives, religion and spirituality have a greater role to play in reminding us of our humanity. What we must do is balance scientific and material progress with the sense of responsibility that comes of inner development."

Most change begins within and requires openness. It involves continually practicing and refining our balance, and also returning to a balanced state whenever we are temporarily knocked from it. It spirals out from each balanced individual to touch and move us toward the One Mind.

Epidemiological data tells us the three most important factors in longevity and healthy living are nutrition, fitness, and meaning and purpose. Do you know which factor has the most impact? Meaning and purpose, as I also pointed out in my discussion on the blue zones in Chapter 16. "Even though the realms of religion and science in themselves are clearly marked off from each other, nevertheless there exist between the two strong reciprocal relationships and dependencies. . . . The situation may be expressed by an image: Science without religion is lame, religion without science is blind," the great physicist and thinker Albert Einstein said.

Intention & Intuition: In 1972, Dr. Candice Pert discovered the opiate receptor. She knew it was densely populated in the limbic brain, known to be where our emotion develops.[58] However, she also found these receptors populated every other part of the body. The implication? Emotion, or bliss, is *not* generated by the brain. It is generated by the body and *processed* by the brain. Scientists later confirmed Dr. Pert's thesis when they discovered a similar distribution of the endorphin receptor, the source of the well-known "runner's high" or "blissed out" state we feel after exhilarating hikes. The research then expanded to neuropeptides, neurotransmitters, hormones and what came to be known as informational substances. The point is we carry this bliss and the ability to receive it throughout our bodies.

Dr. Pert and others found high concentrations of these informational substances in focal locations throughout the body, including the brain, neck, heart, gut, genital and anal regions—corresponding to the locations of our chakras, or cerebrospinal spiritual centers. Anatomically, we know these areas are filled with neuronal plexuses. It's quite easy to see a connection between the body, mind and spiritual/emotional aspects of things. In the nearly 50 years since Dr. Pert's revolutionary finding, millions of yoga practitioners and others have come to understand how energetic blocks in particular chakras cause corresponding physical problems. In all cases, the opiate receptors are blocked, too.

Intuition: What if doctors were intuitive? What if we had access to a simple yes-or-no answer to any question we wanted to ask? Or more advanced or complex information? I say we do. I taught the first class on medical intuition to medical students at UCLA. I could sense at first they were thinking, *Really?* And after our simple exercises they were thinking, *Oh yeah, this is valuable and real!*

The beauty of Western medicine is that we can check it out. We can do a test and find out if our hunch is right. But what if everyone had this access? David Hawkins, a well-known author and expert on mental processes, described these phenomena when referring to consciousness and ways to access it. He spoke of a "wormhole" between physical, the mind and the spirit.

Drs. Norman Shealy, Caroline Myss, Christine Page and Judith Orloff all have done a great deal of work in what is now known as intuitive medicine. They say we all possess this gift of inner self-diagnosis, of listening to our bodies and attuning to the messages it sends us. It is just a matter of using it. Like any other muscle we're awakening back into shape, we need to start slowly and flex it, then gradually practice more and more. Practice makes for deeper attunement.

Goodness: The HeartMath Institute published numerous studies to support the fact that the heart is not just a simple pump.[59] Doctors know from medical school that the heart communicates with the central nervous, endocrine and peripheral nervous systems and vagal nerve. However, did you also know that there are bioelectromagnetic interactions between your heart and the brain waves of those around you?

In their studies, HeartMath showed a profound positive effect of acts or feelings of goodness on perceptions, emotions, behaviors and health. Not only do they impact us individually, but collectively, in a way that can turn health-care issues around in this country and world. We need it. The negative effect (anxiety, depression and unhealthy stress) costs US employers over $300 billion per year in absenteeism, tardiness, worker's compensation and health insurance costs, according to the University of Massachusetts Lowell. Furthermore, depressive illness, commonly associated with work stress, results in almost 10 sick days per worker per year.[60]

HeartMath developed what they call the Freeze-Frame technique, a sophisticated method of teaching people how to sustain a continually appreciative heart. We can all do this in our own way. Think of an image or thought that puts you into that state of complete and utter appreciation. Try to sustain it for five minutes. What happens? We experience less stress, greater joy and feeling of purpose and self-worth, and diminished susceptibility to disease. The immune system *strengthens and improves* for six hours, measured by a rise in IgA, a marker for immunity. It is the first line of defense on our mucosal surfaces from mouth to gut.

The information technology services division of a state agency wanted to adopt a complete change in management and technology. They taught 54 employees Inner Quality Management (IQM) to deal with stress and to focus on active engagement while in a positive emotional state (feeling good). The really wonderful thing about this technique? It can transform inefficient mental and emotional reactions in the moment. What do you think happened? Employees reported fewer symptoms of stress, such as anger, depression, sadness, fatigue, anxiety, body aches, indigestion, and rapid and irregular heartbeats. At work, their performance and productivity levels jumped—as did their job satisfaction, clarity of goals and effective communication.

Compassion: David Hawkins once described an amazing result that happened with thousands of desperate people that came to him. He focused on compassion in his work and invited his patients to practice it with others and themselves. He observed how, over and over again, this compassion recontextualized each patient's reality to experience healing on a level that transcended the world and its appearances. They elevated above their own suffering, and started attuning to the suffering of others, a pure example of the Dalai Lama's words: "Our compassion must stem from recognition of their suffering."

Through this technique, they achieved inner peace, an unintentional state of spiritual or psychological calm despite stress or homeostasis. "Compassion refers to the arising in the heart of the desire to resolve the suffering of all beings. The inner peace in which I existed encompassed us both, beyond time and identity. I saw that all pain and suffering arises from the ego and not from God," noted Harvard scientist and *Be Here Now* author Ram Dass said.

During the past 20 years, as complementary medicine and deeper spiritual paths have taken some hold, many articles have addressed the benefit of compassion. In an *Archives of Internal Medicine* article, "When the Spirit Hurts: an Approach to the Suffering Patient," Emil Patrick Lesho, DO, discussed how the mere acknowledgment of pain in a patient tended to improve symptoms and lessen discomfort.[61] A 2003 randomized controlled trial published in the *Journal of the American Medical Association* demonstrated the importance of *patient-physician communication in patient outcome.*[62]

Awareness: During the late 1960s, Ram Dass touted a philosophy of "Be Here, Now," which became an anthem for spiritual and higher consciousness seekers among the Baby Boomer generation. Besides speaking to the fact that the only true point of our personal power is in the present, he opened an increased focus on presence and awareness. Two decades later, Dr. Jon Kabat-Zinn, a student of several Zen Buddhist teachers, including Thich Nhat Hanh, carried it into a new perspective on the millennia-long practice of mindfulness. Kabat-Zinn was one of the first to integrate these teachings with a scientific approach.

Kabat-Zinn is founder of the Mindfulness-Based Stress Reduction (MBSR) program at the University of Massachusetts Chan Medical School. In 20 years, he treated 11,000 patients and more than 2,000 health-care professionals. He and his colleagues showed without a doubt that mindfulness meditation can help or cure any disease, especially those related to anxiety and pain. He wrote many bestsellers including *Wherever You Go, There You Are*, *Full Catastrophe Living* and *Meditation Is Not What You Think*. These books and others are especially relevant as we deal with the aftermath of the pandemic.

Another key concept for practitioners is to live in awareness of the moment, which reminds the physician of the sacred doctor-patient bond of trust. Unfortunately, this is sometimes a distant memory in our current Western medicine world, where doctors tend to spend less time seeing patients. Even though it is not financially beneficial, I am opposed to this "see more patients in less time" approach. I want to take the time my patients need from me. This is intricately related to the practitioner's willingness to be present and listen. Recent literature by Lesho in the *Archives of Internal Medicine*, and Detmar and others in *JAMA*, the *Journal of the American Medical Association*, report on the importance of listening.[63] When the practitioner acknowledges the suffering of the patient, that patient's perceived suffering lessens. They feel safer from the attention.

Love: In *Power vs. Force*, David Hawkins said of his many end-stage patients, "I saw how love changed the world [the patients] each time it replaced 'un-love.'"[64] Buddhist and yoga practitioners have known about this for thousands of years.

Civilization could be profoundly altered by focusing this power of love at a very specific point. Whenever this happened, history branched out new roads and new ideas.

Mindfulness: Buddhism [spirituality] and science are not conflicting perspectives on the world, but rather differing approaches to the same end: seeking the truth. In Buddhist training, it is essential to investigate reality, and science offers its own ways to go about this investigation. While the purposes of science may differ from those of Buddhism, both ways of searching for truth expand our knowledge and understanding.

Let's revisit the earlier mentioned study regarding monks and meditation. The Dalai Lama decided to work with a group of brain scientists to study the effects of compassion, mindfulness and spiritual practices on behaviors, brain function and their underlying biological basis. These scientists included Richard Davidson, Daniel Goleman and others from the HealthEmotions Research Institute at the University of Wisconsin. Their work with the Dalai Lama and his monks resulted in Daniel Goleman's book *Destructive Emotions.*

Buddhists have a 2,500-year history of working with emotions through mindfulness practices. They have learned how to modulate negative or destructive emotions. In *Destructive Emotions,* Goleman reported on studies which used quantitative electrophysiology, PET and fMRI studies to quantify brain function.[65] They found the Dalai Lama's monks to have the highest activity in the left prefrontal lobe compared to non-monks. Then they taught 40 corporate employees to meditate for 45 minutes per day, six days a week. In only eight weeks, those employees showed a marked increase in left prefrontal lobe activity, similar to the monks. It was associated with more positive emotions and increased immunity and persisted for another four months after testing. As a saying by the Dalai Lama states: "What science finds to be nonexistent we should all accept as nonexistent, but what science merely does not find is a completely different matter. An example is consciousness itself."

An interesting example of this comes from my work with a woman I met on social media. Although a positive encourager on Facebook, she was growing weary of social isolation during the coronavirus quarantine. She was getting depressed. There were underpinnings of the loss of a son and her move to the Los Angeles area, away from her grandchildren. They used to visit her on Easter before he passed away.

"I am disoriented under the pressure of isolation. I'm lonely, Dr. Randall," she said. "They used to visit before. All my life, there were traditions and get-togethers. That can't happen now. All that energetic buildup of the season is pulsating in me . . . just sayin'."

"Maria, I miss my kids too," I replied. "I am going to do a Facetime dress-up Easter with them, bunny ears and all. I'm also going to meditate on the importance of this Passover Easter and pray about it. Do you meditate?"

"Yes, I do, and I should. It will probably help. I'm going to try that Facetime Easter thing, too. I don't have ears, but I will figure something out."

After Easter, I spoke to Maria again. "My depression has lifted," she said. "You got me back to my meditation and I had a great visit with my grandkids."

"My pleasure, Maria. You did it. I just pointed the way and reminded you that you are not alone."

A study at the UCLA Neuropsychiatric Institute, published in the September 2003 issue of *Psychosomatic Medicine*, showed that a group of older men and women who took Tai Chi courses for 45 minutes a day, three days a week, showed an increase of up to 50 percent of memory T cells, immune system cells, that recognize and attack the varicella herpes viruses that cause shingles.[66] Each of us is vulnerable to shingles if we ever contracted chickenpox (which most children did before 1995 before a vaccine was available), because the responsible virus can remain dormant in nerve cells indefinitely. With age, immunity often weakens, allowing the virus to reactivate. The result is Shingles a disorder that frequently causes blisters on the skin and can be extremely painful. Although increased numbers of vaccinated individuals have also contracted Shingles because of waning immunity from the vaccine. Tia Chi seems to be a good preventative according to the results of this study published in September 2003 of *Psychosomatic Medicine*.

Wellness Is Our Own Responsibility

We are responsible for our wellness. Doctors, practitioners and healers are expert guides for patients in unfamiliar territory. We treat symptoms with medicines, instruments, surgical procedures and technologies, but our larger job is to find the root causes of an illness and help patients find their way to wellness. We are trail guides on that path of discovery and recovery, but true healing is always dependent upon the willingness of the individual to open and receive the healing, as well as to put the work into making it happen.

Each of us has a specific genetic code that determines our physical expression. We also seem to be born with unique topographical maps that determine the mental, emotional and spiritual work we are to do in this life, "the work we agreed to do when we came in this time," as my teachers put it. When we fall off or choose to leave our authentic path, something happens in our lives to slap us back onto the correct path. If we get sick, for example, and discover the gift of the illness, we move back onto our path and become whole once again.

No one can fully heal another person. Even if we could, we would rob patients of the opportunity to evolve by dealing with and learning the lessons from their own disease. We all must take responsibility for our own healing process.

To that point, if we doctors are asking you to take responsibility for your process, then it's only fair that we *return the power to patients* for their own well-being. The healer's job is to empower through unconditional love and education. Some practitioners will try and control their patients by getting them to believe they would not be able to stay well without their treatments. That is a misuse of power. A true healer will teach us how to stay well ourselves. One of the key essentials of effective healing is authentic self-discovery. This process is imperative for the continuation of self-healing after the healer is gone. We must take responsibility for our own process and self-care.

There are many techniques that can lead us to discovering our authentic selves. Some include journaling, counseling, meditation, hypnosis, rebirthing, prayer, energy work and ceremony; there are many others. All of these techniques attune the body's energy closer to the understanding of self. The closer our perception of self and the authentic truth of who we are, the more self-healing power we possess.

The healer can only guide the patient as far as their readiness to acknowledge their work with the truer, more authentic image of self. This must be done without judgment and preconceived notions. The healer must be sensitive to not force too much truth onto the patient at once, or a healing crisis could result. Not all patients will be ready for such an undertaking. We healers need to honor that and remain in support for the day when the patient is ready. Forcing patients to face things when they are not ready can cause more damage than good. Like Kenny Rogers sings in "The Gambler," you need to know when to act or walk away.

Part of returning to health involves learning to trust our own inner teacher and the truth that comes from within. We need to remember that we have access to inner guidance and then learn to trust it. One way is to directly communicate with the consciousness of our bodies through guided meditation. Get into a quiet space and frame of mind, and tune into the part of the body causing trouble. Ask a number of questions without stopping to think about the answers. Just write them down or "hear" them. For instance: Is it hot or cold? Angry or sad? Old or new? Emotional or spiritual? What color? Smooth or rough? Hard or soft? The answers may begin to paint a picture.

A simple way of communicating with ourselves is to go to a quiet spot in a garden, the beach or lake, mountains or desert, or wherever we feel safe. Ask a simple question of our inner guide, something like, "Would exercise be good for me today?" Usually, a resounding "Yes!" from within will lift our hearts up, while a "No!" will cause a sinking feeling in our chests or a dull pain in our gut. Then you know. The first answer we receive during meditation is usually our guidance. If your mind is flipping back and forth, clear your mind by breathing deeply in and out, and try again.

All humans are gifted with the innate ability to heal ourselves. With the right treatment combination and use of this power, we can ultimately rise from almost any ailment or disease that afflicts us.

CHAPTER 23
Covid-19: Past, Present and Future

What happens when we do all of this healing work, feel alive and thriving in the world, our purpose renewed and our dreams taking shape again—and then the world seems to come crashing down?

In early December 2019, we all watched in horror as a new coronavirus broke out in Wuhan, in the Hubei Province of China. People literally dropped like flies, dying quickly and at an astounding rate. By February 2020, when the world began to get a grip on the potential extent of this novel virus, it had already spread throughout the planet, on its way to killing millions and infecting tens of millions more, including more than 930,000 Americans who have died as of February 21, 2022. Experts said it would be one and a half to two years before an effective vaccine could be created and distributed—which sent the world into a tailspin. Also as of January 2022 there have been nearly 250,000 new coronavirus cases in LA County alone due to Omicron. Many of which have occurred in vaccinated and boosted individuals.

We are not done yet—but there is a much different way to look at this than the persistent drumbeat of fear and questionable (at times) information the media and government officials continue to produce.

During this pandemic, I've seen great acts of compassion and kindness and people opening up their hearts to a better way. I've also seen terrible behavior such as prejudice and bias against the infected and unvaccinated and vice versa. Which reminds me of the time we were hit with the AIDS pandemic just as my medical career was beginning.

As a medical intern in 1982, I witnessed and treated the first outbreaks of HIV. We didn't even have a name for it yet. Many of these people, mostly young men, would present to us with Kaposi's sarcoma, a type of cancer that manifests as blood-red liver spots on their faces and bodies. When others saw these spots, they immediately feared, hated and ostracized the victims. We used to put the HIV patients in confinement and isolation, in-hospital quarantine, and we wore hazmat suits, gloves, hats, booties and masks like we're seeing today with COVID-19.

What did all this paranoia, fear and resulting hostility toward the suffering come from? In part, a simple lack of basic knowledge of how the virus behaved and how it was contracted and transmitted. The vast majority of these men, and some women, were so ill that we knew they were not going to make it through. None of the HIV medicinal cocktails existed that, today, are not only keeping people alive, but allowing them to carry on with normal lives. In fact, we had no real treatments at all.

I remember one gentleman who suffered from Kaposi's sarcoma on his face and in his lungs. I was called *emergently* (yes, it was both an emergency and urgent—that dire) to find him bleeding into his chest cavity from one of the Kaposi's sarcomas. I obtained the equipment to place a chest tube so that he could breathe, and to get the blood drained from around his lung before it took his life. Sweat beads appeared on his brow and his eyes shone with a pleading fear. I found the spot and made the plunge. The blood rushed into the tube and was collected in the bag. He relaxed, as did I. The next day, when I returned to his room, he was so grateful—but I could tell he was worsening overall. That's when I moved into compassion mode. I moved closer into his room and sat on his bed. I took off my mask, because I knew that may be one of the last faces that he ever laid eyes on. Also, I intuitively felt that whatever the causes were of contracting this virus that was attacking primarily gay men, it did not happen from simply having a face-to-face conversation. So as a compassionate and loving person, I did my best to make him feel human and cared for one last time. As I spoke with him, I felt no fear. I was not afraid of the virus; I just wanted to know how we could treat these people.

As it turned out, the reason the mass public was so afraid and acted so hatefully, and out of fear, was because they did not understand this virus nor how it behaved. At that time, neither did medical researchers and doctors. We since discovered that it's not dangerous until it gets inside your body; for that to happen, it requires a blood-to-blood or sexual contact with another person who's infected. Also, since we've found the drugs and created highly effective cocktails to treat it, you rarely hear about people dying of HIV in 2022. We are now 40 years removed from that day in 1982 . . .

Why Are People Afraid of COVID-19?

Now let's get back to the novel coronavirus, or COVID-19. Why are people afraid? Acting out in fear and hostility? Expressing hatred toward one another? And fighting themselves and others over whether or not to get the vaccine? People have polarized over a difference in their choices of what to do—vax or don't vax? Mask don't mask. A person's decisions about their body needs to be a personal choice, best if guided by a physician. However, we need to respect each other's diversity and understand we don't have to agree. As a physician in a pandemic, I highly recommend masks and vaccines. However what has been left out of the equation by the government and health officials for the most part is the importance of health, vitamin D levels and good nutrition. Statistics have shown us people with chronic diseases, depression and low vitamin D levels are more likely to be hospitalized for COVID-19.

When I heard about this virus, I pulled together the entirety of my experience and knowledge in dealing with other epidemic- and pandemic-level viruses like EBV, herpes type one or type two, HIV, CMV, and stealth organisms like Lyme disease. I warned people about hand washing, against touching their nose or going into crowded places and cautioned about traveling at the time. I also recommended a healthy diet free of refined carbohydrates and a good sleep schedule.

Of note, I have treated hundreds of people with COVID-19; most were unvaccinated when we started. However, there are a variety of conditions which increase the risk of death with COVID-19. The majority of people who have died after contracting the virus had one or more preexisting conditions or comorbidities, including diabetes, heart disease, obesity, hypertension, cancer, pregnancy, or mental health disorders, including anxiety and depression. Unfortunately, over half of the US has a preexisting condition—including 42 percent of American adults with obesity. There's also an increased risk of hospitalization and death for older adults. Another factor is vaccination status. According to the Centers for Disease Control and Prevention, unvaccinated vaccinated Americans are 14 times more likely to die from COVID-19 than those who are fully vaccinated, and 97 times more likely to die than those that have received a booster dose.

Just like HIV, COVID-19 is a weak virus—until it gets inside you. Its Achilles' heel is the fatty envelope within its structure. If you use an agent such as alcohol, soap or vinegar, you will cut through that fatty envelope and kill it. Honestly, soap and water are all you really need. Because of the rush to stay safe, people turned to hand sanitizers, which can be very unhealthy

. . . and even dangerous. You are better off putting alcohol or vinegar in a spray bottle and using that. Dangerous chemicals found in hand sanitizers include methyl alcohol, also known as methanol or wood alcohol. This type of alcohol is extremely poisonous and even deadly if swallowed. Also 1-propanol has been found in hand sanitizers. It is included in industrial cleaning agents and can also cause death when swallowed. Most sanitizers are made of ethanol or isopropyl alcohol.

The problem with any of these products is that they destroy your microbiome by killing off the good or beneficial bacteria and can cause eye and skin irritation. I had a patient that was spraying sanitizers in his nose, which explained his resulting sinus problems and dry eyes. The CDC recommends washing with at least a 60 percent alcohol solution, and preferably using soap and water when possible.

So how does coronavirus spread? It starts with respiratory droplets, like all other cold and flu viruses. That's why it is so important to wear a mask and gloves or wash your hands. If we get it on our hands, and touch our nose, then we're exposed. If the virus gets inside our nostrils, that is direct exposure. Generally the mask stops the virus before it can get inside your mouth or nose; it benefits both the wearer and others. N-95 and KN-95 masks are best.

The bottom line? Take the safest measures you can—which do give you a great deal of safety. Wash with soap suds that cut through the viral membrane, or use alcohol or vinegar.

I also have voiced concerns with the term "social distancing" since officials started using it in March 2020. Social distancing should really be called "physical distancing." People need their families and communities, no matter what, but especially during a shutdown pandemic. So I advise my patients, and advise you, *not* to socially distance. Stay in touch often with your friends, loved ones and community, even if the situation requires you to remain physically apart. It is very important not only for you, but for your family and community. Research tells us how important family, community and friends are for our health.

What about this fear and stress that has gripped the country since COVID-19 landed on our shores? Let's address that. The first thing is to always take care of yourselves, and not to be frightened or stressed out—because that impacts and weakens your immune system. When an uncontrolled pandemic-level virus sweeps around the world, you want the strongest immune system and the most positive attitude possible, because they definitely work hand-in-hand to fight off unwanted viruses.

We might also want to consider some deeper-seated factors that contributed to the unleashing of this novel coronavirus. We have been mistreating animals and the planet for a long time. Some of our worst treatment of animals takes place in feed lots and slaughterhouses—the heart of how our meat is processed. Feed lots are very toxic places where animals are crowded and mistreated, filled with disease and pestilence; even the massive quantities of growth hormones and disease-preventative antibiotics that fill livestock troughs cannot stop it all. Packing houses are even worse. Animals are diseased and inspectors have approximately 17 seconds to inspect a *full-sized beef cow* as its carcass passes by on conveyor belts. Discovered abscesses are punctured, which leads to pus being sprayed everywhere. Many abscesses are missed. Conditions are crowded for animals and meat-packing employees—which led to a horrifying COVID-19 outbreak at packing centers throughout the country in 2020, directly impacting the people handling our meat supply. This is all a set up for breeding and spreading more mutant viruses.

What is the likeliest origin source for the virus? While the media focuses on a lab in Wuhan, I focus on the meat markets in that city—also a possible origin spot. And one that makes more sense to me is our misguided relationship with animals and the environment, and the way we raise the livestock we eat, as in the practices of "The Big Four": Tyson, Cargill, JBS and National Meat. This does not refer to regeneratively farmed animals and some high-integrity grass-fed ranches. However, as mentioned before, their practices are hard to sort out. This poor treatment of animals and shady production of meats may have caused a viral reaction that brought the people and planet to its knees. But as bad as COVID-19 is, it also gives us an opening to heal ourselves and the planet, and to learn and consider new regenerative approaches to life and our relationship with the earth, health and food.

Finally, let's look at the overall fatality rate of COVID-19. In the beginning of the pandemic, we didn't know what to expect or how many would get sick and die. Since then, it has acted like a true pandemic. As of January 2022, over 300 million people worldwide have contracted the virus, and 5.47 million have died. That amounts to 1 in every 26 people testing positive, and 1 in 1,417 people dying globally. In the United States, 58.5 million cases have been reported, and now more than 939,000 people in the US have died thus far of 78.6 million cases.

Overall, this adds up to a recovery rate of about 98.2 percent per WebMD. And, the seemingly disproportionate number of cases in the US reflects how strong the testing and reporting has become after a rocky start—and how much further testing needs to be distributed in other nations, especially developing and underprivileged countries.

Now for the news that might surprise you: the chances of dying from any of the winter influenza strains that come around are significant but lower than COVID deaths 2019–2020. COVID deaths have risen to 10 times those by influenza.

Most recently we experienced a global setback with the Omicron variant of COVID-19, and it seemed like a complete repeat of the original COVID-19 pandemic. With an infection rate of roughly four times that of the Delta strain (itself about two times as infectious as the original strain of COVID-19), infections, deaths and hospitalizations soared. However, because of vaccines, long-term immunity from T and B cells, and it being a less virulent strain, Omicron was not as bad clinically on an individual level. There have been other negative effects, however. People had already been isolating and suffering socially since 2020, and it added to mental health issues, anxiety, isolation and had detrimental effects on merchandising. Grocery prices increased by 30 percent and the workforce fell by 50 percent in the medical field and across the board. So Omicron was damaging. In a surprise move many cities and states lifted COVID-19 restrictions, mask and vaccination rules. Although seemingly paradoxical, it may increase the functioning of our societal infrastructure and economic status in general. Time will tell.

My personal opinion is that COVID-19 will go from being a pandemic to more endemic. Like the flu, it will still exist but long-term immunity in the population will keep it from ever being as bad as it was in the beginning. The real mystery is whether other pandemics will arise because of poor practices around animal rendering or other misguided ways we deal with food on the planet.

CHAPTER 24

Regeneration: the Key to Healing Ourselves— and Our Planet

Never in my 40-plus-year career in medicine has it been more crucial for us to understand the connection between our own health and the health of the planet. Today, we find ourselves at a crisis point in both areas, the human health crisis, not just in this country but globally, and planetary health—climate change crisis—facing the sixth mass extinction.

When I initially wrote *Soul Doctoring: Heal Yourself, Heal the Planet*, I saw the book as a combination of my life experiences as a young woman, doctor and healer and a powerful tool for self-healing. It was the blending of treatments and practices from more than 20 traditional and integrative modalities that affirmed for me how the connections between self-healing and the planet are critical for all of us. Not only to move medicine into the future but to see the continuity between the health of humanity and the health of the planet. *Soul Doctoring* evolved into exactly what we need now to restore full balance: healing ourselves, and in so doing, contributing to the healing and regeneration of all humanity and the planet. Nothing could be more important!

I have been attuned to the relationship between our bodies and planetary regeneration for four decades. Thankfully, hundreds of millions of people and much of the business world are now catching up. For example, Sustainable Brands is a consortium of 100 full corporate partners and several thousand participating companies focused on bringing sustainable, environmentally and socially conscious practices to business: treating the earth as a *source*, not a resource. That's a regenerative philosophy. At the SB '21 conference in San Diego, Nestlé CEO Aude Gandon coined the term "Generation Regeneration."[67] I love this term! I also love its deeper context: that Nestlé, long a company with, shall we say, not so friendly environmentally or socially conscious practices, has turned a sharp corner and become a leading voice for both in the corporate world. This is huge—and so necessary. They are following their CEO's lead and have joined "Generation Regeneration."

As I've said on my Friday night Instagram TV shows, social media and *Soul Stories* podcasts for years, robust restoration and regeneration requires focus on mental, emotional, physical and spiritual self-healing. And new business practices. Through these practices, we will see a wave of movement toward the "one humanity, one planet" path.

My book really began its 25-year trajectory with the Sundance vision I was gifted in New Mexico in 1997. The vision showed me the connections between personal self-healing and the planet. In addition, it guided me to actively participate in the regeneration of our planet's health by holding sacred every life choice we make. Only then can we begin to mitigate and reverse the various climate, societal and cultural challenges with which we are faced.

So, how do we go about this? How do I, as your host on the *Soul Doctoring* journey, further empower you to bring your health and that of the planet into full integrated focus? By starting with the answer: *"We are the solution."* The true regenerative lifestyle takes regeneration into account with every living choice we make. I want to emphasize that small steps by each of us can result in great changes on our planet—and our own health. From self, to family, to community, all humanity can be healed with these regenerative lifestyle practices. Yes, science is great, but we do not need to wait for "them," the government or scientists, to fix it for us when we are already the solution to the problem. *We* caused it. We can resolve it.

How do we bring regenerative practices into our own lives and make them central to our daily routines? And what does *regeneration* even mean? How do we get people to "look up" when they feel overwhelmed and disengaged? We need to help people understand that all regenerative actions are helpful no matter how small or big. We need to show people that doing these things is easy and we can collectively bring about big changes. That way when people choose well and start doing things like growing their own food, buying local food, composting, buying sustainable clothes, repurposing clothes or giving back to nature or community, it has a positive effect both personally and planetarily. It feels good, you become healthier and happier.

Paul Hawken's book *Regeneration: Ending the Climate Crisis in One Generations* is an amazingly inclusive book covering all aspects of climate change and the spread of regeneration globally.[68] It also has a very specific section addressing what to do and how to start addressing climate change in every way. A brilliant, inspiring, necessary guide in dealing with the climate change crisis.

First, let's examine our food choices. Changing the food system is, without a doubt, one of the biggest game changers that we can become involved in to slow down the health and the planetary climate change crisis. I always tell my patients, "Vote with your dollar" when talking to them about organic, regenerative food. Eat foods that benefit us, our land and the planet at the same time.

If we are to regenerate ourselves and the planet, we need a fully regenerative food system. This is the single greatest healing action that can restore our environment and climate, while reversing the chronic disease epidemic and provide additional benefits to the economy. The current food system is one of the largest contributors to global warming, destruction of the rainforest, poisoning and desertification of the land (removes all microorganisms from the soil), and destruction of the oceans. It is also the cause of inflammatory-based diseases (diabetes, heart disease, stroke, obesity, autoimmune disease, some forms of cancer) due to contamination with glyphosates, other toxins, hormones, unhealthy animal fats and generalized lack of nutrients in foods grown in soil devoid of microorganisms and nutrients.

We need to further consider regeneratively grown food and meats. Measures need to be taken to completely eliminate growing poisonous glyphosate tainted grain to feed our livestock. The CO2 from tilling the soil to grow the crops to feed the livestock contributes as much carbon to the atmosphere as all the combustion engines on the planet combined. This poisonous meat is fed to our families, children and most of the people in lower economic strata. In my view, this is equivalent to a slow genocide, and should be outlawed. Also we need to move people away from meat-packing plant practices, fast foods and reliance on our sick food supply system and standard American diet (SAD), which is killing our people and our planet. Regenerative practices also help to avoid the run of pandemic inception and spread by eliminating the need for conventional meat-packing practices.

Regeneratively raised livestock is another subject. Livestock raised on grass alone are healthier and happier. They are allowed to graze in one area for a limited period of time before ranchers mimic the predator-prey relationship and move them to another hectare of land before the grass is eaten halfway down. This strengthens the grass and makes it more phytonutrient rich. The grasses also cool the earth and the regenerative ranching process keeps the soil probiotic rich, *reduces* carbon emission and provides clean, hormone- and toxin-free food. This is also true of regeneratively raised food crops and vegetables. The no-till method of regenerative gardening and farming eliminates massive releases of carbon from the land. Any regenerative planting draws down carbon, fixes nitrogen and releases oxygen, thus combating and helping reverse global warming.

Another big carbon consideration is how we receive our food—usually trucked or sent by train from farms hundreds or thousands of miles away. That's a lot of road miles, and concomitant carbon emission. Source regenerative foods near you. Buying foods locally from farmers markets or growing your own are good choices. The fewer miles your food travels from ground to table, the better for the planet and you. Look in your community for a community-supported agriculture (CSA) plot, which supports your food and the community.

If you live in an apartment or urban home without available ground you can grow and raise sprouts inside, which are 10 to 50 times more nutrient dense than lettuce and vegetables grown indoors for you daily salads. If you have a deck—plants love planters and pots. You can grow tomatoes and cucumbers from hanging pots in or around your home!

One final thought on food: can you imagine how much we can contribute to regenerating our planet, and whole plant-based food sources, by teaching our children or grandchildren to garden? There is a growing movement in school districts across the country to replace an elective class with one semester of home gardening. If we teach children now, they may avoid chronic inflammatory diseases that currently plague the majority of people in our nation. Can you think of a better gift and legacy?! Gardening gives us good exercise, clean air, improves our microbiome, reestablishes the relationship with the earth our ancestors had and emulates the regenerative lifestyle of indigenous peoples.

We need to take other types of shopping into account when looking at how we can actively participate in regenerating ourselves and our planet. Clothing is a big one. The so-called "fast fashion" industry knocks off the latest styles put out by high-fashion moguls. Companies copy these styles within days, fly the products to more than 5,000 stores around the globe and sell them for cut-rate prices.

Our clothing consumption is egregious. The average American buys nearly 68 new outfits a year today; back in the 1970s, it was 12 per year. Many of these garments are never worn and the average American disposes of 80 pounds of clothing per year. It is tremendously wasteful—not to mention the consumption of water, fuel and other resources to produce and transport these clothes.[69]

We need to buy more durable clothes, repurpose items—or shop in our own closets! Also, take some extra time to research the growing number of high-quality sustainable fashion companies. These manufacturers take sourcing, available resources, transportation, materials, and impact on climate and environment into consideration with everything they do.

For example: Boody makes durable organic hypoallergenic clothing from plant sources that include bamboo, cotton and hemp. All plants made into yarn are grown in accordance with the established international organic standard, as well as the USDA National Organic Program. Each bamboo stalk is 100 percent free of any chemical pesticides. The woman-owned company Nube turns recycled plastic into responsible and fashionable activewear using recycled polyester. Their dyes are non-toxic, low impact and lead-free, and their shipping materials are 100 percent recycled and recyclable. Nearly three-quarters of Patagonia's massive clothing line, which brings the company more than $800 million in annual revenue, is made from recycled materials.[70] All of the virgin cotton used in production is either grown organically or recycled.

You may want to look at your computer technology and devices. My former IT consultant, closetotheearth.com, advised that we make our devices last as long as possible. Computers contain heavy and precious metals, making them simultaneously valuable and toxic to dispose. They can be upgraded, updated and sped up, and we don't always need to buy a new device. When you do need to buy new, recycle your old devices by giving them to someone who needs them.

To think regeneratively, you need to research and source anything you want to buy. Look for the miles on your product, the source materials, how they were transported, where they came from, and the interaction of the company with suppliers and employees.

When considering transportation, reduce high-fuel-consumption plane flights and drive whenever possible. Carpooling is a good old-fashioned way to save fuel and reduce your carbon footprint. Also choose a low-energy-consumption automobile, and if feasible consider hybrids and electric. Mass transport on trains, buses and subways is best.

We need to come up with new outside-the-box regenerative lifestyle practices. For instance, I live near the ocean and watch the container ships go out with clock-like regularity. During 2020 all around the globe, we witnessed miracle returns and even evolution of species previously nearing extinction. Watch David Attenborough's astoundingly beautiful documentary *The Year Earth Changed*. Whales began to communicate with each other in whole new languages because they could hear each other in absence of any human- or ship-generated noise. Baby turtles were able to make their dash for the ocean for the first time in decades without people obstructing their path, which resulted in an increased young turtle population. What if a law was passed to close the beaches and surrounding waters to accommodate animals and give them a chance to feed, communicate and breed? What if laws were passed to keep ships to a certain schedule, such as sending them out in batches, giving animals and sea creatures a chance to interact, breed and feed? Would that hurt us? Quite the contrary, I believe. These are small differences that could bring about large transformations for our planet and her animals.

We need to remember we are one humanity, one planet! We are all in this together, no matter color, sex, religion, country of origin, ethnicity! Just like with farming, more diversity brings more unity! What is good for us is good for the planet.

Small steps we can all do to be part of the solution (and feel good about it!):

1. Stop using single-use plastics.
2. Take your own cloth or other grocery bags to store.
3. Do not use plastic bags offered in grocery stores for produce. You can buy net bags or make your own out of repurposed cloth and clothes. Or be brave and put your produce right in the cart.
4. Repurpose clothing into mosaic tops or dresses—adorable!
5. Turn the water off while you are brushing your teeth, soaping up in the shower or washing your hair. Then rinse.
6. Put a large vessel such as a bucket or pot to catch extra water in your shower. Plants don't mind a little soap; it may even repel bugs and pests.
7. Keep a compost receptacle in your kitchen. Add vegetable and plant scraps to your main compost pile once a week or so. Gardens love it!
8. Turn heat down at night in the winter. Turn air conditioner temp up in summer.
9. Do not leave lights on in rooms you are not occupying. I hardly use lights at all. I have battery-operated candles placed around my living area to avoid using excess electricity. They are on a timer and turn on at sundown and run for about 4 hours (or however long you set them for).
10. Do not leave doors to refrigerator open when you are doing other things.

11. Do not turn oven or stove on until you are ready to cook. It not only wastes energy but is toxic with gas appliances.
12. Recycle plastic (try not to use any), glass and paper.
13. Try to buy liquids like oil and vinegar in glass bottles.
14. Store things in mason jars like rice and dried goods. Looks attractive in your kitchen as well.
15. Use bamboo or other non-paper towels, paper plates and napkins. They are easy to find. Or do not use them at all. Use ceramic dishes, cloth napkins and cloth towels.
16. Wash in cold water. Use environmentally friendly soap. You would be shocked at the environmental toxicity of laundry detergent, fabric softener and dryer sheets.
17. Use EWG (Environmental Working Group)-approved cleaning products and cosmetics.
18. Avoid takeout or delivery. Reduces carbon debt by decreasing fuel use and disposable eat-ware and plastic bags.
19. Cook at home instead—it is healthier and better for family time and community.
20. Grow your own food or buy food that has been grown locally to reduce miles your food travels.
21. Do not use outside lights when you are not going anywhere and no one is coming over.
22. Use solar lights when possible. I have several outside solar lights which are effective and beautiful. They turn on when the sun goes down and off in the morning.
23. Walk, bike or take public transportation instead of driving.
24. Think of your own planet-saving habits. Remember, we are the solution!

CHAPTER 25
One Mind—One Planet

The vision for this book came a quarter-century ago, in a flash of inspiration—my 1997 Sundance vision. I was told to write a book about applied integrated healing and pull together the wisdom, knowledge and practices from all directions to help heal the planet and her people. Personally, I had the philanthropic desire to bring you with me to experience some of my powerful journey and wonderful healing modalities. Interestingly, at the time of the vision, I had not mastered all of the modalities I am trained in yet, making the vision not only inspirational but also prophetic.

Most of all, I wanted to share the essential pieces to create a healthy environment of regeneration, inside and out, for you to heal. By sticking with me this far in the book, you may well be more awake and aware of medicine, health, healing and staying healthy, than ever. That is the true precipice of healing, not only for us and the human race, but also the planet.

I have always held a heightened awareness and sense of Oneness with the planet, its animals, plants, humanity and other beings. For instance, several months before the devastating 2019 Amazonian fires broke out, I felt an inferno inside my heart. My already deep passion for the earth exploded. Even before teen environmental activist Greta Thunberg hit the international scene, Jane Fonda started her Friday environmental fire drills and Leonardo DiCaprio's campaign took off (all of which are fabulous herculean efforts), I was deeply moved to talk to almost everyone about our planetary crisis. I started a website and Facebook and Instagram accounts called Pledge 4 Planet. I attempted to contact President Barack Obama and his wife Michelle Obama, Jane Fonda and Leo DiCaprio. I felt passionately that, if we could get enough people on the same page, change could be quickened. These were the leaders that could bring together the masses. They actually did step in, a little example of one-mindedness. Now, we all see that the coronavirus has done that quickening for us.

During this time, my older sister informed me that I'd been speaking about saving the planet since I was a little girl playing with her four-legged friends in the Nebraska pasture. Maybe it was the near-death experience I had when I was born, or the love, compassion and caring I felt from *the kind ones* outside my little newborn body that ignited my soul to the "All" and "One" and gave me the foresight to see the future threat to our earth. Or maybe I was just born that way.

Before the Amazon forest and the Australian bushfires, what I felt inside was impending, horrific destruction, the heat of devastating fires and fear of a worldwide pandemic moving through me as it moved through my connection with the All, a touching of cosmic consciousness that pushed me further. "We are the first generation to feel the effects of climate change, and the last generation that can do something about it," then-President Obama said. I felt it at every level of my being.

The awakening happens for all of us at different times. This book has hopefully been another agent of quickening and awakening for you. The first step in healing is awareness, and how to heal and maintain wellness through it and maybe because of it.

Renewed Focus on Environment and Climate

It is shocking that humans physically occupy less than 10 percent of the world, yet we have leavened all this damage. After all, 70 percent of earth is water, 10 percent desert and 10 percent inhospitable mountains and waste-lands. How can we unleash nearly 100 percent devastation despite only 10 percent occupancy? Are we the stewards and keepers of the earth, as we originally agreed to be? Or are we a destructive pestilence that should be yanked out and treated with antibiotics? At what point did our near-ancestors decide that our planet and its creatures and plants were material resources to be plundered for industry and profit, rather than living beings connected together, treating the earth as a source of energetic connection to be honored and tended? Is Mother Earth a resource? Or a source?

The fateful decision to treat the earth as a resource for our Industrial Age, manufacturing- and construction-based lifestyle not only opened the door to harm our planet, but also unleashed the beginning of a health-care crisis that shows no signs of letting up, unless we take firm command of our own health, diets, lifestyle, relationship to the planet and how we treat others.

The pandemic forced us inward—into our homes and into ourselves. We learned that, once we step out of the way (or are forcibly sidelined), the planet can heal more quickly than we ever imagined. Many people can work at home. Living a hygienic, clean life is not that hard. Much of the media spews out a lot of nonsense which distracts, often misinforms and disturbs peoples' peace. Health-care professionals are undervalued and should be regarded as highly as actors and sports heroes. Animals in captivity probably feel like we do in quarantine. Oil is worthless in a society without drive for consumption; in fact, on April 20, 2020, the price of oil dropped *below zero* for the first time.

Life is valuable and fragile and needs to be treated with great care and gratitude. The best motto is to treat others with kindness and compassion.

Become a Benevolent Guardian of the Planet

I believe that, with the awareness that comes from healing ourselves, we can and will become the truly benevolent guardians of our planet once again. Some of us have served in this role for decades; others are just now coming to it. I believe it is time for *all* of us to take on this responsibility. When we shift our perspective, we become aware of cosmic consciousness, or the One Mind.

What happens when we awaken in this way? For one thing, we can't look at a piece of plastic the same. We can't ignore waste and the toxins we're ingesting in our food, or feel the same about taking drugs with toxic incipients manufactured by Big Pharma. It is crucial for the earth that we continue to evolve into a compassionate, caring, loving race that realizes our deep interconnection with each other and everything surrounding us. This allows a direct route to Oneness, to being on the same page and bringing about change in a quickened way. Social media can help, as well as group-form demonstrations and rallies.

However, the most important thing is achieving Oneness.

Some may doubt that this form of walking through life amounts to an actual spiritual, personal, healing or life path. I submit that we have great evidence of this being a truly great path, one we can all walk when we launch our courage and change our perspective. Going back to the "normal" that existed pre-coronavirus (before March 2020 in the US) is a bad idea. "Normal" is not working. Now that we're opened back up, sadly, most are trying to cling onto that old "normal." By doing so, we are losing the deeper teaching of the past two years.

Instead, we are being called to rise up to transform and treat each other and the planet better.

From Social Activism to Spiritual Activism

We made huge changes in how races are treated during the Civil Rights Movement. That same decade, millions of Baby Boomers turned on to the Love Generation, opening their hearts and souls to an infusion of cosmic consciousness and the spiritual and healing knowledge of ancient cultures never seen before in the West. Not to mention the massive opening of minds to new ideas and ways of living. The 35 million people who practice yoga in the US today can thank we "flower children" Boomers for giving the age-old practice from India a foothold here. In 1975, we brought our brothers, sisters, sons and daughters home from the Vietnam War through voicing our protest and collective connection. We got on the same page.

Now, there are a huge number of organized spiritual gatherings for developing Oneness, like the million-person meditation on April 4, 2020, the 21-day meditation co-hosted by Deepak Chopra and Oprah Winfrey, and many others. But we can achieve greatly on a local level, too. During the 1980s, a group of women, including me, kept the Los Angeles wild-life corridor open in the Santa Monica Mountains by gaining the support of celebrities like Barbra Streisand, Jack Nicholson, Magic Johnson, Merv Griffin, Don Henley of the Eagles, Carrie Fisher, Warren Beatty, Annette Bening and others. As the LA Urban Wilderness Coalition, we teamed up with the Santa Monica Conservancy. A former opponent of ours, then-LA City Councilman Zev Yaroslavsky, began to use the words from our letters: "For All the People. For the Grandchildren." He later ran successfully on an environmental platform. If we could turn him around, what about everyone else? This effort saved many parks and preserved hundreds of square miles of open space for wildlife and people alike. It remains in the public domain today.

How did this happen? Experiences with Cosmic Consciousness or Universal Mind are more common than many think. As we wore our eco-warrior hats in the Hollywood Hills during the 1980s, we were attempting to save several ancient oak trees from destruction. All were huge and looked every bit of their age. We took turns sitting in the trees to prevent developers from chopping them down. This forced the developers to negotiate with us. We climbed down and gathered our papers, showing the lead developer our demands.

Almost on cue, a swarm of bees started buzzing around us. I have always been intrigued by the sacred nature of bees. What one bee knows, they all know—and they know it well beyond their hives. They are very altruistic. Bees are known to leave or move their hive if their keeper dies and they are not informed. In this case, three bees lit gently on my chest and began to walk around. The lead developer, a large Persian man, was visibly shaken. He started to sweat, and his eyes twitched as he pointed at my chest. "Lady, lady, you have . . ."

"I know," I said calmly. "The bees do not want to lose these ancient trees. They are part of their home and ecosystem."

He stammered out a few words in Persian; I'm pretty sure he was cussing. He turned away, never to return. By unnerving him as they did, the bees helped to save the precious trees.

Another time, I was preparing to head to New Mexico for my Sundance ceremony. I packed my car with a light, joyful heart, so happy to make a sacrifice in this way to bring new visions and life to the planet. I spread out my arms in the driveway as though I were a giant hawk, dance-flying in my way to fetch more stuff for my journey.

Out of seemingly nowhere, a gigantic red-tailed hawk swooped down, touching his right wingtip to the fingertips of my left hand. In awe, I watched him sweep up and circle four times overhead before flying away. *Thank you, Brother!* Then I realized *he* was thanking *me* for embarking on the Sundance!

Many times, I have had premonitions or dreams about patients before seeing them. This is a perfect example of a Cosmic Consciousness connection, or *One*-mindedness, as I discussed more thoroughly when I talked about dream doctoring in Chapter 18.

Experiences such as these leave no doubt that we are all individual pieces of a large, infinite consciousness much greater than the sum of its parts. This new way of thinking is, in so many ways, a return to the ancient, indigenous way. It is defined by what we call holistic, regenerative, biomimicry and sustainable practices in concert and partnership with natural processes. The pre–COVID-19 way sets up man as a force over nature and science as God, and the altar from which we draw our intentions and tools.

Many of you have other words for what I am calling Cosmic Consciousness and One Mind. You may call it the Universe, God, Jesus, Allah, Higher Power, Source, Adonai, El Shaddai (All-Sufficient One), Jehovah, the Void, or Absolute and many others. The name is not as important as awareness of an all-knowing greater than we are, one that holds answers for everyone. We are individuals allowed to interface with it, if we come from love, caring, compassion and respect for all beings and things. We heal ourselves and make ourselves ready for the ultimate connection.

Planetary Lessons from My Journeys to Africa

All of my journeys to Africa were amazing experiences, woven with connection to Source. On one trip, I was lucky enough to have my own tent rather than sharing with a roommate. On the third day, I mentioned to my friend and guide Sekongo, "I miss the lions. I haven't heard them at night as we usually do."

"Oh, they are here," he replied.

"OK." I still wondered why I hadn't heard them, as I had on my previous trips.

The night grew chilly, as it usually does that time of the year. Our summers are their winters, making the trips to Africa even more magical. I snuggled up to my woven cloth-covered hot water bottle that the beautiful women of Macatoo placed in our beds to keep us warm. Under a multitude of stars too numerous to count, I fell into a deep sleep inside the canvas tent.

Soon, I heard the characteristic, repetitive grunt of a lion at my back, not two feet from where I lay! Like all cats, lions have different sounds and calls for different needs or to command their cubs. First, almost startled, I opened my eyes wide. I say "almost" because I felt the love of the lioness and her call: *"Hunh! Hunh! Hunh! Hunh!"* It immediately lulled me back to sleep, and I was so grateful she answered my longing and came to sleep by me.

Then next morning, I stepped outside the tent to investigate. I took pictures of her paw prints and body outline in the sand where she'd lain down and sang to me. When I showed Sekongo, he said, "You know, they only sleep with their pride. You must be lioness!"

A little, I thought, happy for this gift of awe and connection.

On another occasion, in Botswana, elephants were on my mind. I pined for contact with them. Elephants are extremely bright, sensitive, intelligent beings that honor their dead and care for each other's children. One day, I stayed back from riding horseback safari. Much to my delight, an entire matriarchal herd came to my tent and encircled it. They were making their happy sounds, growling more than the trumpet warnings we're accustomed to hearing in nature films. They ate, crunched and growled for hours.

After watching through tent windows for a long time, I walked outside onto my little front porch and sat on the edge to get a closer look at the eight or nine mothers and their babies. One of the mothers walked slowly but decisively over to me, her calf in tow. She stretched out her enormous trunk and softly caressed my face and hair. Her breathy puffs made some of my white-blonde hair fly up. It reminded me of the first time I went to visit the horsies when they blew their caring breath on my little face in Nebraska. This elephant was in the wild, not domesticated or tamped down by zoo or circus. She was sharing the love, honoring me in a way she knew. I was so humbled and grateful. We shared in the Oneness together.

Since I first found my way to the horses at age three, I've known that animals respond to love, caring and compassion. These happen to be the very qualities that we respond to deeply as well, that allow us to interface with the Cosmic Consciousness, the One Mind—the face of God. Gentle compassion is a key for the interface. This uncanny knowingness is the same as what allows a family member or concerned friend to know when another is in trouble.

Intuition Is Critical: Treating Gary

One Monday, I felt called to go into my office. I usually spend Mondays out of the office, catching up on paperwork, writing or other projects. Why did I feel so compelled to go in this time? I didn't yet know, but convinced myself I was bringing lunch to my team. I headed over the Santa Monica Mountains from my Malibu house and arrived at my office. Soon after my arrival, while chatting with the team, we heard a loud crashing sound. "Sounds like an elephant doing a somersault," I said.

We ran outside. Gary, the building's owner, had fallen down the outside stone stairs. His face was smashed into the second-to-bottom stair, his neck twisted toward the wall. His left foot was wedged into the space between the sixth stair up from the bottom and the wall. His left leg and torso were contorted, his belly down and against the stairs.

Something stepped up inside me. I saw everything in an instant. I went into auto-drive in front of a growing crowd of concerned observers at the scene who were unsure what to do. "Call nine-one-one, Rhonda," I said. "Gary, are you OK?"

"Yes," he said. Blood dripped down the stairs.

"Monica, call his wife." (Monica is his secretary). A young man stepped up to help. "Take off his left shoe, slowly," I said.

I turned to Gary. "Can you feel your arms and feet?"

"Yes," he said.

Three more young men offered their assistance. Gary was a very large man. Normally, you don't move someone with a potential neck injury, but the information I was receiving inwardly, and through training, told me it would be worse to leave him with all his weight on his face with his neck twisted.

Time to move him. "You, you and you . . . brace him and slowly, ever so slowly allow his legs, then his body to lower down toward the bottom," I instructed the men. They began their work, a bit eagerly at first. "Slowly . . . slowly," I reiterated. Then I looked at Gary. "Tell me if anything hurts."

"I'm OK," he said.

Soon, Gary sat at the base of the stairs. "Any numbness anywhere? Can you move everything?" I asked.

"Yes."

I turned to the men. "OK, prop him up against the wall."

Then I saw Gary's face more completely. Part of it was smashed and his nose was broken, leaving a significant pool of blood on the steps. "Gary, you should go with the paramedics and get looked at," I said. "You hit your head and broke your nose." I sensed resistance, despite the dramatic fall and injuries.

"No, I did not," he protested.

"Yes, you did."

Before his stubbornness could go any further, his wife arrived, as did the paramedics. He reluctantly agreed to get checked out at the hospital.

Two days later, Gary walked into my office, barely recognizable from all the swelling. He'd been released from the hospital the previous day. Tears rolled down his swollen, bruised cheeks. "I wanted to come see you and thank you for saving me," he said. "I cleaned up the best I could and took a shower." We both giggled a little through the tears.

I smiled. "Of course, Gary."

"Out of all those people who were there, you were the only one who acted. You knew what to do."

"My pleasure."

"Turns out I just have a broken nose and severe bruises. You were right. My brain and neck are OK on the scan," he added.

"God is amazing, Gary, and you are tough," I said, being sure to affirm one of his qualities. He hugged me and left.

Afterward, I reflected on the experience. I knew it was the Source, or God, that compelled me to drive to the office that day—and to be in position to assist Gary to safety.

There is a great deal of scientific data supporting the existence of Cosmic Consciousness. I was a friend of the late Jeanne Achterberg, who I met at Rancho La Puerta while serving as executive director. Jeanne was a prominent psychologist known for her therapeutic application of guided imagery and creative visualization. She was also president of the Association for Transpersonal Psychology. Her last of three books, *Imagery in Healing; Shamanism and Modern Medicine*, came out in 2013. She kept me abreast of her research, as she knew of my keen interests in remote healing, energy healing and shamanism. She also knew of my early association with Valerie Hunt, one of the first to measure the energy and auras of both healers and patients. Jeanne showed, without a doubt, that remote healing in the form of positive intentions, and purposeful prayers, was measurable with fMRI measurements of recipients' brains.

Although the interfacing with Source or Cosmic Consciousness is usually spontaneous, it is the prepared soul that receives "preferential" access. The healed body, mind, spirit and emotional being can more easily access the One Mind.

This is my call to action for all of us: heal ourselves. Connect with Oneness. One Mind—One Planet. This is indeed a bold call. However, these are troubled times that call for bold words and actions. It is the most direct rapid way to effect change. If we wake up and, despite our cultural and religious differences, realize we are One People—One Planet and that our planet is in trouble, then a critical mass of people with common intention can effect global change immediately. Think back to the Civil Rights Movement and the Vietnam War. *Heal yourself, heal the planet.*

Personal and Planetary Health Go Hand in Hand

Personal and planetary health go hand in hand. It starts by placing your positive intention into healing the earth and changing your own behavior in every way possible. Conserve water, don't waste food, start a compost pile, carpool, recycle, drive an electric or hybrid car, use solar or other alternative energy sources, start your garden, plant trees, stop single use plastics, use washable net bags for produce, or cloth bags to carry your groceries. Demonstrate, sign petitions. Eat organic, local produce. If you eat meat and dairy, choose from regenerative farms that absorb CO_2 from the environment and restore the soil (see Chapter 14).

All farming needs to move toward regenerative or aeroponic indoor farming, but this will take time to change over from the industrial farming system backed by governmental financing and mostly an entire planet population addicted to industrially raised foods.

There is a bright light on the food production horizon: aeroponic and vertical indoor farming. These are controlled, automated farming systems like no other. They conserve the earth's resources through almost unimaginably efficient farming practices that use up to 99 percent less water and land, and produce zero runoff or environmental contamination. Aeroponic crops require no poisonous herbicides, pesticides or fungicides. Since the operation is robotically operated and controlled, the product never interacts with humans or the environment, removing the risk of contamination and disease. This controlled environment also allows artificial intelligence to alter the plant's experience by adjusting the lights, temperatures, day lengths, etc. The plant can be grown to accentuate most desirable properties, nutrient density, size, color, smell and taste.

This creates the ability to personalize fresh food production. For instance, kidney patients may need food with less potassium, heart patients may need less sodium or pregnant women may need more vitamin A. These farms will be responsive to our health goals and needs, in pursuit of eliminating the diet-related diseases that currently plague our society. In the near future, we will all own a plot in our own local farm and achieve year-round access to the highest quality produce the planet has ever seen.

I was honored to be part of the advisory board for such a brilliant initiative, Willo. It is so badly needed right now on our planet. It has been birthed by the genius of John and Sam Bertram, in amazing alignment with One Mind—One Planet. It is another future farming option. This type of farming will make real the truth of food as medicine.

Dr. Larry Dossey's book *One Mind: How Our Individual Mind Is Part of a Greater Consciousness and Why It Matters* rang so true with me and this whole visionary concept. Years ago, I had the honor of meeting and spending some time with Larry and his wife Barbara at Rancho La Puerta. I will always have gratitude in my heart to Deborah Szekely, who introduced us. I had always followed Larry's works and teachings, and meeting him was a great privilege. I met him after I had finished a first version of what became this book. He found it engaging. It took 25 years to finish it; I had not experienced all that was needed to pull it to a close and be the guide for moving into the future. Plus, it was written for *right now*! As we put our foot on the precipice of climate change destruction—together we can change it. Reverse it! Regenerate our planet. All we have to do is decide together.

Looking back on my Sundance vision 25 years ago, it is all there. Larry's book drew me in because I was heading for the One Mind—One Planet goal so desperately needed right now. And I saw the same qualities and One-Mindedness in his words. Very moving. Thank you, Larry, for driving me and the planet even stronger forward.

Paradoxically, it is the COVID-19 virus that is giving us the greatest push to come together in the Cosmic Consciousness and do earth-centered things as we move forward in our lives and the planet's life. We need to be aware that we all come here to serve other souls with the gifts and talents we have. It is truly time to come together in love, compassion, and awareness and transform back into the true guardians of our planet. To reunite as one people-one humanity. No matter what race, ethnicity, gender, religion, gender or sexual orientation we are all people. We need to come together with that in common and respect each other's diversity. Unity through diversity with regenerative healing ways for humanity and the planet. One humanity—one planet. If a critical mass of people can achieve this, we can make a huge difference in beneficial planetary change.

One of my teachers, healer Howard Wills of Hawaii, said:

> For more than six thousand years, humanity has been scourging itself, all life forms, and the earth through pollution, greed, hatred, jealousy, judgment, and a sweeping and persistent ignorance. It is time for humanity to move into higher levels of intelligence, choosing life over death, by taking responsibility for all of our actions, and by allowing ourselves to grow into the consciousness of what we are—in the image and likeness of the Infinite. We are children of the Infinite, and as we awaken to what we are and to our creative and potential realities, we move individually, globally and universally into higher levels of intelligence. As we take responsibility for the health of our planet, for all life forms, and for ourselves—we can and will become the guardians and protectors we were designed to be, reawakening the essence and beauty of our earth, all life, and ourselves. Let us join in the creation and sharing of heaven on earth, individually, globally and universally. The time is now . . .

Meanwhile, Doctors Bruce Lipton and Rashid Buttar and the International Association for a Disease-Free World (IADFW) broadcast a daily call to think of health, harmony, love and gratitude. They focus on the presently unsustainable condition of our planet, the "sixth extinction," caused primarily by humans this time. If our behavior does not change, we will surely perish.

In their urgent call to action, the doctors offer a silver lining. The scientific reality is that our thoughts really do and can shape our existence. We know through quantum physics, the most valid science on earth, that consciousness is creating our life reality. That means there is a group, or collective reality through collective consciousness. There is a new technology that reads brain function better than EEG; it shows our thoughts are not contained in our heads, but rather are literal projections of energy. The more individuals that share a thought, the more power behind it. Satellites have shown that the electromagnetics of the world can be changed with collective thinking.

The more that people share a belief system, the more likely it will unfold into reality. Let us change the electromagnetics of the planet by joining together in our common thoughts through collective consciousness to project and feel compassion, love and a brave new world of improved planetary and collective health.

Howard Wills reflects on our thoughts as well:

> Action is the last leg of the triune creation process: thoughts, words and deeds—to create the present and the future. The actions that we and others take in life affect our well-being, the well-being of those around us, and the well-being of our planet. By partaking in positive and blessing actions, we are creating blessings for everyone in our presence—and what we do to others, we do to ourselves. So by blessing others through positive actions, we are also blessing ourselves and helping ourselves to feel better and have greater well-being.

I invite and challenge you to walk with me into the future, and to collectively align our intentions and thoughts and prayers to regenerate ourselves, contribute to the regeneration of our families and friends, be a change leader in our communities, and work hard to help regenerate our planet. Let us connect with each other to help the planet through the One Mind, God, and agree to save our Mother Earth for our grandchildren and all our relations! Let's do it as people living our most healthy lives, helping each other, and understanding that by being healthy and keeping our planet healthy we are at our best to serve our God and each other. That is the essence of *Soul Doctoring*.

REFERENCES

CHAPTER 3

Page 45

1. Ayurveda defines health as…

    Basisht, Gopal, *Exploring Insights Towards Definitions and Laws of Health in Ayurveda: Global Health Perspective,* AYU: International Quarterly Journal of Research in Ayurveda, Oct-Dec. 2014 https://www.ncbi .nlm.nih.gov/pmc/articles/PMC4492016/

Page 47

2. I think of the late mythologist-storyteller Joseph Campbell's classic work, *Hero of a Thousand Faces.*

    Campbell, Joseph, *Hero with a Thousand Faces,* New World Library (3rd edition), 2008.

Page 48

3. I was reminded of this when reading *Un Do It! How Simple Lifestyle Choices Can Reverse Most Chronic Diseases,*

    Ornish, Dean, MD, *Un Do It! How Simple Lifestyle Choices Can Reverse Most Chronic Diseases,* Random House, New York, 2019.

Page 49

4. Years ago, Richard Davidson and his colleagues at the Health/ Emotions Institute in Madison, Wisconsin, asked to study Tibetan monks to practice meditating.

    Lian, Dian, "Study shows compassion meditation changes the brain," *University of Wisconsin-Madison News,* March 25, 2008. https://news .wisc.edu/study-shows-compassion-meditation-changes-the-brain/

CHAPTER 4

Page 63

5. I explained how the Women's Health Initiative Study, published in 2002, villainized estrogen.

    Rossouw, Jacques E. MBChB, MD, National Heart, Lung, Blood Institute, et al, "Risks and Benefits of Estrogen plus Progestin in Healthy Postmenopausal Women: Principal Results from the Women's Health Initiative Randomized Control Trial," *Journal of the American Medical Association,* July 17, 2002. https://jamanetwork.com /journals/jama/fullarticle/195120

CHAPTER 5

Page 73

6. Years ago, studies by David McClelland at Harvard showed that medical students who watched three different movies before exams had three different immune system readings...

    McClelland, David C., Ph.D., "The effect of motivational arousal through finals on salivary immunoglobin A," *Psychology & Health* 2(1): 31-52, January 1988. https://www.researchgate.net/publication/247532754 _The_effect_of_motivational_arousal_through_films_on_salivary _immunoglobulin_A

7. Dr. Dean Ornish writes, "Our survival depends upon the healing power of love, intimacy, and relationships. Physically, emotionally, spiritually. As individuals. As communities. As a country. As a culture. Perhaps even as a species."

    Ornish, Dean, MD, *Love and Survival: 8 Pathways to Intimacy and Health,* William Morrow, New York, 1999.

8. The famous Nurses' Health Study from Harvard Medical School, an annual tradition started in 1976, found that the more friends women had, the less likely they were to develop debilitating physical problems later in life. Instead, they would lead joyful, fulfilling lives...

    The Nurses' Health Study today featured 121,700 married women participants in 1976, when the aforementioned study was made.

    Colditz, G.A., Philpott, S.E., Hankinson, S.E., *The Impact of the Nurses' Health Study on Population Health: Prevention, Translation, and Control.* American Journal of Public Health: Sept 2016, Vol. 106, No. 9, pp. 1540-1545.

9. Similarly, in July 2016, a Harvard Men's Health Watch survey of 127,545 men on marriage and health found that married men were far healthier than unmarried men.

> "The Workplace and Health: Poll Report," T.H. Chan School of Public Health, Harvard University, Robert Wood Johnson Foundation and NPR, July 2016. https://legacy.npr.org/documents/2016/jul /Workplace-Health-Poll.pdf

Page 75

10. In the 1990s, I began using Sanesco neurotransmitter hormonal testing and therapy intensely when I was one of the first physicians to take holistic functional integrative medicine into the inpatient addiction recovery world, which helped change the conversation in addiction therapy...

> Richard, Ramona, MS, NC, "Neurotransmitter Testing: What It Could Mean For You," Sanesco Blog, July 25, 2018 https://sanescohealth .com/blog/neurotransmitter-testing/

> This is a more recent, updated blog that summarizes experiences including my own from the 1990s and forward.

CHAPTER 6

Page 93

11. "Respect is love in plain clothes," said Frank Byrnes, the President of Human Potential Consultants.

Frank is the head of Human Potential Consultants, Inc., which provides values-driven training, facilitating, coaching and consulting services worldwide, and a former Irish radio host. https://hpci.net

> https://www.passiton.com/inspirational-quotes/5409-respect-is-love -in-plain-clothes

CHAPTER 7

Page 98

12. As medical intuitive and author Dr. Caroline Myss wrote in *The Creation of Health, Intuition is so natural, so ever-present, that it is accepted without question when it comes in the form of a symphony or a great painting...*

Myss, Carolyn, Ph.D., *The Creation of Health: The Emotional, Psychological, and Spiritual Responses that Promote Health and Healing,* Harmony: Three Rivers Press, 1998.

13. In her book, *Dr. Judith Orloff's Guide to Intuitive Healing,* Dr. Orloff defines intuition as: *A potent form of inner wisdom not mediated by the rational mind. Accessible to us all, it's a still, small voice inside—an unflinching truth-teller committed to our well-being...*

   Orloff, Judith, MD, *Guide to Intuitive Healing: Five Steps to Physical, Emotional and Sexual Wellness,* Harmony, 2001.

Page 99

14. In 1990, the death rate was nearly 100 percent, according to the Centers for Disease Control and Prevention.

   "Current Trends Mortality Attributable to HIV/Aids Infection, United States, 1981-1990, *MMWR Weekly,* Centers for Disease Control & Prevention, Jan. 25, 1991.

15. In 2020, according to UNAIDS, the death rate was less than 6 percent of all HIV cases worldwide.

   "Seizing the Moment: Tackling Entrenched Inequalities to End Epidemics," UNAIDS, July 6, 2020. https://aids2020.unaids.org/report/

Page 100

16. Dr. Orloff makes a comment in her guide to intuitive healing that speaks to both the awesomeness and subtlety of our intuitive power: *We all possess within us an intuitive healing code that contains the blueprints for health and happiness, and for the survival of everything that is good here on earth...*

   Orloff, Judith, MD, *Guide to Intuitive Healing: Five Steps to Physical, Emotional and Sexual Wellness,* Harmony, 2001.

Page 102

17. In *The Creation of Health,* Caroline Myss writes: *Traditional medicine and holistic health represent more than just two different approaches to healing disease. They illustrate two essentially different paradigms of reality...*

   Myss, Carolyn, Ph.D., *The Creation of Health: The Emotional, Psychological, and Spiritual Responses that Promote Health and Healing,* Harmony: Three Rivers Press, 1998.

Page 103

18. In her book *Infinite Mind: Science of the Human Vibrations of Consciousness*, she describes how we all have intuitive ability and a vibration.

> Hunt, Valerie, *Infinite Mind: Science of the Human Vibrations of Consciousness,* Malibu Publishing, 1996.

CHAPTER 8

Page 107

19. *When humans participate in a ceremony, they enter a sacred space...*

> This saying by the great Ojibwe teacher and writer Sun Bear (Gheezis Mokwa) has appeared many times, more recently in the Live Oak Chicago Blog "Rites of Passage," by Jeff Levy. https://liveoakchicago.com/rites-of-passage/

Page 111

20. As Joseph Campbell once said, "Your sacred space is where you can find yourself again and again."

> Campbell, Joseph, *Reflections on the Art of Living: A Joseph Campbell Companion,* Harper Perennial, 1995.

CHAPTER 9

Page 119

21. *There are only two days that nothing can be done. One is called yesterday. The other is called tomorrow.*

> Dalai Lama, notable quotes https://www.goodreads.com/quotes /735245-there-are-only-two-days-in-the-year-that-nothing

Page 120

22. Statistics from the Centers for Disease Control and Prevention are frightening: in 1970, the adult obesity rate in the US was 15 percent. By 2018, it had increased to an official total of 42.5 percent...

> "Overweight & Obesity: Adult Obesity Facts," Centers for Disease Control and Prevention, https://www.cdc.gov/obesity/data/adult.html

Page 124

23. In a revealing 2013 interview with famed TV news anchor Dan Rather on AXS-TV, Rock & Roll Hall of Famer Roger Daltrey of The Who addressed this point to then 16-year-old pop superstar Cody Simpson, who was also being interviewed...

https://www.axs.tv/channel/the-big-interview-with-dan-rather
/the-big-interview-with-dan-rather-season-1/video
/roger-daltrey-cody-simpson-1/

Page 129

24. In the December 31, 2017, issue of *Psychology Today*, Stephanie Sarkis, PhD, listed out four ways to achieve meaning and purpose in your life...

   Sarkis, Stephanie, Ph.D., "Four Ways to Achieve Meaning and Purpose in Your Life," *Psychology Today*, Dec. 31, 2017. https://www .psychologytoday.com/za/blog/here-there-and-everywhere/201712 /4-ways-achieve-meaning-and-purpose-in-your-life

CHAPTER 10

Page 130

25. "Ultimately we know deeply that the other side of every fear is a freedom."

   From Ferguson, Marilyn, *The Aquarian Conspiracy*, The Tarcher Group, 1980 (reprinted 2009).

Page 133

26. "It takes a lot of courage to release the familiar and seemingly secure, to embrace the new..."

   From Cohen, Alan, *Spirit Means Business: The Way to Prosper Wildly Without Selling Your Soul*, Hay House, 2019.

CHAPTER 11

Page 139

27. Between January 2019 and July 2020, about one in ten people reported anxiety and depression—an alarming enough number. Since then, however, that number has jumped to four in ten, or 40 percent.

   From De Angelis, Tori, "Depression and anxiety escalate during COVID," American Psychological Association report, Nov. 1, 2021. https://www.apa.org/monitor/2021/11/numbers-depression-anxiety

CHAPTER 12

Page 146

28. According to the University of Massachusetts Lowell, job stress costs the US economy and corporations $300 billion per year in the form of health costs, absenteeism and poor performance. . . .

"Financial Costs of Job Stress: Total Worker Health for Employers."
Accessed May 16, 2022. https://www.uml.edu/research/cph-new
/worker/stress-at-work/financial-costs.aspx.

Page 147

29. Today's middle school students are 10 years away from entering a
workforce in which up to *50 percent of the jobs and careers they will
apply for do not yet exist...*

From *Tech Cat* by Lori Schwartz, edited by Robert Yehling, unpublished
manuscript (reprinted with author's permission).

30. "The days of going to college, getting a degree, putting in 40 years as
a loyal employee and leaving with the pension are basically over—
especially for people in school today. It doesn't work that way anymore."

From Yehling, Robert, "Cara Santa Maria: Correspondent, National
Geographic Channel," *STEM Today magazine*, Fall-Winter 2019,
Online Edition.
https://innotechtoday.com/stem-today-fall-winter2019/

Page 151

31. "Our 'spirits' are longing to be recognized as legitimate, meaning they
are every bit as real as our physical selves. . . ."

From Myss, Carolyn, *Anatomy of the Spirit,* Three Rivers Press, New York,
1996.

Page 152

32. "Even our physical bodies cannot contain us, because our spirits can
step out of our bodies and spirit-travel..."

From a talk given by Frank Fool's Crow (1890-1989), ceremonial chief
of the Oglala Sioux. Further information can be found at https://
windspeaker.com/news/footprints/holy-man-lived-hollow-bone
-philosophy

Page 155

33. According to the American Psychological Association, if you
express pure gratitude or joy for 90 seconds, your immune system is
strengthened for *up to 24 hours*. However, if you express pure anger for
90 seconds, it is weakened for *up to 8 hours*.

From "How to recognize and deal with anger," American Psychological
Association report, 2012. https://www.apa.org/topics/anger/recognize

CHAPTER 13

Page 162–163

34. Farmers have grown and fed grains to their livestock and families in the larger region for more than 5,000 years. Archaeological digs show the earliest farmers were cultivating the land in parts of what is now Turkey, Syria and Lebanon up to 8,000 years ago . . .

> Many sources are available for historical agricultural statistics. A good common source, and the source for this information, comes from "The Dawn of Agriculture," available through the Khan Academy. https://www.khanacademy.org/humanities/world-history/world-history-beginnings/birth-agriculture-neolithic-revolution/a/where-did-agriculture-come-from

CHAPTER 14

Page 166

35. If we in the United States merely replaced meat with beans, we'd mitigate much of the *world's* greenhouse gas and global warming problem.

> From "What If Everyone Ate Beans Instead of Beef?" *The Atlantic Monthly*, Sept. 25, 2017 video https://www.theatlantic.com/video/index/540765/beans-instead-of-beef-methane/

36. Standard livestock production accounts for *14.5 percent* of all human-caused emission.

> Ibid. From *The Atlantic Monthly*, Sept. 25, 2017 video. https://www.theatlantic.com/video/index/540765/beans-instead-of-beef-methane/

Page 176

37. Functional medicine expert Dr. Mark Hyman, author of *The Food Fix*, minces no words. He calls sugar a "recreational drug."

> From Hyman, Mark, MD, *Food Fix: How to Save our Health, Our Economy, Our Communities and Our Planet—One Bite at a Time*, Little, Brown, Spark: 2020.

Page 178

38. I spoke with Kentucky-based regenerative farm pioneer Timothy Kercheville. I was so moved by his efforts that I invited him on my *Soul Stories* podcast. Timothy went beyond merely restoring farms to their natural states, even incorporating what's good about regular industrialized farming.

My discussion with Timothy Kercheville is from a transcript of *Soul Stories,* my weekly podcast conversations with individuals changing the world through living their purposes and soul-directed missions in life. You can find all *Soul Stories* episodes by going to https://www .drgmrandall.com/contents/soulstories-podcast. To listen to the full 56-minute podcast with Timothy: https://podcasts.apple.com/us /podcast/soul-stories/id1546395044?i=1000525320270

Page 179

39. Recently I had the great opportunity and privilege of talking to and working with Charles Dowding.

My discussion with Charles Dowding is from a transcript of *Soul Stories,* my weekly podcast conversations with individuals changing the world through living their purposes and soul-directed missions in life. You can find all *Soul Stories* episodes by going to https://www.drgmrandall. com/contents/soulstories-podcast. To listen to the full 50-minute podcast: https://www.buzzsprout.com/1488061/10364197-soul -stories-charles-dowding-renown-no-till-innovative-pioneer

CHAPTER 15

Page 181

40. The Organic Consumers Association, University of Texas Department of Chemistry and Biochemistry, and a number of European studies show that soil mineral content has depleted by 60 to 80 percent since 1930—right before industrialized farming entered our food supply along with World War II.

From "Soil Depletion, and Why We Need Multivitamins and Minerals More Than Ever," July 25, 2020 report, Bliss Pharmaceutiks, UK. http://blisspharmaceutiks.com.pk/2020/07/25/soil-depletion-and -why-we-need-multivitamins-minerals-more-than-ever/

Page 184–185

41. According to the American College of Cardiology, more doctors take and administer antioxidants than aspirin to help prevent cardiovascular disease and heart attacks.

From Meyer, Joseph, MD et al, "New Data on Aspirin Use in the Era of More Widespread Statin Use," American College of Cardiology, Sept. 28, 2018

Page 185

42. In 1998, US consumers spent $2 billion on vitamins, immunity and herbal supplements combined, according to *Nutrition Business Journal.*

From "Supplement Business Report – New Hope Network", as originally reported in the *Nutrition Business Journal*. https://www.newhope .com/sites/newhope360.com/files/2016%20NBJ%20Supplement %20Business%20report_lowres_TOC.pdf

43. In 2020, according to industry research analyst IBISWorld, that figure was *$35.7 billion* in the United States alone and almost $150 billion worldwide.

From "Vitamin & Supplement Manufacturing in the U.S.: 2005-27," IBIS World https://www.ibisworld.com/industry-statistics/market-size /vitamin-supplement-manufacturing-united-states/

44. MarketWatch estimates that, by 2026, total sales will reach $349.4 billion.

From "Global Dietary Supplements Market Trends and COVID-19 Impact Report... 2022 to 2026" MarketWatch. https://www .marketwatch.com/press-release/global-dietary-supplements-market -trends-and-covid-19-impact-report-competitor-landscape-in-depth -104-pages-report-with-types-applications-sales-and-forecast-till -2022-to-2026-2022-04-26

CHAPTER 16

Page 188

45. I first heard about blue zones in a November 2005 *National Geographic* story, "The Secrets of a Long Life." In the article, they identified five blue zones associated with people that live 90 to 100 years, and sometimes up to 150 years.

From "The Secrets of a Long Life," *National Geographic,* Nov. 2005 https://www.bluezones.com/wp-content/uploads/2015/01/Nat_Geo _LongevityF.pdf

Page 189

46. Dan Buettner writes about a few more common characteristics: the people hold strong life purpose, and they don't overstress— and in fact practice stress reduction just by their daily routines.

From Buettner, Dan, *Blue Zones: 9 Lessons for Living Longer from People Who've Lived the Longest*, National Geographic, Second Edition, Nov. 6, 2012.

Page 191

47. "Once I live to 75, I'm not going to do anything to end my life, but I'm not going to do anything to prolong it anymore, because after 75,

more than one half of people get cognitive decline and biologically disintegrate . . . I've never seen anyone after the age of 75 do anything positive."

> This shocking comment, with which I could not personally disagree more, is from Dr. Ezekiel Emmanuel, "Why I Hope to Die at 75," *The Atlantic,* October 2014. https://www.theatlantic.com/magazine /archive/2014/10/why-i-hope-to-die-at-75/379329/

Page 192

48. What about being 100 years old and still making a difference, like the elders among the blue zone populations? In 2021, I featured two such centenarians on my *Soul Stories* podcast. The first was Dr. Gladys McGarey, the mother of holistic medicine in the United States . . .

> My discussion with Dr. Gladys McGarey is from a transcript of *Soul Stories,* my weekly podcast conversations with individuals changing the world through living their purposes and soul-directed missions in life. You can find all *Soul Stories* episodes by going to https://www. drgmrandall.com/contents/soulstories-podcast. To listen to the full 63-minute podcast with Dr. McGarey: https://podcasts.apple.com /us/podcast/soul-stories/id1546395044?i=1000529185954

CHAPTER 17

Page 199

49. Dr. Michael Gershon, chairman of the Department of Anatomy at New York Presbyterian Hospital and author of *The Second Brain,* wrote, "The second brain doesn't help with the great thought processes . . . religion, philosophy and poetry are left to the brain in the head."

> From Gershon, Michael, MD, "Think Twice: How the Gut's 'Second Brain' Influences Mood and Well-Being," *Scientific American,* Feb. 20, 2010.

Page 202

50. Another is SIBO (small intestinal bacterial overgrowth), first described in 2004 by Dr. Mark Pimentel at Cedar-Sinai.

> All of the information on SIBO cited for *Soul Doctoring* on this page can be found in "Small Intestinal Bacterial Overgrowth and Irritable Bowel Syndrome — An Update," by Will Takakura and Dr. Mark Pimentel, Front Psychiatry, 2020, National Library of Medicine. https://pubmed.ncbi.nlm.nih.gov/32754068/

Page 204

51. "A gut microbial analysis from a simple stool sample [through an RNA or MAP test] could become one of the most powerful screening tools in health care . . ."

> From Mayer, Emeran, MD, *The Mind-Gut Connection: How the Hidden Conversation Within Our Bodies Impacts Our Mood, Our Choices, and Our Overall Health*, Harper Wave: 2018.

CHAPTER 18

Page 207–208

52. Connie Kaplan, my teacher and author of *The Woman's Book of Dreams*, says it best about dreaming: "Truth presents itself in dreaming and later exposes itself in form. The dreamer must simply learn to read and track the energy. Dreaming can only be spoken indirectly in metaphor. Nothing is precise about dreaming, yet to be a dreamer, one must be extraordinarily precise in living the dream."

Connie Kaplan has written several books on dreams, and I have had many interactions with her. The basis of my dream work comes from her first, *The Woman's Book of Dreams*, originally published in both trade paperback and workbook form in 1999.

> From Kaplan, Connie, *The Woman's Book of Dreams*, Beyond Words Pub Co., 1999.

Page 210

53. The work of psychologist Patricia Garfield also promotes healing through dreams. In *The Healing Power of Dreams*, she describes dreams that demonstrate all phases of healing, from diagnosis to cure.

> From Garfield, Patricia, *The Healing Power of Dreams*, Fireside, 1992.

CHAPTER 19

Page 220

54. In 2002, while presenting a workshop at a future-thinking spiritual and social conference, I participated in a wonderful experience of miracles in action with my dear friends at the Sierra Dove Healing Center.

This was a great personal experience for me. I was invited to keynote a conference by the Sierra Dove Healing Center, an organization of healers, seers/visionaries, educators and creative powerhouses in southeastern New Mexico, led by Native seer Jozef Dominguez and educator Julia Price. From that keynote came many long-standing friendships and spiritual relationships, a healing of me, … and a big leap forward in the creation of *Soul Doctoring.*

CHAPTER 20

Page 229

55. As of 2022, there are more than five million people with Alzheimer's and other forms of dementia in the US. Those are just clinically recorded cases. By 2050, that number is expected to grow to 16 million.

Statistics from the Centers for Disease Control and Prevention. https://www.cdc.gov/aging/ag-info/alzheimers.htm

Page 230

56. According to international neurodegenerative disease expert Dr. Dale Bredesen, cognitive decline and the impending onset of Alzheimer's and dementia occur due to six major causations…

The six major causations listed by Dr. Dale Bredesen, which I break out further with my additional findings throughout Chapter 20, are the basis of his important 2020 work, *The End of Alzheimer's Program: The First Protocol to Enhance Cognition and Reverse Decline at Any Age,* Avery, 2020.

Page 236

57. In their book *Brain Wash,* David Perlmutter and his son, Austin, talk about the importance of empathy to deal with the cognitively affected.

From Perlmutter, David, MD and Perlmutter, Austin, MD, *Brain Wash: Detox Your Mind for Clearer Thinking, Deeper Relationships, and Lasting Happiness,* Little, Brown Spark, 2020.

CHAPTER 22

Page 256

58. In 1972, Dr. Candice Pert discovered the opiate receptor. She knew it was densely populated in the limbic brain, known to be where our emotion develops.

Candice Pert's work was seminal to many first-general integrative medicine practitioners, doctors and researchers – myself included. I build on her findings in this chapter, much from her classic *Molecules of Emotion: The Science Behind Mind-Body Medicine,* Simon & Schuster, 1999.

Page 257

59. The HeartMath Institute published numerous studies to support the fact that the heart is not just a simple pump.

> The HeartMath Institute does great work concerning the heart, and is a wonderful source of information, which I have utilized for years.

60. The negative effect (anxiety, depression and unhealthy stress) costs US employers over $300 billion per year in absenteeism, tardiness, worker's compensation and health insurance costs, according to the University of Massachusetts Lowell. . . .

> "Financial Costs of Job Stress: Total Worker Health for Employers." Accessed May 16, 2022. https://www.uml.edu/research/cph-new /worker/stress-at-work/financial-costs.aspx.

Page 258

61. Emil Patrick Lesho, DO, discussed how the mere acknowledgment of pain in a patient tended to improve symptoms and lessen discomfort.

> Dr. Lesho discusses this in *Archives of Internal Medicine* article, "When the Spirit Hurts: An Approach to the Suffering Patient. https://www. researchgate.net/publication/9015375_When_the_Spirit_Hurts_An _Approach_to_the_Suffering_Patient

62. A 2003 randomized controlled trial published in the *Journal of the American Medical Association* demonstrated the importance of *patient-physician communication in patient outcome.*

> From Ihler, Elizabeth, "Patient Physician Communication", Jan. 1, 2003, https://jamanetwork.com/journals/jama/fullarticle/195694

Page 259

63. Recent literature by Lesho in the *Archives of Internal Medicine*, and Detmar and others in *JAMA*, the *Journal of the American Medical Association*, report on the importance of listening.

> Ibid., "Patient Physician Communication", Jan. 1, 2003, https:// jamanetwork.com/journals/jama/fullarticle/195694

64. In *Power vs. Force*, David Hawkins said of his many end-stage patients, "I saw how love changed the world [the patients] each time it replaced 'un-love.'"

> I build on a few principles of Hawkins' in this chapter. All come from his book *Power vs. Force: The Hidden Determinants of Human Behavior*, Hay House, 2014.

Page 260

65. In *Destructive Emotions*, Goleman reported on studies which used quantitative electrophysiology, PET and fMRI studies to quantify brain function.

> A decade before he wrote the seminal book *Emotional Intelligence*, Dr. Daniel Goleman, wrote another vitally important book as well, *Destructive Emotions: A Scientific Dialogue with the Dalai Lama*, Bantam, 2004.

Page 261

66. A study at the UCLA Neuropsychiatric Institute showed that a group of older men and women who took Tai Chi courses for 45 minutes a day, three days a week, showed an increase of up to 50 percent of memory T cells, immune system cells, that recognize and attack the varicella herpes viruses that cause shingles.

> Published in the September 2003 issue of *Psychosomatic Medicine*. https://organizations.dgsom.ucla.edu/psychsig/pages/psychosomatic

CHAPTER 24

Page 270

67. At the SB '21 conference in San Diego, Nestlé CEO Aude Gandon coined the term "Generation Regeneration."

> Aude Gandon was a keynote speaker at the SB '21 San Diego, the annual world conference of Sustainable Brands, an association of businesses large and small, influencers and innovators committed to creating 100% sustainable business practices in the world. https://sustainablebrands.com

Page 271

68. Paul Hawken's book *Regeneration: Ending the Climate Crisis in One Generations* is an amazingly inclusive book covering all aspects of climate change and the spread of regeneration globally.

> From Hawken, Paul. *Regeneration Ending the Climate Crisis in One Generation*. Penguin Books. 2021.

Page 273

69. Our clothing consumption is egregious. The average American buys nearly 68 new outfits a year today; back in the 1970s, it was 12 per year. Many of these garments are never worn and the average American disposes of 80 pounds of clothing per year.

These statistics come from the website https://www.closetotheearth.com/, a great entry source to gain information on the impact of our clothing purchasing habits and their global impact.

Page 274

70. Nearly three-quarters of Patagonia's massive clothing line, which brings the company more than $800 million in annual revenue, is made from recycled materials.

From "What We're Doing About our Plastic Program," a report on the official Patagonia Website. https://www.patagonia.com/stories/what-were-doing-about-our-plastic-problem/story-72799.html

ABOUT THE AUTHOR

Gayle Madeleine Randall, MD, has been an esteemed physician, scientist, medicine woman, administrator, seminar presenter and writer for more than 40 years. Her passion and thirst for new learning and deep commitment to the health of humanity and the planet reflects her life of raising consciousness and practicing healing from numerous approaches: advocate and pioneer in integrative medicine; indigenous medicine; leader in environmental efforts; and regular women's empowerment and dreaming as a spiritual practice focused on raising consciousness.

After graduating with high honors from the University of Nebraska Medical School, Dr. Randall completed an internal medicine residency and gastroenterology fellowship at University of California, Los Angeles, hospitals and clinics. From 1988–94, while associate professor of medicine at UCLA, she cofounded the first integrative medicine studies program in the country linked to a university's medical school. She also served as the director of the Medical Procedures Unit for the West Los Angeles Veterans Administration hospital. After serving her medical clerkship as the doctor on an American Indian reservation, Dr. Randall's long interest in American Indian and non-conventional forms of medicine, energy healing, dreamwork and spirituality also blossomed.

She integrated multiple modalities in the second half of the 1990s. She was coproducer and participant of *The Healing Connection*, a pilot research project and ground-breaking UCLA study on the integration of Ayurvedic, Chinese, American Indian and Western medicine. She also was a producer for Heaven Fire Productions and appeared twice on NBC's *The Other Side* to discuss holistic medicine. She served as the integrative and holistic medicine co-director of the Malibu Health and Rehabilitation Center, director of integrative health for Miraval Life in Balance, and executive director of guest services at Rancho La Puerta, a health and wellness destination spa in Tecate, Mexico.

During her tenure, Miraval was named the No. 1 for Health Destination Spa in the World by *Conde Nast Traveler* magazine. She continues her medical practice as director at Randall Wellness Malibu in California, while hosting her popular podcast, *Soul Stories*, and continually sharing and teaching on her social media, YouTube and in-person patrons.

Dr. Randall has conducted lectures, workshops, and seminars on holistic and integrative medicine throughout the world. She presented The Science behind Mind, Body Medicine at the renowned MD Anderson Cancer Center in Houston in 2005, and many other esteemed settings. Her writings in numerous holistic publications, educational documentaries and workshops have helped to transform the lives of thousands of patients, clients and attendees by enlightening them to their own healing potential.

Dr. Randall learned her daily practice of prayer and meditation through years of training with American Indian visionaries including mystic Joseph Rael and Soke Takayuki Kubota, founder of Gosoku-ryu style karate, International Karate Association and Mind Like Water meditation. She has a black belt in this style, as well as Japanese Samurai sword.

Dr. Randall reaches thousands weekly through her popular podcast *Soul Stories*, which is available every Monday on all platforms, and her Instagram TV show, which airs on Friday nights from 9–10 p.m. EST. She has a highly engaged following of over 15,000 followers on Instagram.

Dr. Randall is a longtime resident of Malibu, California, where her medical practice, Randall Wellness Network, is also located.

THE RANDALL WELLNESS HEALTH NETWORK

The Randall Wellness Health Network brings together media, promotional and platform tools that promote the message, teachings and work of Dr. Randall, as well as the ongoing promotion of *Soul Doctoring*. She connects with tens of thousands of viewers and followers daily in this highly interactive and engaging platform, which focuses on medical and health topics of concern to individuals, communities and the planet.

The platform combines:

- **The Hub: Website:** Dr. Randall's dynamic site, drgmrandall.com, is the hub of the Network. It incorporates her medical work and professional services with promotional elements of the book, including a Press Kit, *Soul Stories* podcast and other media links, book backgrounder, social media buttons, and information on her many activities and appearances.
- ***Soul Stories* Podcast:** One of the most innovative podcasts in the health and wellness space, Dr. Randall's acclaimed weekly *Soul Stories* podcast has drawn rave reviews. Now in its second year, the podcast has been feted for achieving more than 5,500 official download subscriptions, a number constantly increasing. Dr. Randall focuses on many subjects covered in *Soul Doctoring* as she and her guests discuss their work, and the larger purpose of creating a healthier, cleaner and more beautiful world.

Guests include healing experts, visionaries, futurists and societal leaders that are at the forefront of health and culture, and of living their soul's purpose. Among them are *New York Times* bestselling author Dr. Emeran Mayer; award-winning author Dr. Danielle Delaney (*Expect Delays: How to Reclaim Your Life, Light and Soul after Trauma*); Glenn Brooks, founder of Vibrant Living Network and Programs; Howard Wills, healer; Rebecca Mink of Mink Vegan Shoes, award-winning documentarian and pro athlete Zion Clark (*Zion*); health-care advocate Connie Grauds, Mother of Holistic Medicine; Dr. Gladys McGarey, the 100-year-old founder of the Foundation of Living Medicine; and many more.

Soul Stories is available on all top podcast platforms, including Apple, Buzzsprouts, YouTube, Amazon, iTunes, Spotify, Google, PocketCasts, Anchor, and others.

- **Dr. Gayle Randall YouTube Channel:** New to the Randall Wellness Network, Dr. Randall's official YouTube Channel brings together more than 150 videos of her television guest appearances, talks, *Soul Stories* podcasts and podcast guest appearances, bringing her work to life visually for audiences around the world.
- **Friday Night Live on InstagramTV:** Dr. Randall treats the world, including her more than 15,000 followers, to live 30- to 60-minute shows every Friday night on InstagramTV. The programs, which have a "Fireside Chat" feeling and always feature high participation and engagement, include cutting-edge health, wellness and nutritional subjects of direct interest to their lives. They are also posted on regular feeds. Topics have included:

  - What Is Good for Us Is Good for the Planet
  - Nerves That Fire Together, Wire Together: Rewiring Your Brain
  - What Is a Mediterranean Diet? Why Is It Good for You?
  - Inflammation: How to Avoid Inflammation in Your Body
  - Change Your Diet, Save the Planet
  - Let's Talk about Food Sensibly
  - Heavy Metal Toxicity
  - Cognitive Decline
  - Cancer Prevention
  - Our Planet, Gut, Diet Connection

- **Instagram and Facebook Posts:** Dr. Randall practices strategic posting that focuses on special health, wellness and medical advice; information on our health and the planet; dietary, nutritional and recipe tips; and lifestyle practices that promote personal and planetary health. She posts several times a week, receiving up to thousands of views, and active messaging engagement. Her dedicated followership between the two exceeds 25,000.

- **Monthly Newsletter:** Dr. Randall's monthly newsletter, featuring health, diet/nutrition and wellness tips, as well as a regular excerpt from *Soul Doctoring*, is sent to thousands on her email marketing list, as well as being available to her clinical patients, and listeners on InstagramTV and the *Soul Stories* podcast.
- **Facebook Live:** Dr. Randall participates in occasional Facebook Live broadcasts focused on the issues of the day. In 2020, she appeared on *Natural Remedies for the Human Immune System*, and *What the Media Is Not Telling You about COVID*. She will be appearing in other Facebook Live broadcasts in the coming months and years.
- **Other Podcast Appearances:** Dr. Randall is also a regular participant on the *Better Call Daddy* podcast hosted by Reena Friedman Watts, Brad Swail's *Cultivate Wellness* podcast and Richard Radstone's *Sidewalk Ghost Stories*, reaching audiences exceeding 100,000. She is regularly asked to appear on podcasts, and we will be setting up appearances on leading health/medicine, diet/nutrition/food growing, creative living, visionary/futurist, and general interest podcasts.

You can extend your *Soul Doctoring* experience by tuning in regularly to the Randall Wellness Network and its programs, videos and posts. We will constantly be adding to and further enhancing the book content online, as well as providing regular updates on signings, appearances, promotions and media coverage. On top of that, anything and everything you need for your personal health, and the health of community and planet can be found within its many resources and features.

https://www.drgmrandall.com

INDEX

Manufactured by Amazon.ca
Bolton, ON

27891570R00194